Clubfoot
A Comprehensive Approach
(Past, Present, and Future)

Clubfoot
A Comprehensive Approach
(Past, Present, and Future)

R. L. Mittal
Professor Emeritus
Orthopedic Department
Government Medical College
and
Mittal Ortho Centre
Patiala, Punjab, India

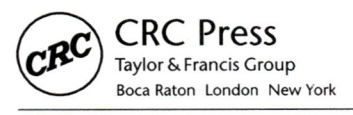

CRC Press
Taylor & Francis Group
Boca Raton London New York

CRC Press is an imprint of the
Taylor & Francis Group, an **informa** business

CRC Press
Taylor & Francis Group
6000 Broken Sound Parkway NW, Suite 300
Boca Raton, FL 33487-2742

© 2019 by Taylor & Francis Group, LLC
CRC Press is an imprint of Taylor & Francis Group, an Informa business

No claim to original U.S. Government works

Printed on acid-free paper

International Standard Book Number-13: 978-1-138-08373-8 (Hardback)

This book contains information obtained from authentic and highly regarded sources. While all reasonable efforts have been made to publish reliable data and information, neither the author[s] nor the publisher can accept any legal responsibility or liability for any errors or omissions that may be made. The publishers wish to make clear that any views or opinions expressed in this book by individual editors, authors or contributors are personal to them and do not necessarily reflect the views/ opinions of the publishers. The information or guidance contained in this book is intended for use by medical, scientific or health-care professionals and is provided strictly as a supplement to the medical or other professional's own judgement, their knowledge of the patient's medical history, relevant manufacturer's instructions and the appropriate best practice guidelines. Because of the rapid advances in medical science, any information or advice on dosages, procedures or diagnoses should be independently verified. The reader is strongly urged to consult the relevant national drug formulary and the drug companies' and device or material manufacturers' printed instructions, and their websites, before administering or utilizing any of the drugs, devices or materials mentioned in this book. This book does not indicate whether a particular treatment is appropriate or suitable for a particular individual. Ultimately it is the sole responsibility of the medical professional to make his or her own professional judgements, so as to advise and treat patients appropriately. The authors and publishers have also attempted to trace the copyright holders of all material reproduced in this publication and apologize to copyright holders if permission to publish in this form has not been obtained. If any copyright material has not been acknowledged please write and let us know so we may rectify in any future reprint.

Except as permitted under U.S. Copyright Law, no part of this book may be reprinted, reproduced, transmitted, or utilized in any form by any electronic, mechanical, or other means, now known or hereafter invented, including photocopying, microfilming, and recording, or in any information storage or retrieval system, without written permission from the publishers.

For permission to photocopy or use material electronically from this work, please access www.copyright.com (http://www.copyright.com/) or contact the Copyright Clearance Center, Inc. (CCC), 222 Rosewood Drive, Danvers, MA 01923, 978-750-8400. CCC is a not-for-profit organization that provides licenses and registration for a variety of users. For organizations that have been granted a photocopy license by the CCC, a separate system of payment has been arranged.

Trademark Notice: Product or corporate names may be trademarks or registered trademarks, and are used only for identification and explanation without intent to infringe.

Library of Congress Cataloging-in-Publication Data

Names: Mittal, R. L. (Rattan Lal), author.
Title: Clubfoot : a comprehensive approach (Past, Present, and Future) / R.L. Mittal.
Description: Boca Raton, FL : CRC Press/Taylor & Francis Group, [2019] | Includes bibliographical references and index.
Identifiers: LCCN 2018031125| ISBN 9781138083738 (hardback : alk. paper) | ISBN 9781315112107 (ebook)
Subjects: | MESH: Clubfoot
Classification: LCC RD783 | NLM WE 883 | DDC 617.5/85--dc23
LC record available at https://lccn.loc.gov/2018031125

Visit the Taylor & Francis Web site at
http://www.taylorandfrancis.com

and the CRC Press Web site at
http://www.crcpress.com

Dedication

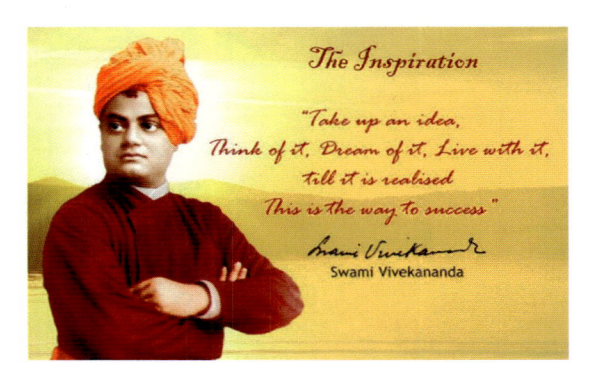

Firstly, I dedicate this book to Swami Vivekananda, a wandering monk and reformer from West Bengal, India, who became famous worldwide after his lectures at the World Parliament of Religions in Chicago in September 1893. He truly inspired me with this lifelong passion.

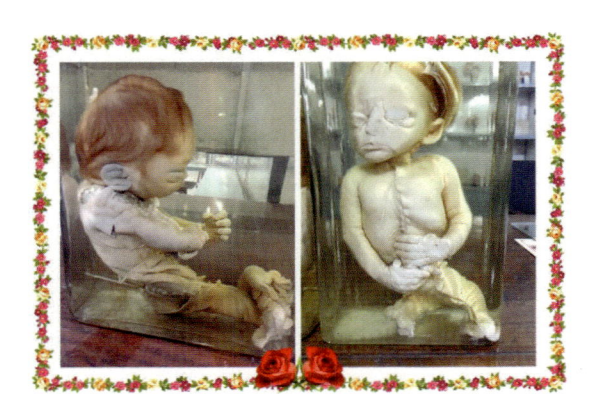

My floral tributes to unknown little angels, stillborn fetuses with clubfoot deformities, from the large collection of the Anatomy Museum of Government Medical College Patiala, with the unique material for this landmark research. They never saw light but have made this book see the daylight. Two of the dissected ones are seen above, "**a cenotaph**."

To my loving parents, I always feel indebted. They always encouraged me to do better next time with their unselfish love, from my schooldays to medical studies, throughout their life. Even now, I can feel their souls blessing me from the heavens.

Contents

Foreword — xi
Preface — xiii
Acknowledgments — xv
Author — xvii

1 Introduction — 1
  1.1 Background — 1
  1.2 This book — 3

2 Epidemiology of clubfoot — 5
  2.1 Nomenclature — 5
  2.2 Classification — 5
  2.3 Epidemiology/etiology — 8
    2.3.1 Intrinsic factors: Ethnicity — 8
    2.3.2 Extrinsic factors — 11
      2.3.2.1 Effect of smoking — 11
      2.3.2.2 Medications — 13
      2.3.2.3 Nutritional deficiency — 14
      2.3.2.4 Maternal diseases—obesity and/or diabetes, hypertension, infections — 16
      2.3.2.5 Amniocentesis and uterine factors — 17
      2.3.2.6 Socioeconomic, maternal age, and environmental factors — 18
    2.3.3 Genetics and clubfoot — 20
    2.3.4 Congenital constriction bands, distal amputations, and deformities, including clubfoot — 22
  2.4 Conclusions — 23
  References — 26

3 Review of literature — 33
  3.1 Historical perspective — 33
  3.2 Ponseti's technique and its pitfalls — 35
  3.3 Other contemporary techniques — 40
  3.4 Ilizarov and allied techniques — 42
  3.5 Older children and adults — 45
  3.6 Talectomy — 48
  3.7 Residual deformities — 48
  3.8 Early surgery — 51
  3.9 Various assessment protocols — 51

	3.10	Imaging techniques: Skiagrams, ultrasonography, CT, and MRI	53
		3.10.1 Skiagrams	53
		3.10.2 Ultrasonography	54
		3.10.3 CT scanning	55
		3.10.4 MRI	55
	3.11	Conclusions	56
		3.11.1 Historical	56
		3.11.2 Ponseti's technique pearls and its pitfalls	57
		3.11.3 Other contemporary techniques	57
		3.11.4 Ilizarov and allied techniques	58
		3.11.5 Older children and adults	59
		3.11.6 Talectomy	59
		3.11.7 Residual deformities	59
		3.11.8 Early surgery	59
		3.11.9 Various assessment protocols	59
		3.11.10 Imaging techniques: Skiagrams, ultrasonography, CT, and MRI	59
	References	60
4	Pathoanatomy of congenital clubfoot	67
	4.1	Normal anatomy of the foot and ankle	67
		4.1.1 The ankle joint	67
		4.1.2 The foot	68
		4.1.2.1 Bones of the foot	68
		4.1.2.2 Capsules, ligaments, and joints of the foot	69
		4.1.2.3 Muscles and tendons of the foot	70
		4.1.2.4 Arches of the foot	71
	4.2	Planes and axes of movements	71
	4.3	Pathoanatomy of clubfoot	71
		4.3.1 Review of literature on pathoanatomy	73
		4.3.2 Author's pathoanatomy study	79
		4.3.2.1 Author's observations on detailed morbid anatomy	80
		4.3.2.2 Biomechanics of abnormal muscles, ligaments, and joints	82
	4.4	Evolution of surgical techniques	83
		4.4.1 Evolution of first-generation surgical techniques on the author's pathoanatomy	83
		4.4.1.1 Skin contractures	83
		4.4.2 Second-generation surgical technique	85
		4.4.3 Third-generation technique with newer pathoanatomical features	85
		4.4.3.1 Each clubfoot is different	86
		4.4.3.2 A generic name	86
		4.4.3.3 Evolution of DOLARZ-E—Adding V-Y plasty to rotation and Z plasty (DOLARZ)	87
		4.4.3.4 Equinus in a new perspective	87
		4.4.3.5 Heterogeneity of scars	88
		4.4.3.6 Deformities at the toes	88
		4.4.3.7 Muscular abnormalities	88
		4.4.3.8 Dorsolateral hump	90
		4.4.3.9 Symptomatic genu recurvatum	91
		4.4.3.10 Numerous unusual pathoanatomical problems with morbidity	91
	4.5	Conclusions	95
	References	97

5	Extreme clubfoot deformities and their management			99
	5.1	Background		99
	5.2	Evolution of triple surgical techniques		101
		5.2.1	First-generation (DOLAR) surgical technique	101
		5.2.2	Second-generation research and the DOLARZ surgical technique	104
		5.2.3	Third-generation research and the DOLARZ-E surgical technique	105
	5.3	Conclusions		158
	References			160
6	Future of clubfoot			163
	6.1	Preventive measures		164
		6.1.1	Control of global population	164
		6.1.2	Controlling epidemiological factors	164
		6.1.3	Genetics	165
	6.2	Therapeutic measures		165
		6.2.1	Pathoanatomy	165
		6.2.2	Various imaging techniques	166
		6.2.3	Orthotics of the future	166
		6.2.4	Complications	166
	6.3	Rehabilitation in clubfoot in the future		166
	6.4	Conclusions		166
	6.5	To summarize		169
	References			171

Index   173

Foreword

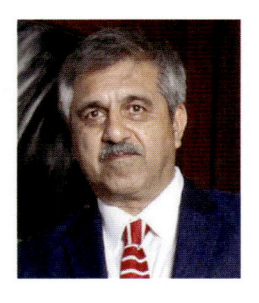

It gives me great pleasure to pen this foreword to this excellent compilation of a lifetime's work, which is now being presented as a book of international standards.

Prof. R. L. Mittal, who retired as the Director, Research and Medical Education Punjab, after serving the Patiala Medical College as a leading orthopedic surgeon, Head of Department and its principal, has not only been my teacher and mentor, but has also introduced me to the science and art of foot surgery. As a postgraduate, I learned what to do, as well as what not to do, by his keen insights into the subject and his extensive work on clubfoot, which at that time in the 1980s was a craft practiced by many, but mastered by few. Prof. Mittal was a pioneer at that time and, I may say, even a visionary, since the concepts for treatment in neglected cases were not clearly laid out. His research attitude and academic acumen can be judged from his recent appointment as Professor Emeritus in the orthopedic department at the Government Medical College Patiala, after 23 years of his retirement from here only to actively participate in research, teaching, and academic programs.

About 25 years ago, when Prof. Mittal became the President of the Indian Orthopaedic Association, he became a role model for all young orthopods in India. His passion and his zeal, along with his single-minded quest for achieving excellence in any sphere he takes up, has allowed him to pursue his work on clubfoot, especially neglected cases, as a lifetime work which is now being published. Neglected, residual, and relapsed clubfeet are reported in the literature from all over the world with a very high incidence, especially in older children, adolescents, and adults. This book should become a book of the future for orthopedic surgeons all over the world doing clubfoot work.

This comprehensive work includes sections on the epidemiology of clubfoot, nomenclature and classification, as well as discussions on ethnicity and causative factors, which perhaps are discussed, for the first time, in one place.

The section that reviews the literature and discusses the pathoanatomy, focuses on anatomical dissections done by the author himself, which led to a breakthrough in the understanding of the problem and gave insights into evidence-based discovery of skin contractures as a significant causative issue; this subsequently led to the development of Prof. Mittal's unique surgical technique, DOrsoLAteral Rotation skin flap (DOLAR) in the first phase of this research. There were two further phases in this research. In the second phase, he incorporated Z-plasty in that incision (DOLARZ) for more severe deformities, while in the third phase, VY-plasty was added in the same incision as 3-in-1 (DOLARZ-E) for the severest ones at all ages, especially older age groups.

This book is an impressive compilation of his experience and personal work on difficult cases of clubfeet, which perhaps are no longer encountered in the developed world, but are a common occurrence in Asia, Africa, and other low and middle-income countries (LMICs). His work on Trimorphic Extreme clubfoot deformities and triple surgical skin expanders, along with his explanation of the other techniques, would thus help surgeons worldwide. A significant feature in his research is that a well-shaped, longer, flexible, better-functioning foot without arthrodesis can be achieved.

I wish Prof. Mittal all the best, and I hope that there will be many more insights on this subject, which he has made his own, in the future. This is an essential book that needs to be kept in all institutional libraries for the benefit of both students and surgeons, as well as a proud possession for clubfoot enthusiasts.

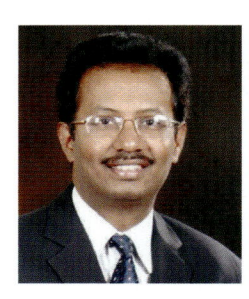

To my teacher, mentor, and guide, I wish this book all the success it deserves.

Prof. Mandeep S. Dhillon
MBBS, MS (Orth), FAMS, FRCS
President, Indian Orthopaedic Association (2018)
Chairman, Research, AO Trauma (Asia Pacific)
Founder President, Indian Biological Orthopaedics Society
Past President, Indian Arthroplasty Association
Past President, Indian Association for Sports Medicine
Past President, Indian Foot and Ankle Society
Professor and Head, Orthopaedics; Head, Physical Medicine Department, PGIMER, Chandigarh, India

It is a privilege and honor to have the opportunity to write a foreword for a monograph on clubfoot by one of the stalwarts in the field and icon of Indian orthopedics, Prof. R. L. Mittal.

Prof. Mittal has been a respected postgraduate teacher and medical administrator in various capacities for more than three decades. His original research work and expertise in the field of clubfoot are well known. The numerous publications, podium presentations, and orations by him on the subject of clubfoot stand testimony to this. It is welcome that his extensive experience and research on this important topic is now being compiled as a book. It is noteworthy that the book consists not only of all the essential elements of the theory of this common pathology, but also the practical aspects of management of this condition. The pearls of wisdom for a successful outcome at all stages of presentation from birth to the neglected or the relapsed clubfoot are clearly elucidated.

This book will be a valuable addition to every library in the field of orthopedic surgery as it has some tips and learning points for every surgeon, from the trainee to the most experienced.

Prof. S. Rajasekaran, PhD
Chairman, Department of Orthopaedic Surgery
Ganga Hospital, Coimbatore, TN, India
President SICOT
Past President, Indian Orthopaedic Association
Past President, Association of Spine Surgeons of India
Past President, ISSLS, Canada
Adjunct Professor, Tamil Nadu Dr MGR Medical University
Hunterian Professor, Royal College of Surgeons England, 2011–12
Chair, AO Spine International Research Commission
Past President, CSRS AP

Preface

Believe it or not, after spending almost half a century of clubbing with clubfoot for this landmark research this book was destined to happen. I have been consistently energized by awards and rewards at National and International levels (see "Author" on page xvii) at frequent intervals and started thinking that the work should be consolidated as a book. However, due to lack of time, increasing age, and searching for a reputed publisher, taking up this high-end, onerous, long drawn-out task of book writing, etc., I did not dare take the plunge. Just then, there was a clincher: an invitation, in the form of an e-mail in February 2016, from Dr. Gaurav Singh, assistant commissioning editor at Taylor & Francis, to explore ideas for a book. This was a God sent motivational opportunity: NOW or NEVER; YES or NO.

The gun was fully loaded (an overflowing mind), and this acted as a trigger to start; just then, in a flash, there was no looking back. Then started the publisher's worldwide, long review process with a go-ahead for writing. That was the culmination of about 6 months of the book proposal and review process. The beginning and turning of this research into a lifetime passion, too, was equally incredible. As detailed in Chapter 1, "Introduction," this intensive research was also destined to happen and, that too, at Patiala. Hard work, initiated with a pinch of inspiration, with frequent motivations by awards and rewards, to pursue this passion, still going on, resulted in landmark success; "Truth Is Stranger than Fiction" is upheld once again.

Chapters 4 and 5, based on the author's own research, makes this book unique and unparalleled, authenticated by its latest publication in the highly reputed SICOT journal, *International Orthopaedics*, in February 2018 (DOI. 10.1007/s00264-017-3741), online first, and now also in its print version in the June 2018 issue.

Extreme clubfoot deformities (severe and rigid, undercorrected, relapsed, or uncorrected) are extremely common at all ages from birth to late age, all over the world (especially in low- and middle-income countries [LMICs]) but have always been neglected. An unusually high incidence of undercorrections and relapses—up to 95% in some reports—are described and the so- called extreme deformities as above have been the target area for lifetime research, innovating triple skin expanding incision.

There are numerous firsts in this book. One of the bizarre cases, given a new name, "OCTOPUS CLUBFOOT," was seen and operated on free of charge in 2016 under the Government of India's National Mission Scheme. The innovative, first ever, 4-in-1 incision had excellent results and was reported in a London (UK)-based newspaper link "dailymail.co.uk/health octopus clubfoot." It is now viral on Google as OCTOPUS CLUBFOOT only, the name given by author due to its resemblance to octopus (photo of this foot and an octopus are shown side by side in this book in Chapter 5). I am sure that this volume will have a global reach for future clubfoot enthusiasts. Some of the reviewers also had a similar opinion. I am also confident that after reading this book, with its encompassing discussion of the intricacies of this deformity, any clubfoot surgeon should become familiar with operating on the rarest of the rare clubfoot deformities as have actually been performed by the author. There is no dearth of rare cases and we will find more than expected.

This is a comprehensive book, with the real content sifted out from the unending, voluminous literature covering all aspects of the past, along with its present status, and a direction for the future. The past was the present a while ago, and the future will become the present a while after now. Therefore, persistent hard work now, with eyes on the target, started with a pinch of inspiration, can make all three glorious, and this is what has been done by the author.

Wishing all the best to the disheartened global clubfoot community of all ages from early childhood to later adulthood, especially in all LMICs, to enable them to get longer, flexible, better functioning, and good-looking feet to improve their psycho-socio-physico-economic outlook, like the rest of their fellow beings.

Prof. R. L. Mittal
Mittal Ortho Centre
Patiala 147001, Punjab, India

Acknowledgments

This is indeed an amazing moment to acknowledge with grateful thanks, the contributions of those who have been instrumental in the stupendous job of writing this unique book. It is indeed incredible, but it was destined to happen.

To my life partner, Prof. Radha Rani Mittal, a popular dermatologist, also a Dr. B. C. Roy National Awardee, my contemporary at Medical College Patiala, and, like me, a devout follower of Swami Vivekananda's organization. Without her consistent whole-hearted support and encouragement, I could never have achieved this.

To my alma mater, Government Medical College Patiala (India), its orthopedic department and other ancillary departments, for their unwavering support, throughout my career and into my retirement, and even now as I have been designated recently as Professor Emeritus.

To the government of Punjab, India, for recognizing my expertise and granting special permission in 2016 to perform free surgeries at Government Mata Kaushalya Hospital Patiala under Government of India's National Health Mission (Rashtriya Bal Swasthya Karyakram project for the poor). Thirty-eight clubfoot surgeries, a record under this project, were performed in one year. There were some unique cases in this series, never reported earlier in the literature, which have been included in this book as an exclusive feature.

To the publishers, Springer *Nature* and JP Brothers for permissions to use my own old published material from their esteemed journals.

To the erstwhile Medical Sciences Commissioning Editor of Global Publishers at Taylor & Francis, whose surprise invitation set the ball rolling, there and then, for writing this book and to the present editorial staff, Mme. Shivangi Pramanik and Mme. Mouli Sharma, for their cooperation and day-to-day help.

To my ever-cooperative patients, who motivated me to innovate newer techniques for their problematic deformities and treat them to their fullest satisfaction.

To Prof. Surinder Lal, for his loving persuasion to put my expertise in black and white.

To Mr. Manpreet Singh for the graphics and computing work in painstakingly setting the manuscript to my satisfaction. He has done a wonderful job in the processing of all the photographs.

To my children, Drs. Arun and Suruchi, Ers. Sanjeev and Pritha, Er. Shaina, and grandchildren, Neha, Arjun, Gauri, and Dhwani, for their loving support.

Prof. R. L. Mittal

Author

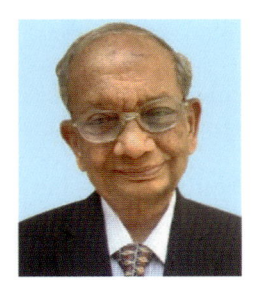

Prof. R. L. Mittal is formerly Professor and Head of the Orthopaedic Department, Principal Government Medical College, Patiala; Dean at Punjabi University Patiala, Punjab, India; as well as Director of Research and Medical Education, Government of Punjab, Chandigarh, India. The author is also an alumnus of this institution. He retired on April 30, 1995, from the government job, although he is still actively involved in teaching and academic activities in various capacities, the latest being as Professor Emeritus in the Orthopaedic Department of the Government Medical College Patiala, his old department. He is presently a practicing orthopedic surgeon at 97 New Lal Bagh Colony, Patiala, Punjab, 147001, India, but is very considerate of poor patients. The author has been the Chancellor's Nominee in the Punjabi University Patiala committee for selection of teachers and also a teacher for M.Sc. and B.Sc. physiotherapy courses at this university. He has also been a teacher for sports medicine courses at the Government of India National Institute of Sports, Patiala.

The author has been a prolific researcher in diverse areas with a large number of well documented works. His special field of lifetime interest has been clubfoot. His innovative, newer concepts in pathoanatomy and surgical techniques in extreme clubfoot deformities, which are prevalent from early childhood to adulthood, especially in low- and middle-income countries (LMICs), including India, have received recognition and won him numerous National and International awards and rewards. This has been a zero-cost research project initiated at the Government Medical College/Rajindra Hospital Patiala that started about half a century ago and is still continuing even after retirement.

Due to his expertise, he was authorized by the Punjab Government, under Government of India's National Health Mission (Rashtriya Bal Swasthya Karyakram), at Government Mata Kaushlaya Hospital Patiala to perform free clubfoot surgeries for underprivileged patients of Punjab. He performed a record 38 surgeries in about a year from 2016 to 2017. He also contributed 12 free surgeries, single-handedly, on August 4, 2016, the National Bone and Joint Day, to the kitty of the Indian Orthopaedic Association, creating a world record of maximum free surgeries by any country with the U.S. World Records Academy.

ACADEMIC ACHIEVEMENTS AND AWARDS

1. One hundred and thirty research publications in reputed scientific journals, about 25% of which were in international journals, many original research works with emphasis on low-cost technology.
2. Skeletal fluorosis research, collaborating for 6 to 7 years with the Indian Council Medical Research (ICMR) New Delhi; received an ICMR National Award in 1991 for outstanding original research in this disease, which was documented in national and international publications.
3. Lifetime achievement for continued research in clubfoot for approximately half a century;

innovated newer concepts in pathoanatomy and evolved new surgical techniques for extreme deformities at all ages with numerous publications in reputed national and international journals. Different aspects of this research have been presented at a large number of international and national meetings.

4. Developed the Patiala Orthopedic Biopsy Needle, a low-cost, simple, and versatile core biopsy instrument, adopted by the Indian Orthopaedic Association in 1985 (published in *Indian Journal of Orthopedics*, Mittal, R.L., Makhni S.S., Sidhu G.S.; "Morbid anatomy of congenital clubfoot," 15 (1981):129–135).
5. Use of a modified low-cost ring fixator (modified Ilizarov technique) successfully for more than 30 years for complicated trauma; presented at many national as well as at the SICOT International Conference at Sydney, Australia, in 1999.
6. Many new orthopedic conditions discovered and published in international journals: traumatic dislocation of tibialis posterior tendon, transcondylar fracture distal humerus, pseudomegadactyly, and so on.
7. New surgical techniques: Besides clubfoot, new surgical techniques for arthrodesis wrist, cock-up deformity of big toe, and hallux valgus (all published in international and national journals).
8. Invented instruments: Scoliometer for mass school screening for scoliosis, Patiala Orthopaedic Biopsy Needle, tropometer (published in *Indian Journal of Orthopedics*),
   a. "School of screening in scoliosis and evaluation of new scoliometer," R.L. Mittal, R. Aggarwal, *International Orthopaedics*, 11 (1987):335–338.
   b. "Diagnostic evaluation of needle biopsy in orthopaedic lesions by a modified simple instrument," R.L. Mittal, *Indian Journal of Orthopaedics*, 19 (July 1985):126–130.
   c. "Evaluation of a modified tropometer for measuring tibial torsion and its significance in congenital club foot," R.L. Mittal, P.S. Dhaliwal, *Indian Journal of Orthopaedics*, 14 (December 1980):184–191.
   d. UNiversal Inter-Locking nail EXtractor (UNILEX), *Punjab Journal of Orthopedics* Vol-XIII, No.1, 2012 and others (published in national and international journals).

UNIQUE DISTINCTIONS AND AWARDS: REGIONAL, NATIONAL, AND INTERNATIONAL

- Senior Commonwealth Fellowship under the British Council (by Health Ministry Government of India); visiting different centers for the study of Medical Education in England—1984.
- Indian Orthopedic Association A.A. Mehta Gold Medal for spine surgery—1985.
- Indian Orthopedic Association Howmedica Fellowship for American Academy of Orthopedic Surgeons conference in Las Vegas, Nevada, USA—1985.
- Indian Orthopaedic Association Silver Jubilee Oration Award for Best Original Research in Club Foot—1988.
- Indian Council Medical Research. New Delhi National Award for Skeletal Fluorosis—1991.
- Appreciation letter by Punjab State Council Science/Technology (1994) for outstanding research during the period from 1990 to 1993.
- Commendation by the Government of Punjab Medical Education Department for outstanding research—1992.
- Member, Medical Council of India, New Delhi—1993–1995.
- President, Punjab Medical Council, Chandigarh—1994.
- President, Indian Orthopedic Association—1994.
- Dr. B. C. Roy National Award conferred by the President of India—1994.
- President, Indian Foot & Ankle Society—2000–2002.
- Dr. B. B. Joshi Oration Award by Indian Foot & Ankle Society—2010.
- Original Research Award, once again for original research in DOLAR (**DO**rso-**LA**teral **R**otation) surgical technique in extreme clubfoot deformities, Indian Orthopedic Association, Golden Jubilee Oration Award—2013.
- Dr. B. N. Sinha Meritorious Award, Indian Orthopedic Association—2013.
- Widely traveled to about 25 countries for conferences as chairman, for guest lectures and fellowships and/or as a visiting professor.

- Life Fellow National Academy of Medical Sciences Delhi since 1995 and member of its advisory panel.
- Life Member, Association of British Scholars, India, Chandigarh Chapter.
- Indian Orthopaedic Association Honorary Fellow Award December 2015.
- Government of Punjab Honour on August 15, 2016, India's Independence Day, for doing free clubfoot surgeries under the Government of India's National Health Mission (Rashtriya Bal Swasthya Karyakram project).
- Recently designated as Professor Emeritus, Government Medical College Patiala for contributing to research and academic activities, including in clubfoot, in April 2018.

RECENT INTERNATIONAL RECOGNITION FOR RESEARCH

- Delivered a lecture on clubfoot at a global Foot and Ankle congress held in China in May 2017.
- Writing this book on clubfoot for Taylor & Francis, USA.
- A comprehensive clubfoot original research article published in *International Orthopaedics* (SICOT), online first in February 2018 and as print version in June 2018." Trimorphic extreme clubfoot deformities and their management by triple surgical skin expanders-DOLAR, DOLARZ and DOLARZ-E (evidence based mega-corrections without arthrodesis)," *International Orthopaedics* (December 2018): 1–10. doi 10.1007/s00264-017-3741-6.
- Indian Orthopedic Association Diamond Jubilee Oration Award to be delivered at IOACON, November 2018 at Coimbatore (TN).

SOCIAL AND COMMUNITY SERVICE

- Volunteered during the national emergency due to the 1971 Indo-Pakistan War, Fazilka Sector, to provide surgical help to war causalties and headed a surgical team at the war front hospital, December 8–18, 1971.
- Punjab State and Patiala District Red Cross Awardee 1985 (life member). Organized a number of Red Cross sponsored orthopedic camps in Punjab providing free surgeries.
- Under a Red Cross sponsored research project, innovated a low-cost mechanical hand for upper limb prosthesis, supplied free to arm amputees of Punjab; this research paper "A low cost functioning prosthetic hand for developing countries," R.L. Mittal, B.S. Brar, A.K. Bansal, *Orthopaedic Journal of Madhya Pradesh Chapter*. It was presented at an international conference at Seoul South Korea—1993, sponsored by the Punjab government.
- School surveys of rural population in Patiala 1987 and 1993 (about 50,000 each) for flat feet and congenital orthopedic anomalies, including clubfoot and scoliosis. Innovated a quick-fix scoliometer, which was also presented at a SICOT International Conference, 1987, Munich (West Germany) (sponsored by the Punjab government) and published as: "Surgical management of resistant congenital clubfoot by rotation skin flap and extensive soft tissue release," R.L. Mittal, *International Orthopaedics* 11 (1987): 189–182.
- Regular yearly contributions to various social organizations: Prime Minister's National Relief Fund, such as Kargil heroes and Uttrakhand disaster, Nepal earthquake, Ramakrishna Mission branches all over India, Help Age India, Patiala Social Welfare Society, Deaf & Dumb School, Patiala Health Foundation.
- Inspired by Swami Vivekananda, running a registered NGO Ramakrishna Vivekananda Seva Samiti Patiala, affiliated with Ramakrishna Mission Belur Math (West Bengal) and financial contributions to its various branches all over India for social services.
- Actively involved in NGO Patiala Health Foundation (Regd), Patiala Medical College Alumni Association charity. With Rs. 3 crores corpus, free medicines to emergency patients, liquid oxygen plant for 24-hour supply, and other services.
- Appointed Professor Emeritus, Orthopaedic Department, Medical College Patiala for contributing to research, teaching, and other academic programs, including clubfoot.
- Will be starting free clubfoot surgeries once again as a research-oriented project.

1

Introduction

1.1 BACKGROUND

Before introducing readers to this unique book on clubfoot, it will be interesting to know about the background of the author's passion for research in this gray area. This is continuing, even now, after 45 years with landmark achievements at the national and international levels (see the author's biography). Work can become a passion when you start getting pleasure out of it in the form of small successes acting as incentives. A pinch of inspiration always works as a catalyst and inspires you more for persistent hard work, which opens the gates for bigger successes. At least, this has actually been the case with this research. The author started from scratch and went on and on and on. This success story should act as motivation for young researchers for hard work, the only way to achieve. Stephen Hawking, the great physicist, said, "No one undertakes research with the intention of winning a prize, but it is the joy of discovering something no one knew before." (Source: brainyquote.com). Thomas Edison, the great researcher with 1,093 patents to his credit, said, "Genius is 1% inspiration and 99% perspiration" (wikiquote.org/wiki/Thomas_Edison). However I feel, if that 1% (pinch of inspiration) also adds to the 99%, you go 100% full throttle. There has been no dearth of great men and women all over the world who have acted as role models and inspired others to follow in their footsteps.

Going down memory lane, this research was destined to happen at Patiala (India) only, because the research material of 15 clubfeet from the stillborn fetuses collection in the Anatomy Museum of Medical College Patiala (a megacollection) could be found here in India. How and from where they arrived here is anybody's guess. Further, the author made three U-turns to the Government Medical College Patiala, full circle; two of these were during the first five years, the first time via Delhi in 1961 and the second time via Rohtak in 1966. After that, he stayed put at Patiala, even after retirement in 1995. The author made the third U-turn recently, in April 2018, being designated as Professor Emeritus at the Government Medical College Patiala to contribute to research and academic activities, including clubfoot, once again.

On the first U-turn, the author took two things from Delhi to Patiala: the inspiration of Swami Vivekananda from two orthopedic surgeons from West Bengal (Dr. RP Chakrabarty, Dr. AK Ghosh) and the idea of clubfoot. Swami Vivekananda (a nineteenth century wandering monk reformer of India) became world renowned after his September 1893 Chicago lectures at the World Parliament of Religions. Within a short span, he founded the Ramakrishna Math and Mission (a worldwide service organization managed by monks) at Belur Math (Howrah) in the state of West Bengal in India. Revered Swami said, "Take up an idea, think it, dream it and live with it till it is realized." (CW: Vol.1, Raja-Yoga, Pratyahara & Dharana). It appears that this idea of clubfoot got ingrained in the author's mind during residency in Delhi, and it is still being realized (Figure 1.1).

A brief chronology of events for the author from January 1961 to the present is given below:

1. Government Medical College Patiala alumnus (1955–1960, third batch).
2. Left Patiala after graduation, January 1, 1961, for New Delhi for a better career. **Orthopedic surgeon by chance, not by choice,** as could not get residency in the popular and competitive subjects of general medicine or surgery at

The Inspiration

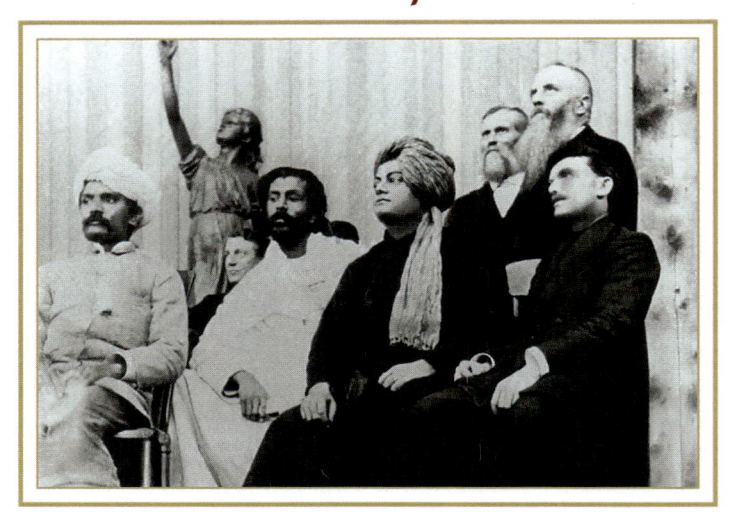

Swami Vivekananda
(seen third from left)
at Parliament of Religions, Chicago, 1893

Figure 1.1 Swami Vivekananda—Wandering monk reformer and a great luminary of India at the Parliament of World's Religions 1893, Chicago, United States.

L.N.J.P. Hospital New Delhi (erstwhile Irwin Hospital in 1961).
3. Residency in orthopedics under two Bengali ortho surgeons, Dr. R.P. Chakrabarty and Dr. A.K. Ghosh, and through them acquaintence with Swami Vivekananda, with first duty in the busy clubfoot clinic, and through them became acquainted with Swami Vivekananda. Every year, India proudly celebrates 12th January, Sw. Vivekananda's birthday, as National Youth Day.
4. The same year, the **first U-turn** to the Medical College Patiala, in the newly created orthopedic department, with a master's thesis on clubfoot, a follow-on of residency.
5. Unwanted transfer to Medical College Rohtak (Punjab State) in 1964. After about 2 years, the **second U-turn** in 1966 and transferred back to Patiala.
6. Discovery of 15 clubfeet from the stillborn fetuses collection in the Anatomy Museum jars, which was indeed a sizable number (a pride mega collection). Study of pathoanatomy, published in *Indian Journal Orthopedics* December 1981. "Morbid anatomy of congenital club foot," R.L. Mittal, S.S. Makhni, G.S. Sidhu, *Ind. Jr. Surgery* 15 (December 1981): 129, a significant and landmark discovery of skin contracture, hitherto ignored, as a potent pathoanatomical factor, setting the ball rolling to continue further.
7. Continuous stay at Patiala and persistent involvement in clubfoot research, sparked by frequent successes, achievements, and motivations.
8. First-Generation Research—the discovery of skin contracture, the evolution of the DOrsoLAteral Rotation skin flap (DOLAR) surgical technique, published in *International Orthopedics* (*SICOT*) in 1987; an Indian Orthopedics Association Silver Jubilee original research award in 1988.
9. Second-Generation Research for severer deformities in older children and adults and more three-dimensional correction by adding Z plasty to rotation flap in the same incision, that is, the DOLARZ technique. Once again, Indian Orthopedics Association original research award in 2013 and an International

Publication in *Journal of Foot Ankle Surgery* (Asia-Pacific) in December 2014.

10. Third-Generation Research–DOLARZ-E (Extended), that is, Rotation + Z + VY plasty in the same incision along with many other innovative ideas, leading to numerous achievements and national and international awards and rewards:
   i. In 2016, under the Government of India's National Health Mission, a record **38 free surgeries** in a year at Government Mata Kaushalya Hospital Patiala.
   ii. Contributed, single-handedly, **12 free surgeries** on National Bone and Joint Day (August 4, 2016) to Indian Orthopedic Association's kitty of maximum free surgeries for a world record by any country at the World Record Academy, USA.
   iii. Lecture at Global Foot & Ankle Congress in May 2017 in China.
   iv. Writing this book, an incredible opportunity, as mentioned in the Preface.
   v. Latest achievement—Original research article in February 2018, online first in *International Orthopedics (SICOT)*. doi 10.1007/s00264-017-3741-6. Now in print in the June 2018 issue: 42(6): 1297–1306.
   vi. Designated as Emeritus Professor, Orthopaedic Department, Government Medical College Patiala to promote research, teaching, and other academics, including clubfoot—this is **the third U-turn** for this research at the same place.

It is notable perhaps that the e-mail from the editorial office sending me the paginated book proofs for review was dated September 11th, the date of the first inspiring Chicago lecture by Swami Vivekananda (my motivator) at the World Parliament of Religions in 1893. Is it a coincidence? Maybe, but it is still worth considering. Certainly, the world does need more dedicated orthopedic surgeons to treat extreme clubfoot deformities, hitherto neglected, as defined in this book, which is a bane of LMICs, with tremendous GBD, and who are looking toward us expectantly. The author feels that this background should have been an interesting read to stress upon young researchers that **perspiration with a catalyst of inspiration can become passion.**

1.2 THIS BOOK

After this background of lifetime work on a single orthopedic problem and with in-depth knowledge of the subject, this book is as comprehensive as possible, covering every aspect of clubfoot, yet it is concise. It is said, **"Add life to years and not years to life."** It is not the number of pages, but the content in it, which should matter. The book should serve its purpose of enabling all concerned to manage clubfoot far better, more so in extreme deformities all over the world. These deformities are prevalent, at all ages, from newborn infants to older age groups, more so in all low- and middle-income countries (LMICs), but have been neglected for want of a tangible solution. This book should prove to be useful for the global clubfoot community. Now we come to the remaining, chapter-wise, content of this book.

In Chapter 2, which focuses on epidemiology, various factors involved have been discussed in detail, and measures to reduce the prevalence are suggested. Each of the factors has been discussed in all its detail. Different settings of the factors responsible for greater prevalence of clubfoot have been separately discussed, with their relative importance. After that, the measures to control them have been outlined. If the prevalence is reduced by the concerted efforts of all responsible, it will improve the socio-economic status by reducing the global burden of disease (GBD) with respect to clubfoot. With reduced prevalence, management of the remaining problem will become easier.

Chapter 3 is a review of the literature. The literature on clubfoot is voluminous, especially with the advent of the Internet. Unbridled writing has made this subject even more confusing. It is a maze. It is an extremely difficult job to sift out the requisite authentic content from the plethora of literature. Effort has been made to present the most authentic literature, divided in different subsections for the convenience of the readers. This book should enable them to find their desired material easily in the subsections, spending much less time and energy and enabling them to understand the problem from their point of view and do a better job.

Chapter 4 discusses the pathoanatomy of clubfoot, to which the author attaches a very high importance, because it is unique and its incomplete understanding has been at the root of all failures and incomplete successes. Typical normal anatomy has been described in the beginning of this chapter, so as to understand morbid anatomy better. Planes of axes of movements have been explained in a simple, innovative way. The author had studied the detailed pathoanatomy by anatomical dissections in 15 deformed feet in the mid-1970s and compared them with the normal, and this was the second largest reported series in the literature until that time. As has been stressed previously, these deformed feet gave insight into this myriad, faceted, enigmatic disease. A large number of innovative ideas on morbid anatomy were supplemented during clinical experience over all these years, and numerous newer pathoanatomical features have been added in all their detail. Newer ideas are still emerging and are being added. A highly significant fact of pathoanatomy is that **"Each Clubfoot is Different"** and is a great discovery, proved on abundant evidence. This has been discussed in great detail, because it will help readers to diagnose better and treat better. It is because of this fact that you will go on finding new things.

Chapter 5 is also based on the author's research innovating new surgical techniques, which have been need-based in a distinct timeframe, with some overlap, during more than last the 45 years. Extreme clubfeet deformities are very common, but remained neglected due to incomplete understanding. This chapter is devoted to the treatment aspect in this gray area. It has been divided into three phases: first- to third-generation, that is, GEN 1–3. All extreme clubfoot deformities are trimorphic with three hierarchic grades 1–3. To correct these, triple surgical skin expander techniques have been innovated with long-term follow-up. All these techniques have been discussed in detail with numerous unique examples, which is an exclusive aspect of this book. This comprehensive research has been authenticated by its publication in the globally reputed *International Orthopaedics (SICOT)* hybrid journal, online first in February 2018 and now in its print version in the June 2018 issue. "Trimorphic extreme clubfoot deformities and their management by triple surgical skin expanders- DOLAR, DOLARZ and DOLARZ-E (evidence based mega-corrections without arthrodesis)." doi 10.1007/s00264-017-3741-6.

Chapter 6 discusses the future direction of research in clubfoot so that it can be managed in a better way than what was being done in the past and what is being done now, especially the extreme clubfoot deformities as discussed here. Increasing population and decreasing resources are the biggest catalyst of all health problems, including clubfoot. The disease is much more prevalent in LMICs, with poor resources creating physico-psycho-socioeconomic problems. The importance of preventive measures has been stressed, besides the necessity for more research in epidemiology and genetics to improve that aspect. Genetics and epidemiology are interrelated also through many known and many unknown ways, which need to be explored. Creating a dedicated work force in LMICs, where this is much more of a problem compared with developed countries, is also stressed in this chapter. One method of treatment cannot be the solution for every clubfoot, because each case is different. There are numerous methods of treatment, and each one can succeed with proper case selection, depending upon one's experience. Extreme clubfoot deformities are a class in themselves at all ages, which need special care by newer techniques, innovated by the author, and more new ones yet to be invented. Research never stops.

It is also worth mentioning that clubfoot, without qualification and by convention, means congenital clubfoot. All other types need a prefix to designate the type, of which there are so many. Most of the principles of treatment used for congenital clubfoot will apply to others as well, except that, in these, tendon transfer and arthrodesis procedures are needed much more often than in congenital versions. This is because of the fact that, in other varieties, paralysis of muscles, whether spastic or paralytic, or fibrosis of muscles leading to their impaired function, is an important feature of such cases.

Lastly, there are repetitions in many places in this book, which is deliberate because of numerous innovative ideas. This has been done to make available that particular point there only, rather than searching in the Index, which is inconvenient, time consuming, and impracticable. Therefore, this has been considered an essential feature. The author is confident that after reading this book, clubfoot management should improve and become easier, more so in extreme deformities at all ages from birth to later adulthood. The author hopes the readers enjoy reading this book. There may be some lacunae, expected in such a work. He offers his apologies for the same.

2

Epidemiology of clubfoot

2.1 NOMENCLATURE

Before describing its epidemiology, it is important to know what exactly congenital clubfoot, or talipes equinovarus is and various names associated with it.

It is the most common foot deformity in which the foot is plantar flexed, adducted, and inverted, whereas varus obviously stands for both adduction and inversion. These three components of the deformity are present in varying proportions of severity and rigidity. However, there is a fourth component of deformity also, that is, cavus, invariably present in varying severity and rigidity, but in the nomenclature (equinovarus), it does not find a place. To be exact, it should be called equino-cavovarus, but by convention, it is called equinovarus only. This is an anomalous situation, cavus being an important component of composite deformity and remaining neglected by name. This component of the deformity also requires correction in order to achieve a good functional and cosmetic result. In this book, this has been handled with a new perspective in Chapter 4, which also discusses its pathoanatomy. There is yet another omission in the nomenclature. Among its various types, idiopathic variety is by far the most common type, from very mild to the most severe. Technically, it should be known as idiopathic congenital clubfoot, being present since birth and of unknown etiology. However, it is simply called clubfoot, and it has continued to be named as such since ancient times, being a short and simple name. When we say clubfoot, it means idiopathic; all others have to be addressed along with their cause. There is a tremendous variation in the deformity from case to case, and **each clubfoot is different** with regard to severity and rigidity. The equinus deformity, viewed in a different perspective, has been a significant part of research by the author and is discussed in detail in Chapter 4, proving its veracity on numerous evidences. This is a highly important fact, taken care of in the treatment of extreme clubfoot deformities.

2.2 CLASSIFICATION

The congenital form of clubfoot is the most common foot deformity, yet it can result from many uncommon, acquired causes. Therefore, it can be classified into various types according to the primary cause. Out of all congenital varieties, the idiopathic type is by far the most common, accounting for more than 90% of these cases. Classification is essential to defining the various groups, and makes it easy to remember and not confusing. There are many ways of classifying clubfoot. In the congenital variety, they can be broadly grouped under two headings:

I. As an isolated clubfoot deformity only or a part of a syndrome
   A. *Isolated clubfoot*: In this group, clubfoot is the only congenital defect. This may further be subclassified into familial and nonfamilial.
   B. *Syndromic clubfoot*: These are associated with various syndromes and are genetic in nature. Some examples are Moebius syndrome, Klippel–Feil syndrome, Turner syndrome, and many others due to chromosomal defects.
II. Another simple and easy way of classsification can be according to its cause, that is,

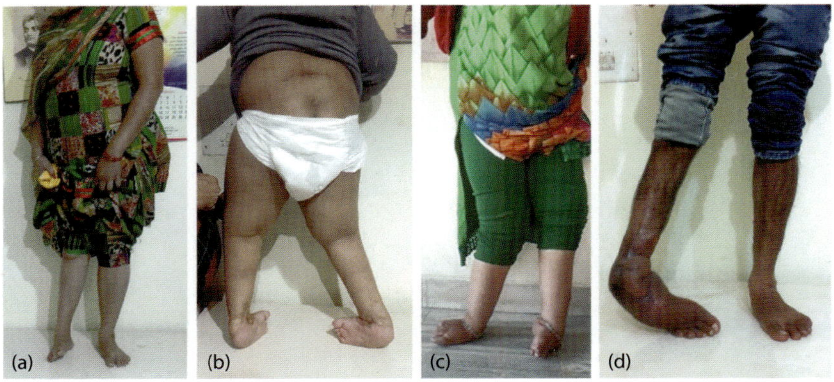

Figure 2.1 (a) Post-polio paralysis with equinovarus deformity right foot in a female patient of 35 years with wasted leg. (b) Paralytic equinovarus deformities of both feet (right more) due to spina bifida (operated) in a 10-year-old male child. (c) Equinovarus left and valgus right foot in a 25-year-old female patient due to myopathy. (d) Traumatic equinovarus deformity in the right foot due to an old crush injury in a 25-year-old young adult male.

depending upon primary involvement of tissues: idiopathic, neurological, muscular, or osseous. All of them may be congenital or acquired.

Congenital

1. *Idiopathic variety*: The exact cause is not known. This is the most common type of clubfoot, as stated above, and the most common congenital defect too. All of the tissues, from the skin, fascia, muscles, bones, and joints, are affected.
2. *Neuropathic variety*: This variety is due to involvement of neurological tissue from the central to the peripheral nervous system, and depending upon the site of involvement, there are many types. The lesion may be an upper motor neuron lesion from the brain to just proximal to the anterior horn cells or a lower motor neuron lesion from the anterior horn cells to the neuromuscular junctions, leading to spastic or flaccid paralysis, respectively. Both may be present since birth or may be acquired after birth (Figure 2.1c). The upper motor lesions are spastic and lower motor lesions are flaccid in nature.
    A. **Upper motor neuron paralysis** with spastic clubfoot may be congenital or acquired.
        i. *Congenital*: Due to cerebral palsy involving only lower limbs with clubfoot, hemiplegia, or all four limbs with varying degrees of severity and, if more severe, may be associated with varying degrees of mental retardation. Causes of cerebral palsy may be brain injury or brain malformation which occurs during pregnancy, premature delivery, or hypoxia during difficult labor. Severity of this will determine the severity of signs and symptoms. The other congenital rare causes of upper motor lesion with clubfoot are congenital ataxias. There are other heredo-familial genetic ataxias with clubfoot, progressive in nature, which manifest later in childhood.
        ii. *Acquired*: Due to encephalitis with postencephalitic sequalae with spastic clubfoot in early childhood or, in later life, due to cerebral stroke causing hemi- or monoplegia or due to some rare hereditary causes in the brain.
    B. **Lower motor neuron paralysis** with flaccid paralytic clubfoot can also result from both congenital and acquired causes.
        i. *Congenital*: Spina bifida occulta/meningocele or meningomyelocele present since birth with unilateral or bilateral involvement with both sensory and motor affliction of varying degrees. Trophic ulcer may also be present along with paralytic

clubfoot with involvement of sphincters (Figure 2.1b).
ii. *Acquired*: Cause is post-polio paralysis, with a lesion being in the spinal cord at the anterior horn cells due to polio virus, resulting in only muscular paralysis without any sensory features. There is usually partial recovery after onset and post-polio sequelae with residual post-polio paralysis varying in severity with partial involvement of one limb or, in the severest form, involving all four limbs and spine. It has become rare due to preventive measures. Post-polio equinovarus deformity of the foot is a common deformity after poliomyelitis. Other acquired causes of clubfoot can be radicular or peripheral nerve lesions like common peroneal nerve paralysis (Figure 2.1a).
3. *Muscular variety*: Due to involvement of muscles in different ways; present since birth or genetic but developing and progressing after birth.
   A. *Arthrogryposis*: Multiplex and distal, mostly due to amyoplasia with hypoplastic muscles having fibrous and fatty degeneration of muscles, leading to multiple joint deformities called arthrogryposis multiplex congenita. There is another type, called distal arthrogryposis, involving only the hands and feet, sparing proximal joints; this is due to a specific genetic defect.
   B. *Muscular dystrophy*: Cause of this is due to muscular degeneration, which is progressive, inherited, and genetic in origin. This affects male children, and females act as carriers.
4. *Osseous variety*: This can manifest in many ways, and the majority are present since birth, but some may be acquired also.
   A. *Congenital variety*: Clubfoot may be due to absence of bones or absent and extra bones due to duplication, associated with isolated extra foot bones only complicating the deformity, or associated with osseous coalitions of tarsals only or tarsals with metatarsals further complicating the deformity. The acquired variety can result due to trauma with or without infection, leading to fusion of foot bones after crush injuries.
   i. *Absent bones*: Congenital absence of tibia and absent great toe ray is invariably associated with clubfoot and is extremely rare. Club hands also may be present, which may be unilateral or bilateral.
   ii. *Absent and excess bones*: This is due to fibular dimelia associated polydactyly and clubfeet, usually bilateral.[1] Upper limbs may also be affected with ulnar dimelia and polydactyly affecting all four limbs.[2]
   iii. *Tarsal coalitions*: In still others, clubfoot may be associated with variable tarsal fusions,[3] which may be fibrous, cartilaginous, or osseous, magnetic resonance imaging (MRI) may be able to detect all and they have reported 11% incidence of fusions. Digital X-rays can only show osseous coalitions.[4]
   iv. *Polydactyly bones and fusions*: There may be others, but uncommon, associated with polydactyly and tarsal coalitions with polydactyly. I have seen a unique case, the first case of its kind, unilateral, with eight toes, intertarsal and tarsometatarsal and intermetatarsal coalitions, 2⅓ inches shortening, hypoplasia of affected lower limb, wind swipe deformities of both knees and flexion deformity of right knee, walking on lateral border with about 3 inches apart double callosities, X-ray picture resembling an octopus and hence given it the name of octopus clubfoot. This will be shown in Chapter 5 along with the first of its kind surgery in such a case.
   B. *Acquired*: Trauma can complicate a congenital clubfoot secondarily, or clubfoot can result due to crush injury in a normal foot and thus be completely acquired (Figure 2.1d). In congenital clubfoot, the deformity may become more severe due to ischemic changes after crush injuries to the leg. In the acquired variety, clubfoot deformity could result due to a severe crush injury to a normal foot or leg involving muscles, peripheral nerves, or even bones,

which may produce a very severe and rigid clubfoot, leading to problems of correction. All of the above varied forms of clubfoot have been seen by the author, corroborated in literature.

Some of the photographs of the acquired causes of clubfoot are given as in Figure 2.1a–d.

2.3 EPIDEMIOLOGY/ETIOLOGY

To my mind, deliberation on the epidemiology, at length, of any disease is very important, because it gives the complete picture of the magnitude of the problem and various causative factors including genetics. This is important to prevent the disease and also plan the treatment for the whole clubfoot community for improving the physico-psycho-socioeconomic conditions of the patients and thereby of the community.

The origin of epidemiology can be traced to more than 2,000 years ago.[5] In 400 BCE the Hippocrates classic referred to the plague epidemic and environmental factors influencing the occurrence of diseases. The earliest reference to epidemiology can be traced to 1400 BCE in the Babylonian text referring to a cough epidemic. The word epidemiology is derived from Greek words, namely, *epi*, meaning on or upon, *demos*, meaning people, and *logos*, meaning the study of. It is defined as the study of any disease, meaning thereby the study of its distribution in a specific population with various ethnic, socioeconomic, and environmental factors (intrinsic and extrinsic) influencing it, as well as the measures adopted to control it. It is data based and involves a systematic unbiased collection, analysis, and interpretation to arrive at a logical conclusion. Originally, it was confined to study the communicable and non-communicable infectious diseases only. However, with the development of many more investigative tools, it has expanded to cover even birth defects, chronic diseases, and many more areas[6–8] in order to improve the preventive and curative methods. Over the years, epidemiology is no longer a branch of medicine exploring epidemics only and treating them, but it has expanded its horizons to cover every discipline of morbid conditions, including even plants and animals.

Whereas etiology is only the cause and is therefore limited in scope, epidemiology is broad, covering multiple aspects. There are a large number of factors that play a role in the epidemiology of clubfoot: they are ethnicity, genetics, a large number of external and internal environmental factors, and others.

There are many intrinsic and extrinsic factors affecting the incidence of congenital clubfoot. There may still be many more unknown factors, epidemiology being a highly complex subject.

2.3.1 Intrinsic factors: Ethnicity

Dobbs and Gurnett[9] reported prevalence in most of the studies as 1:1,000, and it is the most common congenital deformity. Clubfoot is associated in 20% of cases with distal arthrogryposis, congenital myotonic dystrophy, myelomeningocele, amniotic band sequence, or other genetic syndromes such as trisomy 18 or chromosome 22q11 deletion syndrome. In the rest of the cases, it is isolated with unknown etiology. They are commonly associated in unilateral cases with thinner calf/leg bones and smaller feet, with limb-length discrepancy, which are clearly appreciated in unilateral cases, but in bilateral cases, this discrepancy is less obvious. However, there are no significant histological or electrophysiological differences, and muscle biopsies from clubfoot lower extremities typically show nonspecific abnormalities histologically. Mild limb-length discrepancy may also be present in some cases.

Dobbs and Gurnett further argued in favor of a strong familial and polygenetic association in clubfoot. In isolated clubfoot, this is supported by many arguments. Firstly, about 25% of cases show positive family history in isolated clubfoot patients. Secondly, there is a consistently higher concordance rate in identical twins (33%) than fraternal twins (3%). Thirdly, there is a gross difference in prevalence in different ethnic populations (reporting from a study in Hawaii because of its mixed, stable, and multi-ethnic population). Prevalence of clubfoot varies widely in different races/ethnicities: it is lowest in Chinese at 0.39:1,000 and highest in Hawaiians and Maoris at 7:1,000 live births with a constant male:female ratio, that is, 2:1 in different ethnic groups. However, the exact genetic factors responsible are not yet clear, but it appears to be multifactorial and polygenic, rather than a single gene mutation. The incidence of clubfoot varies between countries and populations and may be related to numerous endogenous and exogenous factors. As the inheritance pattern is complex, isolated clubfoot is more likely to be multifactorial and polygenetic rather than a mutation in a single gene. Sex discrepancy, males being more commonly affected than females, is a strong argument against a single gene mutation. A polygenic inheritance model with a dimorphic sex threshold for the affected phenotype would explain this discrepancy. The Carter effect is also positive.

Noonan et al.[10] have attributed limb-length discrepancy to decreased foot height, as a result of surgical treatment in unilateral clubfoot. Three patients who underwent extensive posterior, medial, and lateral release were noted to have an average discrepancy in foot height of 2.1 centimeters, with a range of 2.0–2.3 centimeters.

Ching et al.[11] in a study from Hawaii with a mixed population corroborating the above contention of Dobbs and Gurnett, found that risk is the greatest in pure Hawaiian ancestry, less in Asian ancestry, and least in Caucasians. Prevalence has been found to be 5.67, 11.21, and 68.12 per 10,000 births in unmixed, Asians/Caucasians, and Hawaiians, respectively. Racial differences are considered to be due to a predominantly multifactorial inheritance mode.

Pompe van Meerdervoort[12] carried out a South African hospital-based prospective study from 1989 to 1992 to determine incidence and types of neonatal congenital anomalies. They found that incidence of externally visible congenital anomalies was 14.97:1,000 live births, which was 26.2% of the total, which could be diagnosed by five years of age, which reached 57.14:1,000. The cumulative incidence from all third-world countries was reported to be 84.85:1,000 by five years of age; neural tube defects (NTDs) was 3.55:1,000 and Down syndrome was 2.10:1,000, which are both preventable by prenatal screening. They concluded that managing these problems is possible by appropriate prenatal genetic, family planning, and pediatric facilities in the public health delivery system.

Yamamoto[13] in a study from Tokyo, Japan, hospitals, found in 1,600 births during 1973 to 1976 an incidence of 0.87:1,000 live births, family history in 185 patients from 1960 to 1976, male:female ratio of 2:1 with an equal number of bilateral:unilateral patients. The author also agreed that clubfoot is compatible with multifactorial inheritance.

Boo and Ong[14] in a study of newborns in Malaysians, found clubfoot to be prevalent as 4.5:1,000, bilateral and unilateral left foot were twice more commonly affected. Low birth weight was significantly common. They favored a multifactorial genetic influence.

Mittal et al.[15] in a door-to-door survey of a rural Indian population of 50,055 for detection of congenital orthopedic anomalies reported an incidence of 2.25 cases per 1,000 people, and clubfoot was found to be the most common anomaly at 0.9 per 1,000.

Shaw et al.[16] reported a population-based case-control study of risk of NTD in women of Mexican descent and white women out of 708,129 births from June 1989 to May 1991 in California hospitals. They concluded that the risk of NTD in newborns is twice as much in Mexico-born Mexican parents than for white parents, which is consistent with earlier reports for Latinos. The authors also commented that nearly 20% of new births in California are to Mexico-born Mexican mothers, and this increased risk is relevant to the population burden of NTD.

Chapman et al.[17] in a study in a New Zealand Polynesian population with 287 clubfoot families of Maori Pacific Islanders, found a high incidence of clubfoot in the New Zealand Maoris, with prevalence between 6 and 7 per 1,000 (with similar birth prevalence in the Hawaiian and the Tongan populations), with a major genetic role and multifactorial inheritance in the etiology of clubfoot. They found this population to be the best genetic model for clubfoot study due to a single dominant gene with a penetrance of 33% and a predicted gene frequency of 0.9%. The likelihood of affected subjects carrying a copy of the gene is sufficiently high in this population, which predisposes to clubfoot, and any family with multiple affected members is almost certain to carry a copy of this gene.

Barker and Macnicol[18] in a retrospective study of three years, from 1994 to 1996, reported a prevalence of idiopathic congenital talipes equinovarus as 0.64–2.5 per 1,000 live births in a Scottish population and also found it more common in births during March and April.

Krogsgaard et al.[19] analyzed the incidence of clubfoot as 1.2:1,000 in all of Denmark over a long period of 16 years from 1978 to 1993 and found it to be significantly more in counties with higher population density, indicating the influence of environmental and other exogenous factors. There were both isolated and syndromic types. Prevalence of isolated clubfoot was found to be 1.2:1,000 (1,126 isolated clubfoot out of 936,525 births), whereas syndromic clubfoot was 0.22:1,000. Male:female ratio was 2.2:1 in the isolated and 1.4:1 in the syndromic variety. The incidence of clubfoot with a higher population density (more than 500/km^2) was higher, especially the isolated clubfoot, indicating the effect of exogenous factors rather than genetic factors.

Da Silva Costa et al.[20] in a study from Brazil, found a prevalence rate of 1.7% for congenital malformation out of a total of 9,386 births, consisting of major and minor defects, in the city of Rio de Janeiro. Major defects were in the central nervous system (CNS, neural tube including spina bifida), whereas minor defects forming 66% of total defects with polydactyly and clubfoot were most common. In Brazil, folic-acid supplementation in wheat and corn flour with folic acid has been mandatory since June 2004, as there is strong evidence of folic-acid deficiency in the etiology of congenital defects, in general, as well as in clubfoot cases.

Wallander et al.[21] in a prospective multicentric study in 44 clinics in Sweden found that prevalence of clubfoot to be 1.4:1,000 live births, male:female ratio as 3:1 bilateral:unilateral as equal, and more in the southern than northern part of Sweden, which may be due to an extrinsic factor of smoking.

Li et al.[22] in a population-based survey of birth defects in four counties of Shanxi province of China during 2003, found an incidence of 160 NTDs in 11,534 births. The rates of anencephaly, spina bifida, and encephalocele were 65.9, 58.1, and 14.7 per 10,000, respectively, with spina bifida at second place. This was more in mothers of 20–30 years of age and with lower education, and only six out of 143 NTD mothers used folic-acid supplements.

Cardy et al.[23] reported a case-control study of 194 cases with 60 controls from the United Kingdom. The male:female ratio was 2.1:1, and bilateral cases were slightly more than unilateral cases with right more than left. There were 10 twin pregnancies and nine were nonidentical (fraternal). They found a significant association of clubfoot between paternal smoking family history during pregnancy, an interaction between smoking and unknown genetic relationship.

Siapkara and Duncan[24] reported that clubfoot is prevalent in Europe as 1.2:1,000 live births, and males are affected twice as often as females. Compared with the general population, first-degree relatives have a significantly higher risk. A father with clubfoot has a 2%–4% greater chance of having a clubfoot child. However, if a child and another family member of both parents have the deformity, the risk is increased further.

Mathias et al.[25] reported the prevalence of congenital clubfoot in Uganda from a study of a total of 110,336 live births in eight regional hospitals during the period from March 2006 to October 2007; they found the incidence at 1.2:1,000 live births over a 20-month period, with males affected 2.4 times more than females. Such a study is important to estimate the resources required to give early treatment in this deformity.

Nguyen et al.[26] found the prevalence rate of clubfoot in a Vietnamese population to be 1:1,000, with a male:female ratio of 2:1, a unilateral:bilateral ratio also of 2:1, and left foot:right foot ratio of almost 1:1. A strong association of clubfoot incidence was found with breech presentation and younger maternal age as compared with normal births.

Pavone et al.[27] analyzed a Sicilian population from 1991 to 2004; during those 14 years, there were 827 cases of clubfoot out of 801,324 live births, a prevalence of roughly 1:1,000, and male:female ratio of 2:1, with the right foot affected slightly more often than the left. There was a statistically significantly positive family history in clubfoot patients compared with controls, a difference in birth weight in clubfoot newborns compared with controls (3.013 and 3.903 kilograms, respectively), and a positive history of maternal smoking with clubfoot newborns.

Palma et al.[28] reported a study from Lima, Peru, with 72 clubfoot patients and 103 controls. The male:female ratio was 2:1, unilateral:bilateral was also 2:1, left:right showed no significant difference; parent age and education were both lower in clubfoot patents. History of both parents smoking and household smoking of others in the family was significant.

Werler et al.[29] reported the largest population-based series of confirmed clubfoot cases in North Carolina, Massachusetts, and New York from 2007 to 2011. In mothers of 677 clubfoot cases and 2,037 non-malformed controls, controlling for various factors, they found a strong association of obesity in mothers with high body mass index (BMI), more than 30%, increases the risk by 10%–20% with a positive family history risk, but the risk decreases significantly in second and third-degree relatives. There is further association of increased risk with factors resulting in fetal constraints (oligohydramnios, breech delivery, bicornuate uterus, plural birth) and family history in first-degree relations.

Wu et al.[30] in its first population-based reliable study from Kenya on surgical congenital anomalies, observed clubfoot at a prevalence at 2.9:1,000 and an overall prevalence of other congenital surgical anomalies at 6.3:1,000 out of 5,559 children surveyed door-to-door. Being a door-to-door survey, it is more reliable than data from hospital figures, which do not include all cases. The most prevalent condition was clubfoot, and spina bifida had the highest burden of disease.

Gili et al.[31] in a collaborative study in Latin American countries of South America for more than 40 years presented their data. They found a total of 25,082 deformed neonates from 2,557,424 births at 129 hospitals between 1995 and 2012. They looked for 17 deformities, including foot anomalies. Native and African people with high consanguinity were more susceptible.

Sitkin et al.[32] highlighted the high prevalence of congenital anomalies in LMICs with high GBD and distressing 25.3–38.8 million disability-adjusted life-years (DALYs) worldwide (DALY is one healthy year of life lost due to disability or premature death). They further state, quoting a World Health Organization (WHO) document, that congenital anomalies rank seventeenth in causes of GBD, and further, this is not the complete picture due to incomplete data. In addition, the facilities of treatment are not adequate and not accessible for various reasons.

In Argentina, Groisman et al.[33] identified a higher incidence for eight selected specific congenital anomalies (CAs) including clubfoot (anencephaly, encephalocele, spina bifida, diaphragmatic hernia, talipes equinovarus, omphalocele, cleft lip with or without cleft palate, and Down syndrome) from 703,325 births, in 133 maternity hospitals during a particular period from 24 potential provinces. There was a statistically higher prevalence rate, which could be due to a high referral rate there.

Tracey et al.[34] published a comprehensive review, the first of its kind, of a systematic search of six databases comprising 48 studies, which reported prevalence of clubfoot in LMICs. They provided data from 13,962,989 children in 20 countries over 55 years (1960–2015). The study included all kinds of clubfoot, that is, isolated as well as syndromic. The region-wise average prevalence per one thousand births found was 1.11 (0.96, 1.26) in Africa, 1.74 in the Americas, 1.21 in Southeast Asia (excluding India), 1.19 in India, 2.03 in Turkey (European region), 1.19 in the Eastern Mediterranean region, 0.94 in the West Pacific (excluding China), and 0.51 in China, varying from 0.51 to 2.03 in LMICs. However, a standardized uniform approach is required to find out the exact figures, as many may have been missed.

2.3.2 Extrinsic factors

2.3.2.1 EFFECT OF SMOKING

Maternal smoking, before conception and during pregnancy, especially during the first trimester, has been known to have deleterious effects on the fetus. There are a large number of direct publications in the literature about the harmful effects of smoking, while many indirect ones quote these specific studies carried out by others.

Van den Eeden[35] studied the effect of maternal smoking during pregnancy on congenital malformations, including clubfoot, in newborn babies in a population-based case-control study from 1984 to 1986 of Washington state birth records. This was done in 3,284 affected babies and compared with a similar group of 4,500 control babies. They concluded that maternal smoking is a potential risk factor in the etiology of specific types of defects like microcephaly, cleft lip/palate, and clubfoot.

A WHO book titled *Tobacco or Health: A Global Status Report*[36] reported the tobacco epidemic from 190 countries and published the trends of the last two decades. According to this book, there are about 1.1 billion smokers worldwide, comprising about one-third of the world population aged 15 years and older. Eight hundred million smokers live in developing countries, with 300 million in China alone, with a far higher incidence in developing countries than affluent ones. It is not only active tobacco use but also passive tobacco exposure, that is, living in a smoking area, that can have a deleterious effect. Tobacco use can lead to cancers, cardiovascular disease, chronic obstructive pulmonary disease (COPD), and various developmental defects of the skeleton. Tobacco is a mixture of approximately 4,800 compounds, with approximately 100 being carcinogenic chemicals. Genetics can go a long way in the prevention of the effects of tobacco through future research on animal models interacting with human genetics. However, the production of tobacco also must be controlled to get relief from this menace.

Werler[37] observed that exposure to cigarette smoke is a major hazard on reproductive health, resulting in birth defects, in view of the myriad publications on the subject in the literature and the fact that 15% of women smoke during pregnancy. Cigarette smoke contains hundreds of toxins and there are many pathways of their harmful effects: nicotine with its major metabolite cotinine is a vasoconstrictor and reduces placental and fetal circulation; thiocyanate (cyanide) is a known marker of smoking; carbon monoxide depletes maternal and fetal oxygen supplies; excess cadmium has been found in the ovaries, follicular fluid, and placenta of smokers; lead along with some other aromatic hydrocarbons are also known to have damaging effects. Because of the presence of all of these poisonous elements in the maternal fetal blood circulation, there is a strong risk of congenital malformations. The author collected evidence on the effects of maternal smoking from the already published literature and affirmed that smoking does produce important deleterious effects on newborn infants.

Honein et al.[38] reported a case-control study in Atlanta, Georgia, of 346 infants with isolated clubfoot and 3,029 infant controls without defects born from 1968 to 1980. They defined smoking as smoking during the first three months of pregnancy and family history as a first-degree relative having clubfoot. They found a statistically significant effect of smoking in the first trimester of pregnancy, this being the critical period for development of clubfoot. They found strong evidence of the effect of smoking in isolated clubfoot, and it is much more in cases with a positive family history of first-degree relatives with a potential smoke:genes interaction. The mechanism of action may be through nicotine, which is vasoconstrictive, and higher level of carbon monoxide and many other volatile compounds in leading to fetal hypoxia or leading to vascular disruptions compromise or some other unknown way of genetic interaction.

Woods and Raju[39] conducted a cohort study of 1943 mothers who smoke from January 1998 to December 1999 and looked at 22 types of congenital defects, including foot deformities. There was statistically significant evidence for a premature birth and congenital heart diseases. However, other defects were found to be more common than in controls, but this was not statistically significant.

Saha et al.[40] reported that there are innumerable publications on the ill effects of smoking on the reproductive health of mothers and structural birth defects. They quoted from the Office of the Surgeon General of the United States Health Service review of more than 7,000 research articles on the topic of smoking and health, and publicly recognized the role of smoking in various diseases, including lung cancer. They also reported that about 15% of women smoke throughout pregnancy. Tobacco contains hundreds of toxic chemicals. They investigated the relationship between tobacco use and human health and confirmed the definite association with its use. Modern genetics has been making good progress in finding the association between tobacco use and development of diseases in human beings.

Dickinson et al.[41] in a North Carolina study of 443 clubfeet and 4,492 controls, also found consistency with others regarding the harmful effect of smoking on the etiology of clubfoot. Werler et al.[42] investigated the effect of maternal consumption of cigarette smoking, alcohol, and coffee in a population-based study of isolated clubfoot in Massachusetts, New York, and North Carolina from 2007 to 2011 with 646 patients and 2,037 controls. They concluded that cigarette smoking is positively associated with increased incidence of clubfoot, but for alcohol and coffee, they observed that the risk increased only with a higher level of intake.

Sommers et al.[43] observed that clubfoot is a common defect and that it affects 135,000 children worldwide. Maternal cigarette smoking during pregnancy is the only environmental factor that has been consistently associated with clubfoot all over the world. If there is a family history along with this, this risk increases 20 times. Metabolism of chemical compounds in the smoke occurs through a xenobiotic metabolism pathway affecting the eight genes which they studied. They concluded that the xenobiotic pathway is affected in some way to produce the deformity.

Hackshaw et al.[44] in a comprehensive meta-analysis of 172 articles published from 1959 to 2010, with a total of 173,687 malformation cases and 11,674,332 controls, found a significant association of maternal smoking with congenital defects, including clubfoot. Congenital clubfoot was one of the major congenital malformations due to maternal smoking. They also suggested that, to increase awareness, such material should be included in the public health educational materials to encourage quitting smoking.

The U.S. surgeon general,[45] in a book from 2014, reports comprehensive details of smoking and its health hazards producing diseases. Smoking affects all reproductive aspects producing infertility and affecting pregnancy and fetal development, including all organs, clubfoot and other skeletal developmental defects, and causing various developmental defects.

Werler et al.[42] carried out a population-based case-control study of clubfoot in Massachusetts, New York, and North Carolina from 2007 to 2011 and studied the effect of smoking, coffee, and alcohol intake during pregnancy on the fetus. Mothers of 646 isolated clubfoot cases and 2,037 controls were included in the study. They concluded that women who smoked in the perinatal period had a higher risk of having a clubfoot baby, and the risk was much higher in those mothers continuing to smoke in the later period. For alcohol and coffee, the risk was observed, but only with higher quantities.

Viteri et al.[46] reviewed the literature of 128 articles on the effects of cocaine, marijuana/cannabis, opioids, amphetamines, alcohol, and smoking on pregnancy and congenital malformations. They summarized that drug exposure during pregnancy can increase the risk of congenital anomalies. This is especially true after smoking, more particularly in causing clubfoot.

2.3.2.2 MEDICATIONS

Taking some medicines during pregnancy for other diseases can also have harmful effects on the fetus, causing congenital defects including clubfoot.

Samren et al.[47] analyzed data from five European studies from 1971 to 1990, comprising 896 epileptic mothers taking anti-epileptic drugs (AEDs) and 1,221 children born to them and thus exposed to AEDs, as well as 158 control children born to non-epileptic mothers and thus unexposed to AEDs. They selected a subgroup of 192 exposed children for matching comparison with the 158 unexposed children. There were innumerable variables in age of mothers; type and severity of epilepsy; and type, dosage regimen, and duration of many drugs. In spite of that it was found that, in monotherapy, velaporate (VPA) and carbamazine (CBZ) risk factors were highly significant for major congenital anomalies, including clubfoot, and polytherapies were also harmful.

Veroniki et al.[48] in a recent informative review article from 96 eligible studies from an extensive literature review, reported on common mono- and poly-AEDs used by pregnant women with epilepsy versus control pregnant women with no AED use. The authors reviewed the literature through December 15, 2015, and compared mono- and poly-AEDs in their meta-analysis. They found significantly increased risk of congenital defects, including clubfoot, with the older generation of drugs, but even newer generation drugs are not completely safe as compared with controls. Polytherapies are more harmful than monotherapies. Counseling is important about teratogenic risks when these agents are given during pregnancy, such as switching from poly-therapy to mono-therapy and avoiding use of higher-risk drugs like velproate. A considered decision is important to control the convulsions as well as safety of the fetus.

Louik et al.[49] studied the effects of using periconceptional selective serotonin reuptake inhibitor (SSRI) antidepressants in increasing the risk of birth defects and found no conclusive evidence for the same. However, individual SSRIs may confer increased risks for some specific defects.

Norgaard et al.[50] utilized a Danish birth registry to analyze the effect of fluconazole use in 1,079 pregnant women compared with 170,453 pregnant women who did not use fluconazole. Fluconazole is widely used for candidiasis; the dosages used by these women were 150 mg (74%), 300 mg (22%), 350 mg (2%), and 600 mg (2%). Birth defects, including clubfoot, were found in 4.1% in the fluconazole group and 3.6% in the control group, which was not significant after a short-term treatment. They compared with the results with other similar studies, which also had the same findings. They also concluded that larger studies are needed with long-term use of the drug to completely rule out an effect.

Crider et al.[51] observed, in a population-based study, that use of antibacterial agents in pregnancy are common, whereas sulfonamides and nitrofurantoin are risk factors for many congenital defects, including those of the limbs. The authors concluded from their study that there is a possibility of increased risk for congenital heart defects and recommended quinolones not be used during pregnancy. Whether the infection itself, the antibacterial, or both are responsible is to be investigated.

Allen and O'Brien[52] reviewed the use of misoprostol, which is a synthetic prostaglandin E1 analog commonly used for many indications in obstetrics. Due to its wide use in obstetrics and gynecology, WHO has put misoprostol in its model list of essential medicines. This has been found to be teratogenic and a risk factor for clubfoot and, causing Moebius syndrome, which may be associated with clubfoot and arthrogryposis. However, the estimated risk is only approximately 1%. Still, its use should be with caution and under medical advice.

Callen et al.[53] observed that, after the authentic discovery of the thalidomide episode, increased attention was directed toward other drugs, especially the CNS-active drugs like thalidomide that pass the blood–brain barrier and the placenta, thus reaching the embryo. They recorded their observations in an overview of literature, along with the Swedish reports on drugs from 1996 to 2011, on the effects of opioids, anticonvulsants, drugs used for Parkinson's disease, neuroleptics (antipsychotics and tranquilizers), sedatives and hypnotics, antidepressants, psychostimulants, and some other CNS-active drugs in pregnancy, especially during first trimester. A definite association of use of these drugs in many congenital defects has been found. Continuous use of tramadol has also been implicated to be associated with the clubfoot deformity.

Werler et al.[54] investigated the effect of different medicines taken by the mother during pregnancy in a large-scale, population-based, first of its kind, case-control study from Massachusetts, New York, and North Carolina from 2007 to 2011. Mothers of 646 isolated clubfoot cases and 2,037 controls were interrogated within 12 months of delivery about various medicines used, their timing, and their frequency. Use of antiviral drugs was the most common evidence in isolated clubfoot; others were antibiotics and opioids. Nonsteroidal anti-inflammatory drugs (NSAIDs) and antinausea medicines also had evidence in the etiology. The risk was more for the use of azithromycin and antiviral medications. A greater risk was observed for metronidazole, and slightly higher risks were observed for 2 antinausea treatments: promethazine and ondesetron. Besides the isolated clubfoot, drugs affecting the CNS, which secondarily can cause clubfoot, include opioids, promethazine, other antihistamines, ondansetron, marijuana, and SSRIs and were associated with a somewhat higher risk of clubfoot. However, definite proof of associations and how they act is a subject for further research.

Broussard et al.[55] reported from a U.S. national birth-defects prevention, population-based study from 1997 to 2005 in America that 2.6% out of 17,449 case mothers and 2% of control cases use therapeutic opioids. They reported 3% birth defects out of 3 million births each year, and therapeutic opioid use was reported by 2.6% of 17,449 birth-defect-case mothers and 2.0% of 6,701 control mothers; this was found to be statistically significant and associated with many congenital defects, for example, congenital heart diseases, spina bifida, and others. The mechanism of action of opioids has also been explained.

Yazdy et al.[56] conducted a review of available literature documenting potential harms associated with prescription opioid use, especially codeine during pregnancy for pain management and opioid dependency. They found that, to date, five studies have identified coronary heart disease (CHD) and three studies have proved convincing risk factors on neonate NTDs and congenital clubfoot.

Mitchell[57] observed that adverse drug reactions can also be in the form of drug-induced congenital birth defects in pregnant mothers, and most teratogenic risks can only be found after the drug is marketed and little is known about the fetal safety about most drugs. They can only be known after specific study designs. Caution should always be observed before using any new drug in the periconceptional period.

2.3.2.3 NUTRITIONAL DEFICIENCY

Picciano[58] reported that there is strong evidence that elevated plasma total homocysteine (hyperhomocysteinemia) is a risk factor in coronary, cerebral, and peripheral arterial diseases and other congenital defects including NTDs and clubfoot. It is also well established that periconceptional folic-acid supplementation reduces this risk, but its exact mechanism is not clear.

Vollset et al.[59] in a Norway population-based study of 5,883 women 40–42 years of age, carried out tHcy estimation in plasma (a marker of folate level and a risk factor for CHDs). They found that higher levels of tHcy were associated with most of the pregnancy complications, including congenital defects of cardiovascular system, orofacial, NTDs, and clubfoot. However, there were a large number of variables of various interacting factors requiring further studies.

Karakurt et al.[60] studied the relationship between the plasma total homocysteine level in blood samples of mothers of children with clubfoot (group 1) compared with samples of the control group of mothers of children without clubfoot (group 2). Mean plasma total homocysteine level showed significant statistical difference (16.34 ± 4.78 μmol/L in group 1 and 11.02 ± 1.85 μmol/L in group 2). Congenital idiopathic clubfoot showed a significant association with a high plasma total homocysteine level.

Sharp et al.[61] observed that folic acid is crucially involved in DNA synthesis (the MTHFR gene) and many other metabolic processes, and a low folate status has been found to be a risk factor in clubfoot etiology. The authors carried out case studies in 375 UK cases in 1998 through 1999. According to the authors, this is the first known report of specific genetic proof of an association between clubfoot and folate status. Supplementation with folic acid has been found to reduce the incidence of clubfoot. The authors concluded that folate metabolism is quite complex, involving interaction of so many other nutrients and other factors and thus needs further elucidation.

Molloy et al.[62] commented that low folate during pregnancy is a significant cause of morbidity in mothers, and the role of folic acid preventing NTDs is now an established fact, besides protecting against many other congenital defects. They thus corroborated the strong evidence in the literature regarding the role of folic acid in prevention of NTDs and other birth defects and stressed the need for supplementation with folic acid and vitamin B12.

Czeizel et al.[63] because of the disagreement and doubts about the data in earlier studies in diabetic and epileptic mothers, and in pregnancy with high fever, carried out a large population-based, multicenter controlled trial from 1980 to 1996 in 22,843 cases with different congenital anomalies, including clubfoot and 38,151 controls without any defects. There were 79 diabetic mothers in the congenital anomalies group and 40 received folic acid, while in the control group of 88 mothers, 54 received folic acid, with an average daily dose of folic acid was 3.1 mg in epileptic pregnant women while this dose was 5.6 mg in nonepileptic pregnant women. Risk for congenital anomalies, including clubfoot, was higher in the mothers without folic-acid supplementation. Similarly, the effect of antiepileptic drugs was studied in epileptic mothers, with 95 epileptics in the CA group and 90 in the control group. The same was done for the high-fever group (fever usually due to influenza, tonsillitis, or the common cold). All three illnesses had teratogenic effects and folic-acid supplementation certainly had a protective role. The authors discussed the benefits and drawbacks of four possible ways of using periconceptional folic acid and multivitamins. Under/malnutrition has been an important factor in the etiology of CAs, including NTDs and clubfoot. Supplementation is done in four possible ways: (i) dietary intake of folate and other vitamins, (ii) periconceptional folic acid/multivitamin supplements, (iii) food fortification by folic acid, and (iv) the combining and oral contraceptives with 6S-5-methyltetrahydrofolate ("folate"). These have all been found to be useful in diabetic and epileptic mothers, and in pregnancy with high fever.

In a review article, Czeizel et al.[64] again reported that dietary deficiencies, especially vitamins, are associated with the risk of birth defects, notably NTDs and CHDs. It has been found that about 90% of NTDs can be prevented by multivitamins at least one month before conception and at least two months after conception, while about 70% can be prevented by folic-acid supplementation. CHDs with prevalence of 0.7–1.0 per 1,000 can also be prevented with multivitamins to the extent of about 40%. There are three ways of using this preventive method: (i) dietary intake of folate, (ii) supplementation with folic acid or multivitamins before and during pregnancy (but this simple and cheap method is not possible in an unplanned pregnancy), and (iii) flour fortification with folic acid.

Kaska et al.[65] from Poland, reported that obesity is an important health problem all over the world, more in females than males with about one-third in the reproductive age. In the United States, its incidence was found to be 27%, especially in women of reproductive age. As bariatric surgery is being done more frequently now for morbid obesity in the reproductive age, it poses special problems due to restrictive intake or absorption problems, depending upon the procedure performed. It leads to all-around nutritional deficiencies, especially of micronutrients such as folic acid, vitamin B12, iron, zinc, calcium, and others, and more so in pregnant women. Nutritional deficiency of folic acid can lead to NTDs with consequent paralytic lower-limb deformities. Other micronutrient deficiencies also have their risk factors. Therefore, adequate supplementation is highly important after bariatric surgery.

Gernand et al.[66] discussed, in a review article, the risks of micronutrient deficiencies causing various congenital defects, including clubfoot, and the prevention of these deficiencies during pregnancy, including the overall health worldwide and their intake recommendations. Various micronutrients, including vitamins B6 and B12, selenium, vitamin A, vitamin C, iron, zinc, copper, vitamin E, magnesium, choline, iodine, folic acid, and vitamin D are needed during pregnancy for the mother, the placenta, and fetal development of various organs. All of these are utilized through numerous pathways. There are overall benefits of these nutrients during pregnancy, after pregnancy, and throughout life. Although dietary intake is extremely important through a balanced diet, supplementation of some of the micronutrients is essential during pregnancy, especially in LMICs, and is recommended by WHO.

Gildestad et al.[67] published data from Norway from 1999 to 2013 with a total of 528,220 women with 880,568 pregnancies and 896,674 live and stillbirths and with 270 NTDs. They divided the study into two study periods, from 1999 to 2005 and 2005 to 2013 because of more supplement use in the second period than the first. They found that NTDs were significantly less in the second period, when folic acid use was much higher.

2.3.2.4 MATERNAL DISEASES—OBESITY AND/OR DIABETES, HYPERTENSION, INFECTIONS

Moore et al.[68] reported on data of 22,951 pregnant women with obesity alone or obesity with diabetes about the risk of congenital anomalies including clubfoot. Obesity alone did not increase the risk of congenital defects in the neonates, pre-existing diabetes posed some risk, but both diabetes and obesity, acting synergistically, had a 3.1 times higher risk of congenital defects in an offspring than those who were not obese and nondiabetic. The defects were largely craniofacial and musculoskeletal, including clubfoot.

Allen et al.[69] reported that major structural deformations occur during the third to seventh week of gestation, as detailed in the Canadian document. Pre-existing maternal diabetes; type 1 and 2 and gestational diabetes are important causes of fetal malformations including clubfoot. Their pathogenesis appears to be multifactorial due to nutritional deficiency and toxic metabolites of diabetes, the important one being hyperglycemia. The risk of congenital malformations, resulting in abnormal chromosomes, increases 2–3 times compared to the general population. Risk of congenital malformations, with pre-existing diabetes, is 1.7–3 times higher than in the general population. Glycemic control and folic acid use are beneficial. Gestational diabetes, complicating 2%–4% of pregnancies, has 1.2 times higher risk than the general population. With persistent hyperglycemia, risk of malformations is 3.4 times higher than normal. On the other hand, obesity is an important risk factor for diabetes, and it is established in many studies that obesity along with diabetes has a 3-fold increased risk of congenital deformations. A healthy diet and controlling weight as well diabetes will reduce the risk.

Yazdy et al.[70] studied the observation reported in the literature about risk factors of diabetes and obesity in congenital NTDs. They concluded, from a case-control study of 698 case mothers and 696 control mothers, from 1988 to 1998 at Boston University, that high dietary glycemic index (DGI) and high dietary glycemic load (DGL) increased the risk of NTDs in developing fetuses in nondiabetic women, adding further evidence to the belief that hyperglycemia increases the risk of NTDs.

Cooper et al.[71] commented about other reports in the literature that Angiotensin Converting Enzyme (ACE) inhibitors are contraindicated in the second and third trimesters due to risk of fetopathy, but not in the first trimester. However, they studied, themselves, the use of ACE inhibitors alone during the first trimester in 209 infants, exposure to other antihypertensives in 202 infants, and no exposure to antihypertensive drugs in 29,096 infants. They found ACE inhibitors are not safe even in the first trimester, as compared with other antihypertensives, and can lead to major cardiovascular anomalies, NTDs, and other issues. These drugs, therefore, should be avoided during pregnancy.

Al-Maawali et al.[72] concluded from their study that the use of ACE inhibitors in the first trimester of pregnancy did not increase the risk of congenital malformations. This conclusion was based on a review of the literature of five systematic studies and 19 case reports. They argued that the reports, in opposition to the literature already discussed, were due to inclusion of undiagnosed diabetes and overweight mothers, which are known risk factors. In contrast to that, their use in the second and third trimester is contraindicated due to the risk of congenital malformations in the fetus.

Edwards[73] observed various congenital defects, including neural tube and limb defects following maternal fever and hyperthermia during pregnancy. The actual effect depends upon degree, duration, and stage of pregnancy, and a directly proportional risk is present. The CNS is the most sensitive for anomalies of NTDs.

Luteijn et al.[74] in a meta-analysis of 22 studies from the literature, through July 2013, observed that influenza or influenza-like illness in the mother in the first trimester is associated with increased risk of a number of CAs, including NTDs and limbs defects. However, more research is needed to find out the individual or combined interaction of various factors in influenza, for example, hyperthermia, medicines used for this, or nutritional deficiencies in producing congenital defects.

Rasmussen et al.[75] reported that, since early 2015 when it was first reported from Brazil, Zika virus infection during pregnancy has spread rapidly in America and is associated with skeletal defects like microcephaly and other brain defects. The authors discussed Shepherd's seven criteria suggested as proof of teratogenicity and said that the most essential criteria (1, 3, and 4) are satisfied, which is a sufficient evidence of association of Zika virus in producing congenital defects. Authors have concluded that a causal relationship does exist between Zika virus infection and the above anomalies.

Van der Linden et al.[76] observed a series of seven cases with arthrogryposis with a diagnosis of congenital Zika virus infection during the Brazilian microcephaly epidemic. All seven were positive for brain infection with Zika virus and had arthrogryposis including clubfoot. All seven involved all four limbs, including hips and legs only in one. Clinical, radiological, and electromyographic studies were done in all seven for co-relation. All seven showed brain changes on MRI, arthrogryposis was due to neurogenic in electromyography and of lower motor neuron on spinal MRI. Other infections causing microcephaly can be rubella, cytomegalovirus, and toxoplasmosis. Besides microcephaly and arthrogryposis, there are many other congenital defects, such as hearing and visual, and so it is better to call it congenital Zika syndrome.

2.3.2.5 AMNIOCENTESIS AND UTERINE FACTORS

Nagel et al.[77] in a controlled study, compared the effects of transabdominal chorionic villus sampling and early amniocentesis on fetal mortality and child morbidity. All fetal mortality occurred after early amniocentesis. Clubfoot was seen in 3.1% of cases only after early amniocentesis. The authors concluded that chorionic villus sampling should be the choice for prenatal diagnosis in the first trimester. These authors quoted Sundberg et al. (1997), who also had a similar opinion regarding the evidence of an increased risk of clubfoot with early amniocentesis but none in the chorionic villus sampling group.

In view of many earlier reports of fetal risk and clubfoot in early amniocentesis, Farrell et al.[78] analyzed its adverse effect in the etiology of clubfoot in a review of the largest study by the Canadian Early and Mid-Trimester Amniocentesis Trial group (CEMAT). They were divided into two groups of 2,187 women each: group 1 was the early amniocentesis (EA) group and group 2 was the midterm amniocentesis (MA) group. There were 29 (1.3%) cases of clubfoot in 2,172 pregnancies in group 1 but only two (0.1%) in the 2,162 pregnancies of group 2, that is, 10 times more in EA than MA with the bilateral:unilateral ratio of 52:48. This is well above the overall population risk of 1:1,000. Because of fewer cases, it is difficult to say from this study about the mechanism of clubfoot and whether it is due to or not due to intrauterine position of the foot in early pregnancy which resembles clubfoot (plantar flexed and inverted) and the foot getting straightened as the pregnancy advances. In CEMAT, early amniocentesis is done when the foot is straightening out. There were no structural abnormalities in bones, muscles, or neurogenic tissue in clubfoot occurring in CEMAT, indicating that this is not a primary structural malformation, but is due to secondary disruption owing to a vascular event or deformation due to physical restriction of development and mechanical pressure. Leakage of amniotic fluid after EA and oligohydramnios could be another factor leading to restricted intrauterine space, but it is difficult to confirm. The mother should be informed about this risk when early or midterm amniocentesis is to be offered.

Ercole et al.[79] described often indicated, invasive procedures of amniocentesis, fetal blood sampling (FBS), and chorionic villous sampling (CVS), which provide material for fetal DNA, biochemical analysis, or identification of various infectious agents. They are indicated in cytogenetic and DNA analysis, diagnosing NTDs and identifying infectious agents (toxoplasmosis, cytomegalovirus, rubella, and varicella), and etiology of intracerebral hemorrhage (fetal platelets and coagulation factors). They can sometimes cause complications and should be done only when indicated and with the informed consent of the mother.

Moh et al.[80] in a review article reported on intrauterine growth restrictions (IUGRs) during pregnancy, which means, besides being underweight, the fetus develops with restricted growth. This is multifactorial and may be due to intrinsic as well as extrinsic causes. The normal amount and direction of growth of the fetus, in its different stages of development, requires normal space inside the uterus. The problem arises in 70%–80% later stages of gestation with restricted growth, which may be symmetrical or asymmetrical depending upon the space available for growth, asymmetrical being more common. In growth-restricted infants, this leads to deformities. Biomechanical forces play an important part in the morphogenesis of fetal parts. Various uterine-constraining factors include primigravida; small uterus; uterine malformation like didelphic uterus with duplicated cervix, bicornuate uterus, septate uterus, and arcuate uterus; uterine fibromata; early pelvic engagement of the fetal head; aberrant fetal position; oligohydramnios; and multifetal gestation. Limb deformations can occur due to these, which may be due to intrinsic or extrinsic causes. Oligohydramnios is serious and may occur early or late in pregnancy, leading to deformations including clubfoot. Many preventable and curative measures are available, but more needs to be done.

2.3.2.6 SOCIOECONOMIC, MATERNAL AGE, AND ENVIRONMENTAL FACTORS

Wasserman et al.[81] utilized a population-based, case-control study, to find out whether personal and neighborhood socioeconomic status (SES), as well as of taking multivitamins by pregnant mothers, affects NTDs in newborns. The indicators for lower SES included were education, employment, family income, type of employment, housing, overcrowding, dietary intake, and so forth. They concluded that both types of lower SES, that is, personal and living in a poor neighborhood SES, increased the risk of having an NTD-affected baby. This is directly proportional to the grade of lower SES, that is, the lower the grade, the greater the risk. African Americans were more affected. Their report also substantiated many other similar reports.

Castilla et al.[82] studied the effect of low and high altitude on birth defects in 1,668,722 consecutive births in 53 participating hospitals in South American countries and found that, at high altitudes, there was a statistically significant higher risk of four types of craniofacial congenital defects at highlands, while at lowlands there was a significantly higher rate for other congenital defects, but not so for clubfoot.

Dolk et al.[83] studied socioeconomic effects in 858 cases of congenital anomalies and 1,764 control births during 1986 to 1993 for various types of congenital malformation: CHDs, NTDs, and orofacial clefts (OFCs). They found significantly higher risk for orofacial defects in deprived neighborhoods. Registers from the UK in a multicenter case-control study on the risk of nonchromosomal congenital anomalies near hazardous-waste landfill sites showed that anomalies were found to have increased in incidence.

Carmichael et al.[84] analyzed data from a population-based case-control study of new births in California from 1989 to 1991 in 538 mothers of NTD cases and 539 control mothers and found that physically active women, especially who were taking multivitamins, were at 30%–50% lower risk for NTDs.

Zhiwen Li et al.[85] found that northern China's Shanxi Province has reported the highest incidence of NTDs in the world with 10–20 cases per 1,000. They studied indoor air pollution from coal combustion (commonly used as fuel there) as a possible risk factor for NTDs. They carried out a case-control study, the first of its kind, with 610 NTD cases and 837 controls between November 2002 and December 2007. Increased incidence was noted with indoor heating and cooking with coal, which increased with increased exposure. Compared with women with no air pollution exposure, women with exposure had a 60% increased risk of having a child with an NTD. Most of the mothers were in the younger age group of 20–34 years of age, with a lower education level and no folic acid supplements during the periconceptional period.

Chen et al.[86] carried out a retrospective cohort study in 5,542,861 multifarious young pregnant women and reported that teenage pregnancy increases the risks of congenital anomalies in the central nervous, gastrointestinal, and musculoskeletal/integumental systems, including clubfoot. The exact cause of this is not clear. Some factors could be more prevalent smoking, alcohol, and drugs used in teenagers, lack of prenatal care, and deficiency of multivitamins and folic acid supplements.

Mattison[87] summarized the results of studies exploring paternal/maternal pre-, peri-, and postconception exposures to chemical, biological, and physical agents, for example, air and water pollutants, exposure to various occupational dusts (inhalants or contacts), food chemicals, pesticides, volatile gases, metals, agricultural chemicals, and so forth in causing developmental defects in the fetus. They cause a gene–environment interaction leading to developmental disorders in the newborn by affecting the father, mother, placenta, or the fetus. Therefore, maximum precautions have to be taken in this regard to prevent harmful outcomes.

Lupo et al.[88] in view of several earlier reports, carried out a case-control study to find out the association of air the pollutants benzene, toluene, ethylbenzene, and xylene (BTEX) and the prevalence of NTDs (spina bifida, anencephaly) in newborn infants. This was done from 1999 to 2004 in a Texas birth-defects registry as well as controls of normal births. They asserted that there are potent risk factors in benzene for NTDs, in confirmation of many such previous reports.

Coppola et al.[89] studied the effect of the psychological stress and family support in mothers during pregnancy and prenatal diagnosis of clubfoot, in 17 mothers of clubfoot babies and 17 control mothers. They found that mothers in the affected group were stressed and more depressed than typical and that there was a positive effect of improvement of family support.

Jaikrishan et al.[90] compiled data from government hospital records since 1995, with 142,000 new births and thus a large sample size, in and around the high-level natural radiation areas of Kerala, India, on India's southwest coast where there are natural deposits of monazite sand containing thorium and its daughter products. This entailed 141,540 newborns, in which clubfoot was found in 404 with a prevalence of 2.85%, and this was the most common major congenital defect out of many defects. Among stillbirths, clubfoot prevalence was 20 times higher out of 615 total stillbirths. WHO also stressed the global importance of human studies of the effect of low-dose radiation exposure as an occupational hazard, as well as protective measures.

Lassi et al.[91] carried out a meta-analysis from the available literature and found the effect of preconception usage of caffeine, tobacco, alcohol, and other illicit drugs and exposure to environmental chemicals and radiation can have adverse effects and lead to congenital malformations, besides fetal losses and many other harmful effects. However, there were fewer studies in each section with its own limitations. More rigorous studies with larger sample sizes should continue for firm conclusions.

Padula et al.[92] reported the effects of environmental pollutants and neighborhood socioeconomic factors as risk factors in NTDs after studying the data from a California center from 1997 to 2006. They analyzed the effect of five pollutants and nine socioeconomic factors in the study. They concluded that there is definite high risk with air pollutants, which is further enhanced with these lower socioeconomic factors, and this is more so with spina bifida. The pathway of action seems to be multifactorial.

Zhao et al.[93] found significant seasonal variation in the incidence of clubfoot in eastern and southeastern China; it was higher in autumn in comparison with other seasons, but there was no difference with regard to the severity of the deformity.

2.3.3 Genetics and clubfoot

Human genetics is a study of inheritance of diseases in human beings and it is a vast subject. There are a large number of fields under human genetics, for example, classical genetics, cytogenetics, molecular genetics, biochemical genetics, genomics, population genetics, developmental genetics, clinical genetics and genetic counseling (medical genetics), and so on. All of these aspects are being explored by a large number of investigators all over the world. There is ample progress, but still, there are many gray areas requiring further research. The genetics of clubfoot too, is a highly complex and specialized subject and also multifactorial and polygenic in nature, and investigators are exploring all these possibilities, and some tangible progress has been made herein. To discuss complete genetics of congenital defects in general, and clubfoot in particular, is not the subject of this book. However, some basic aspects will be discussed, which will be helpful in the prevention and treatment of this unsolved common deformity.

There are two well-known varieties of congenital clubfoot: isolated and syndromic. The isolated deformity is much more common and, in this variety, the only defect present in the newborn is clubfoot. There is another well recognized, but much less common, variety, the syndromic variety of clubfoot, in which, besides clubfoot, there are also other associated congenital abnormalities. The isolated clubfoot may, sometimes, have a familial incidence which is much higher in identical twins than in fraternal twins. The familial isolated clubfoot and the syndromic variety are genetic in nature. However, it is not only the intrinsic factors (genes), but also the influence of a large number of extrinsic factors as discussed above (environmental and others), which are responsible for the deformity in innumerable ways, many of which are yet to be explored. There are a large number of syndromes with associated clubfoot deformity, some seen more often, while others are not that frequent. There are innumerable reports in the literature, and some of the important ones have been selected for this book.

Ching et al.[94] reported that the mode of genetic contribution in the etiology of clubfoot is not clear and is highly confusing. The authors quoted references to many hypotheses: autosomal recessive, sex-linked recessive inheritance, heterogenetic/multifactorial due to different autosomal recessive genes, and autosomal dominant gene with reduced penetrance. The authors specifically studied the Hawaiian population for many reasons: a higher prevalence of clubfoot (6.81 per 1,000 live births), a small and stable population numbering only 750,000, good medical care making ascertainment easy, and ease of study of a mixed-racial population. Their study included 232 cases of equinovarus deformity, with complete data during an 11-year period from 1948 to 1958. The incidence of equinovarus deformity increases with increase in Hawaiian parentage, incidence being consistently at 6.8:1,000 for unmixed Hawaiians. All external or intrauterine factors were excluded. Other studies have also reported higher prevalence of clubfoot in Hawaii, increasing consistently with increasing Hawaiian parentage. The authors support a genetic etiology with a multifactorial mode of inheritance.

Dobbs and Gurnett[9] in a comprehensive review of literature, have reported that, besides the common isolated variety of clubfoot, 20% of clubfoot cases are syndromic and are associated with arthrogryposis multiplex, congenital myotonic dystrophy, myelomeningocele, amniotic bands, or other genetic syndromes such as trisomy 18 or chromosome 22q11 deletion syndrome. They further reported many theories in clubfoot pathogenesis: anatomical abnormalities like intrauterine immobility, neurological conditions, and connective tissue fibrosis. Vascular anomalies are very commonly seen, mostly anterior tibial artery hypoplasia. Unilateral clubfoot is associated with a thinner calf as compared to the unaffected limb, but with normal electrophysiological studies of muscles and nerves, and histological muscle biopsies on the clubfoot side show only nonspecific abnormalities. Leg-length discrepancy may also be present in clubfoot. These widespread variations suggest that clubfoot is either heterogenous or due to a single primary cause leading to all of these abnormalities of tissues. The authors have tried to explain pathogenesis of clubfoot on a genetic basis, giving many reasons. In isolated clubfoot: firstly, 25% of all isolated clubfoot cases report a positive familial incidence; secondly, a higher concordance rate in identical twins than fraternal twins (33% versus 3%); and thirdly: variation in the prevalence rate in different ethnic populations. They point out that isolated clubfoot is more likely to be due to multiple factors and/or polygenic. It is unlikely to be due to mutation of a single gene because there is sex affliction discrepancy, with males affected much more commonly than females; in the absence of sex-linked inheritance. A polygenic inheritance with such a sex difference explains this, which is further supported by demonstration of the Carter effect, that is, the less commonly affected sex, that is, females, carry a greater number of susceptible genes than males and are more likely to transmit clubfoot. They also found from many recent studies that there is a key transcriptional pathway, the PITX1-TBX4 in clubfoot etiology, and both PITX1 and TBX4 are expressed specifically in lower limbs, with foot as phenotype along with mutations in these transcriptional factors. The exact mechanisms of these genetic abnormalities producing clubfoot are yet to be investigated, including many other hypotheses regarding its pathogenesis.

Phatak et al.[95] reported a rare case of Patio syndrome (trisomy 13), which occurs in 1:5,000 births and is the most severe of the three autosomal trisomies. The child is born with multiple congenital defects, involving almost every system, including the lower limbs with clubfoot. The majority die within the first month of birth. At ultrasonography, polyhydramnios was detected besides congenital defects of other organs, including clubfoot. Rarely, in a less severe case when the extra chromosome 13, which is usually present in every cell in trisomy 13, is not present in every cell, thus showing mosaicism, which may have a less severe outcome and survival is longer. Clubfoot has been associated with other trisomies also. Chromosomal analysis should be considered when clubfoot is associated with other congenital defects. Many structural abnormalities of soft tissues and bones are present in syndromic clubfoot deformities, given that this is frequently associated with many genetic syndromes.

Alvarado et al.[96] screened cases of familial isolated clubfoot to find any genetic etiology and found that microduplication of chromosome 17q23.1q23.2 is a common cause and provides strong evidence linking it to clubfoot etiology. A recurrent chromosome 17q23.1q23.2 microduplication was identified in 3 of 66 probands with familial isolated clubfoot, which is significant. Osseous abnormalities in the foot bones were also present. The authors also discovered in one of the isolated clubfoot probands a microdeletion at that location. They further found that chromosome 17q23.1q23.2 contains the T-box transcription factor PITX1-TBX4, previously implicated in clubfoot etiology. This chromosomal abnormality therefore appears to be strong evidence in familial isolated clubfoot etiology resulting in abnormal early lower-limb development.

Gripp et al.[97] reported the first long survival of a child with TARP syndrome (talipes equinovarus, syndromic atrial septal defect, Robin sequence, and persistent superior vena cava, as well as many other serious defects), an X-linked condition affecting males. This usually results in death in early infancy. They identified *RBM10* as the disease gene in this genetic disorder and stressed the importance of accurate diagnosis and genetic counseling to prevent recurrence.

McClure et al.[98] reported 23 cases with direct physical examination diagnosis and 96 cases of self-reported diagnosis on survey, the largest series so far, of Moebius syndrome (with bilateral seventh cranial nerve palsy), with an average of 41.7% having clubfoot and the rest with other orthopedic defects. They found clubfoot incidence to be 60% in physical examination cases and 23% in survey cases. Clubfoot was the most common orthopedic defect in Moebius syndrome. Its association with Poland syndrome (unilateral absence of chest wall muscles and webbed fingers) were also present in 17% and 30% of cases in the two series. Klippel–Feil syndrome has also been reported to be associated with clubfoot. The exact etiology is not known, but there are many theories explaining a high association with orthopedic defects. There may be chromosomal abnormalities secondary to teratogenic exposure or a vascular episode subclavian in early pregnancy resulting in decreased blood supply to the brain stem causing such defects. Environmental factors, drugs such as misoprostol, and familial incidence have also been identified in some cases. Early diagnosis is important for proper diagnosis, recognizing the spine defects for anticipated anesthesia problems and timely treatment of orthopedic and other conditions, as well as timely counseling.

Miller et al.[99] reported eight Down's syndrome (trisomy 21) patients with 15 clubfeet with an extra chromosome at the twenty-first location. It is important to know this and explain to the parents that correction of the deformity may be difficult with common surgical procedures.

Cereda and Carey[100] reported clubfoot associated with trisomy 18, also known as Edwards syndrome, which has major defects of the heart and kidney. It is the second most common trisomy disorder after trisomy 21, with infant mortality within the first year around 90%, and only 5%–10% survive beyond first year.

Baty et al.[101] have reported frequent association of clubfoot with trisomy 18 and trisomy 13 (Patau syndrome). Trisomy 13 too is also more commonly associated with serious cardiac anomalies, fatal in early infancy. About 70% death is reported, in both, due to cardiopulmonary causes.

Bosch-Banyeras et al.[102] also reported association of Poland syndrome with Moebius syndrome, the combined features including clubfoot. The Poland–Moebius syndrome is a distinct entity with unknown etiology.

Muir et al.[103] studied this in 94 parents (33 fathers and 61 mothers) of 64 children with severe clubfoot requiring surgery, along with one hundred control parents. They found greater prevalence of the absence of the dorsalis pedis artery in parents of clubfooted children and more incidence of smoking in such parents than control group parents; suggesting thereby poor development of the anterior vascular tree due to genetic factors and smoking. It could be possible that vascular deficiency is primary and clubfoot secondary, resulting from poor blood supply of the anterior compartment with weaker anterior muscles than the posterior group, but not confirmed by histology. However, talus has been found to be consistently abnormal. It is important to remember, while performing posteromedial release on clubfeet, that the posterior tibial may be the main source of blood supply to the foot.

Edelson and Husseini[104] carried out Doppler studies in 40 children with 63 feet and found, in children below 3 years of age with mild-to-moderate deformities, normal anterior tibial arteries, but in severe deformities, it was absent in 2 out of 30 feet under 3 years of age and in 7 out of 18 above 3 years of age, confirming that pulselessness increases with age and severity of deformity They further argued that the anterior tibial may be absent in about 2% of normal cases also. The authors disagreed with some of the earlier reports of 85% incidence in neglected severe deformities. Inadequate populations studied, small series, and variable techniques may be the reason for the higher incidence.

Miedzybrodzka,[105] from a population-based study, suggested a genetic contribution to etiology of idiopathic congenital talipes equinovarus due to positive family history in 24%–50% of cases and sex selection with more males than females. The most likely inheritance is a single major gene operating against a polygenetic background. For mild deformities, uterine pressure as an explanation is a strong possibility. They concluded that genetic and multiple environmental factors are important in the cause of idiopathic congenital clubfoot.

2.3.4 Congenital constriction bands, distal amputations, and deformities, including clubfoot

Choulakian and Williams[106] reported that congenital constriction band syndrome (CCBS) is a sporadic condition present with other congenital anomalies significantly more common in upper limbs and distal parts of limbs, with widely variable prevalence of 1:1,200 after early amnion rupture and epidemiology of 1:15,000 live births. Treatment is given to improve cosmetic appearance and function. Authors have been doing direct closure after excising the band, which is simpler, instead of the age-old Z plasty. They do it in two stages to avoid circulatory problems to the limb. Two theories have been described in its etiology: an intrinsic theory to explain the craniofacial and internal organ defects and the extrinsic theory, due to early rupture of amnion (therapeutic or otherwise) explains the orthopedic defects by oligohydramnios and proliferation of mesenchymal bands and entangling limbs or their parts and causing limb defects including clubfoot or amputations. Patterson classification of four grades is simple and popular: grade 1 is only band, grade 2 is band plus deformity of distal part with or without edema, grade 3 is constriction with fusion of distal part, and grade 4 is intrauterine amputations.

Koskimies et al.[107] studied the spectrum of CCBS in 419 upper-limb and 171 lower-limb defects out of 753,342 births in Finland during 1993 to 2005 and found 71 congenital bands with prevalence of 1:10,600 births. In eight cases, there was congenital clubfoot deformity.

Chang and Huang[108] reported that clubfoot cases associated with CCBS are different than classical idiopathic clubfoot and are more difficult to treat. They described their experience in 11 CCBS cases with clubfeet, treated between 1980 and 1993. Bands were released before correcting the deformities. The casting treatment did not succeed, and all required posteromedial release. Seven of eleven had good results and four had fair results at an average follow-up of 3.8 years. All feet were plantigrade.

Gomez[109] reported their experience in 35 children having clubfeet with constriction bands (Streeter dysplasia); all responded poorly to casting treatment and most required surgery. They also reported a high incidence of abnormal pregnancies with uterine insult.

Moosa et al.[110] described various other names given to a cluster of congenital malformations: Streeter bands or dysplasia, annular grooves or defects, amniotic band syndrome, and intrauterine amputation. Besides other defects, clubfoot may also be present. They reported a case with a band and clubfoot deformity on the right foot, while the left foot had two constriction rings with a rudimentary foot with the absence of the distal tibia and fibula. The right foot was operated on but without follow-up. The authors described the location of bands in four zones: zone 1 is in the thigh, zone 2 is in the leg, zone 3 is between the ankle and metatarsophalangeal joints, and zone 4 is limited to the toes. They also described three grades of severity: grade 1 is up to subcutaneous tissue only; grade 2 is deeper, up to the fascia but without compromised circulation; grade 3 is up to the fascia and compromising circulation, for example, lymphoedema; and grade 4 is congenital amputation.

Aunington et al.[111] reported results of treating 21 clubfeet in 18 patients with ipsilateral constriction bands in the leg during the period 1946–1992. Six had good results, six had fair results, and nine had poor results. Patients with less severity of bands and deformity had the best result.

2.4 CONCLUSIONS

Clubfoot is the most common foot deformity and the idiopathic congenital variety is by far the most common of all causes. It is also called talipes equinovarus, wherein tali means ankle and pes means foot in Latin, equino traditionally means plantar flexion at the ankle and varus includes adduction and inversion. This is the traditional name of the spatial orientation of the foot (down and in position). Besides congenital, there are many acquired, but uncommon, causes. There are also some anomalies in the name: firstly, idiopathic is missing from the congenital variety by convention, in spite of it being the most prevalent cause; secondly, cavus is always present with the other three deforming components in varying proportions, but it is missing from the name; and thirdly, the name does not account for the other four elements of plantar flexion at the heel (heel equinus), plantar flexion at mid-foot cockup deformity of the big toe (extreme medial cavus), and plantar flexion at the metatarsophalangeal and interphalangeal joints, which are parts of the deformity in extreme deformities at all ages. In this book, due to their importance for better corrections and as the newer pathoanatomical features, cavus as well as all five plantar flexions have been discussed in detail in Chapter 4, under a new perspective of equinus. However, age-old traditions are difficult to change, but it is okay, as long as all this is remembered when confronted with the correction of this deformity. All these facts must be remembered while assessing each patient to achieve the best possible result. Practical and easy classifications have been given according to genetic or otherwise; congenital, acquired, or on the basis of involvement of anatomical tissues; idiopathic or involving neural, muscular, or osseous tissues. There is further subclassification into congenital or acquired causes and primarily congenital only or congenital and acquired. It is imperative to know that clubfoot is a three-dimensional deformity, and the typical human foot has a highly complex anatomy provided by nature due to its complex spatial and functional requirements Epidemiology assumes a very important role in the modern era and has become broadly based to include every aspect of etiology, detection, prevalence, magnitude, preventive measures from all angles, and therapeutic measures of various diseases, and this applies to clubfoot also. Various aspects of epidemiology intrinsic and extrinsic factors have been reviewed.

Ethnicity: Dobbs and Gurnett[9] in a comprehensive article, reported that clubfoot has been found to be prevalent at 1:1,000 in most report, with a male:female ratio of 2:1, and almost 20% of clubfeet are either syndromic or associated with other etiologies, while the rest are isolated. When genetic in nature, clubfoot is very often familial and polygenetic in nature. The lowest incidence is in the Chinese at 0.39:1,000 and the highest is in Hawaiians and Maoris at 7:1,000. Isolated clubfoot is more likely multifactorial and polygenetic due to sex differentiation. Ching et al.[11] corroborated this. In regard to other ethnicities, there is a prevalence of 0.87:1,000 in the Japanese, 4.5:1,000 in Malaysians, and 0.9:1,000 in Indians. Chapman et al.[17] reported New Zealand Maoris as the best population model for genetic study. Krogsgaard et al.[19] reported an incidence of 1.2:1,000 for isolated clubfoot and 0.22:1,000 for syndromic clubfoot in Denmark, with a higher incidence with a higher density population due to extrinsic factors. Wallander et al.[21] reported prevalence in Sweden as 1.4:1,000. Siapkara and Duncan[24] reported a 1.2:1,000 prevalence in Europe with the male:female ratio as 2:1. Mathias et al.[25] reported a 1.2:1,000 prevalence in Uganda, with the male:female ratio as 2:1. Pavone et al.[27] reported the prevalence in Sicily as 1:1,000. Wu et al.[30] reported the prevalence in Kenya as 2.9:1,000. Sitkin et al.[32] highlighted the high GBD and millions of DALYs wasted due to congenital anomalies, including clubfoot, worldwide. Tracey et al.[34] published a comprehensive database prevalence in all LMICs varying from 0.51:1,000 to 2.03:1,000.

Besides the intrinsic factors, there are a large number of extrinsic factors in the epidemiology of clubfoot. **Maternal smoking** before and during pregnancy, especially the first trimester, has been uniformly indicated to have harmful effects on the fetus in myriad reports in the literature. Paternal smoking too has an added harmful effect. Nicotine, carbon monoxide, and thiocyanate are the main harmful chemicals, but there are others also. Van den Eeden[35] reported this from Washington state, and a WHO report[36] highlighted 4,800 chemicals of tobacco with their role in causing congenital defects, including clubfoot worldwide, and discussed the preventive measures. Werler[37] highlighted the mechanism of harmful chemicals through the maternal fetal blood. Honein et al.[38] found a statistically significant effect of smoking in the first trimester from an Atlanta case series. Saha et al.[40] reported from the Office of the Surgeon General of the United States Health Service review of more than 7,000 research articles on the topic of smoking and health and reported that about 15% women smoke throughout pregnancy. Dickinson et al.[41] reported that, besides a definite role of smoking, higher intake of alcohol and coffee also has some role in epidemiology of clubfoot. Sommers et al.[42] confirmed that maternal cigarette smoking during pregnancy is the only environmental factor that has been consistently associated with congenital defects, including clubfoot, all over the world. Hackshaw et al.[43] in a meta-analysis of 172 articles published from 1959 to 2010, confirmed a significant association of smoking with clubfoot. Viteri et al.[46] reviewed the literature of 128 articles on the effects of cocaine, marijuana/cannabis, opioids, amphetamines, alcohol, and smoking and reported an increased risk of congenital defects.

Medications: If a pregnant woman has some other chronic disease requiring prolonged use of specific drugs or some acute or temporary illness requiring intake of some medicines, this can also be harmful during pregnancy. Samren et al.[47] and Veroniki et al.[48] concluded from data of five European studies and 96 eligible studies from an extensive literature review, respectively, that in pregnant epileptic mothers compared with an adequate number of controls, monotherapy (velaporate [VPA] and carbamazine [CBZ]) were highly significant risk factors for major congenital anomalies, including clubfoot, but even monotherapies were harmful. Old-generation drugs were more harmful than newer generation drugs. Counseling is important about the risks of these agents when given during pregnancy, including discussion of polytherapy versus monotherapy and avoiding higher risk drugs like velproate. Finding the balance between controlling the convulsions and safety of the fetus is important. Louik et al.[49] concluded that anti-depressant selective serotonin reuptake inhibitors (SSRIs) also increase the risk of birth defects during periconceptional use. Norgaard et al.[50] concluded from a Danish birth registry comparing 1,079 pregnant mothers using fluconazole (for candidiasis) and 158 times more control pregnant mothers not using fluconazole that birth defects were more common in the fluconazole group than the control group. Crider et al.[51] studied the effect of antibacterial agents (sulfonamides and nitrofurantoins) and found them to be positive risk factor when used during pregnancy. Allen and O'Brien[52] studied the use of misoprostol, a common WHO-recommended drug for many indications in obstetrics and gynecology, and still found a 1% risk. Many authors,[53,55,56] knowing the thalidomide episode, reviewed 15 years of literature on the effects of taking various CNS-acting drugs during pregnancy (antipsychotics, tranquilizers, sedatives and hypnotics, antidepressants, psychostimulants, and some others). Definite association of use of these drugs in many congenital defects has been found. Werler et al.[54] studied the effects many other medicines frequently used during pregnancy (antibiotics, opioids, NSAIDS, antinauseas, antivirals, antifungals, etc.) and found that are all associated with risk, some more risk and others less. Mitchell[57] commented that caution is needed while using any new drug during pregnancy, especially during first trimester.

Nutritional deficiency: Many authors[59–68] have affirmed in their own studies or from literature reviews the role of various nutritional deficiencies of various micronutrients during pregnancy, with folic acid being the most important. Others include B1 vitamins B6 and B12, selenium, vitamin D, vitamin A, vitamin C, iron, zinc, copper, vitamin E, calcium, magnesium, choline, and iodine, all of which are needed during pregnancy.

Maternal diseases: Many authors[69–71] from good review of the literature or their own study found obesity with diabetes poses a very high risk of congenital defects, including clubfoot. If the diabetes is pre-existing, the risk increases more than with gestational diabetes. Obesity alone does not pose a risk, but diabetes alone does increase the risk; the hyperglycemic index and dietary load is responsible. Pathogenesis is multifactorial. Authors[72,73] have commented from review of literature and their own studies that ACE inhibitors pose a high risk of congenital defects, including clubfoot, in the second and third trimesters, but not in the first trimester. Many authors[74–77] have reported from meta-analyses of literature reports and their own studies the effect of various viral infections with high fever, including Zika virus, in causing congenital defects with a strongly positive risk factor. The mechanism may be the high fever, medications, and the effect of the virus on the brain, but the association is definite.

Amniocentesis and uterine factors: There are many reports[78–80] regarding early amniocentesis, chorionic villous sampling, and fetal blood sampling, which are done with informed consent due to the risks involved. In early amniocentesis (in first trimester), there is risk of congenital defects and clubfoot to the fetus. Moh et al.[81] reviewed uterine growth restrictions, due to numerous extrinsic and intrinsic factors, and thus multifactorial causes leading to congenital clubfoot and other limb defects. There are many preventable steps and more are needed. Congenital uterine abnormalities are difficult to deal with.

Socioeconomic, maternal age, and environmental factors: Many authors[82] have opined about SES from population-based studies, personal SES, and conditions which are directly proportional to the grade of SES; case-controlled studies have revealed that African Americans are affected more, which is confirmed in other reports. Parameters studied included personal and neighborhood risk factors. Personal risk factors included, for example, education, employment, family income, type of employment, housing, overcrowding, dietary intake, indoor coal combustion, teenage pregnancies, smoking, physical activity, psychological stress and family support, and use of caffeine, tobacco, alcohol, and other illicit drugs. Neighborhood risk factors included, for example, poor areas, high altitude, numerous air and water pollutants, occupational dust, high natural radiation areas, and seasonal variations. All have been found to be risk factors. Vitamin intake in these areas have reduced the risk. The mechanism of action is multifactorial with a genetic effect too. WHO reports suggest preventive measures to reduce the risk of congenital defects including clubfoot.

Genetics and clubfoot: Genetics is a vast and highly specialized subject, but it plays a definite role in clubfoot etiology. Although there has been good progress, still much more needs to be done. Innumerable authors are working on genetic aspects and some of the authentic ones have been selected for discussion. Dobbs and Gurnett[9] report a highly significant extensive review of literature, and they have tried to explain pathogenesis of clubfoot on a genetic basis: 25% isolated variety having familial incidence with males twice as common as females, identical twins having an incidence of 33% with fraternal twins only 3%, and varied ethnic prevalence. Pathogenesis is therefore multifactorial and polygenetic rather than single gene. Ching et al.[94] reported on a Hawaiian population being the best for such a study and supported a genetic etiology that is multifactorial in nature. Many authors, Phatak et al., Alvarado et al., Gripp et al., McClure et al., Miller et al., Cereda and Carey, Baty et al., Bosch-Banyeras et al., Muir et al., Edelson and Husseini, Miedzybrodzka[95–105] have reported on syndromic clubfoot deformities due to different trisomies: 13, 16, 18, 21, Poland, Moebius, Down, Patio, TARP, Klippel-Feil, Patau syndromes all having genetic etiology; there are chromosomal abnormalities. In many cases, a single or more genes have been identified, but a large number of researchers are investigating. This is a highly complex issue due to innumerable factors; whether or not these factors act independently or through the genes is still a gray area.

To summarize, there are many epidemiological factors that definitely have a role in a higher prevalence of clubfoot. Ethnicity is an important factor with more prevalence in some races. Maternal smoking has a definite role, especially in the first trimester. Then there are drugs used in various situations, such as antiepileptic drugs, especially polytherapy with older-generation drugs being more harmful; drugs acting on the nervous system; antifungal drugs; antibacterial drugs; misoprostol; antiviral drugs; antiemetics; analgesics; and many others. In fact, any new drug for any ailment to be given in pregnancy should be done with caution. Malnutrition and deficiency of vitamins and micronutrients definitely increases the incidence of clubfoot. The role of folic-acid deficiency is well established. Diabetes with obesity is definitely a risk factor, but diabetes even alone is harmful due to a high glycemic index. A lot can be done to reduce the incidence of clubfoot by taking all of the public health preventive measures. The rest of the problem of clubfoot can then be managed by various conservative and surgical measures, selecting the best for the particular type of patient. It is highly important to know for the best treatment that **each clubfoot is different**.

Socrates (470–399 BCE, https://en.wikiquote.org/wiki/Socrates), the father of western philosophy, said, "The secret of change is to focus all your energy, not on fighting the old, but building the new." Past researchers in epidemiology did a wonderful job to bring us to the present. Innumerable researchers have been working, since Hippocrates' era, to unravel the epidemiological aspects of this complex problem to enable us to tackle the intricacies of clubfoot. We have come a long way, and there has been significant progress in the knowledge of various intrinsic and extrinsic factors, but more needs to be done. The past was very good and Hippocrates and all others were torch bearers who brought us to the present, and the present generation of researchers will further lead us to the future. We are optimistic that the future will open newer vistas in the prevention and treatment of clubfoot.

REFERENCES

1. Abdalla E, Alaa-Eddin I; Bilateral fibular dimelia with mirror foot: An additional case report; *J Gen Syndr Gene Ther*; 2016;7:2.
2. Nguyen MP, Lawler EA, Morcuende JA; A case report of bilateral mirror clubfeet and bilateral hand polydactyly; *Iowa Orthop J*; 2014;34:171–174.
3. Spero CR, Simon GS, Tornetta P; Clubfeet and tarsal coalition; *J Pediatr Orthop*; May–June 1994;14(3):372–376.
4. Nalaboff KM, Schweitzer ME; MRI of tarsal coalition: Frequency, distribution and innovative signs; *Bull NYU Hosp Jt Dis*; 2008;66(1):14–21.
5. Hippocrates 400 BCE: On Airs, Places, Waters and places; translated by Francis Adams. http://classics.mit.edu.
6. Greenwood M; *Epidemics and Crowd-Diseases: An Introduction to the Study of Epidemiology*. Oxford University Press; 1935.
7. Last JM. editor; *Dictionary of Epidemiology*. 4th ed. New York: Oxford University Press; 2001, P–61.
8. Cates W; Epidemiology: Applying principles to clinical practice; *Contemp Ob/Gyn*; 1982;20:147–161.
9. Dobbs MB, Gurnett CA; Genetics of clubfoot; *J Pediatr Orthop B*. in PMC 2013 Jan 1. *J Pediatr Orthop B*; January 2012;21(1):7–9.
10. Noonan KJ, Meyers AM, Kayes K; Leg length discrepancy in unilateral congenital clubfoot following surgical treatment; *Iowa Orthop J*; 2004;24:60–64.
11. Ching GH, Chung CS, Nemechek RW; Genetic and epidemiological studies of clubfoot in Hawaii: Ascertainment and incidence; *Am J Hum Genet*; November 1969;21(6):566–580.
12. Pompe van Meerdervoort HF; Congenital musculoskeletal malformation in South African Blacks: A study of incidence; *S Afr Med J*; 01 October 1976;50(46):1853–1855.
13. Yamamoto H; A clinical, genetic and epidemiologic study of congenital club foot; *J Hum Genet*; March 1979;24(1):37–44.
14. Boo NY, Ong LC; Congenital talipes in Malaysian neonates: Incidence, pattern and associated factors; *Singapore Med J*; December 1990;1(6):539–542.

15. Mittal RL, Sekhon AS, Singh G, Thakral H; The prevalence of congenital orthopaedic anomalies in a rural community; *Int Orthop*; 1993;17(1):11–12.
16. Shaw GM, Velie EM, Wasserman CR; Risk for neural tube defect-affected pregnancies among women of Mexican descent and white women in California; *Am J Public Health*; September 1997;87(9):1467–1471.
17. Chapman C, Susan Stott N, Port RV, Nicol RO; Genetics of club foot in Maori and Pacific people; *J Med Genet*; 2000;37:680–683.
18. Barker SL, Macnicol M; Seasonal distribution of idiopathic congenital talipes equinovarus in Scotland; *J Pediatr Orthop*; April 2002;11(2):129–133.
19. Krogsgaard MR, Jensen PK, Kjær I, Husted H, Lorentzen J, Hvass-Christensen B; Incidence and geographical variation in Denmark over a 16–year period—An epidemiological study of 936,525 births; *Acta Orthop*; 2006;77:839–846.
20. Costa CMS, da Gama SGN, Leal MC; Congenital Malformations in Rio de Janeiro, Brazil: Prevalence and associated factors; *Cad. Saúde Pública* vol. 22(11) Rio de Janeiro November 2006. http://dx.doi.org/10.1590/S0102-311X2006001100016
21. Wallander H, Hovelius L, Michaelsson K; Incidence of congenital clubfoot in Sweden; *Acta Orthop*; 2006;77(6):847–852.
22. Li Z, Ren A, Zhang L, Ye R, Li S, Zheng J, Hong S, Wang T, Li Z; Extremely high prevalence of neural tube defects in a 4-county area in Shanxi province, China; *Clinical Mol Tetrology*; April 2006;76(4):237–240.
23. Cardy AH, Barker S, Chesney D, Sharp L, Maffulli N, Miedzybrodzka Z; Pedigree analysis and epidemiological features of idiopathic congenital talipes equinovarus in the United Kingdom: A case-control study; *BMC Musculoskelet Disord*; 2007;8:62.
24. Siapkara A, Duncan R; Congenital talipes equinovarus: A review of current management; *J Bone Joint Surg*; August 2007;89–b(8).
25. Mathias RG, Lule JK, Waiswa G, Naddumba EK, Pirani S; Incidence of clubfoot in Uganda; *Can J Public Health*; 2010;101(4):341–344.
26. Nguyen MC, Nhi HM, Nam VQD, Thanh DV, Romitti P, Morcuende JA; Descriptive epidemiology of clubfoot in Vietnam: A clinic-based study; *Iowa Orthop J*; 2012;32:120–124.
27. Pavone V, Bianca S, Grosso G, Pavone P, Mistretta A, Longo MR, Marino S, Sessa G; Congenital talipes equinovarus: An epidemiological study in Sicily; *Acta Orthop*; June 2012;83(3):294–298.
28. Palma M, Cook T, Segura J, Pecho A, Morcuende JA; Descriptive epidemiology of clubfoot in Peru: A clinic-based study; *Iowa Orthop J*; 2013;33:167–171.
29. Werler MM, Yazdy MM, Mitchell AA, Meyer RE, Druschel CM, Anderka M, Kasser JR, Mahan ST; Descriptive epidemiology of idiopathic clubfoot; *Am J Med Genet Part A*; July 2013;161(7):1569–1578.
30. Wu VK, Poenaru D, Poley MJ; Burden of surgical congenital anomalies in Kenya: A population-based study; *J Trop Pediatr*; 2013;59(3):195–202.
31. Gili JA, Poletta FA, Pawluk M, Gimenez LG, Campaña H, Castilla E, López-Camelo JS; High birth prevalence rates for congenital anomalies in South American regions; *Epidemiology*; September 2015;26(5):e53–e55.
32. Sitkin NA, Ozgediz D, Donkor P, Farmer DL; Congenital anomalies in low- and middle-income countries: The unborn child of global surgery; *World J Surg*; January 2015;39(1):36–40.
33. Groisman B, GiliLucas J, Fernando G, Bidondo MP, Barbero P, Liascovich R; Geographic clusters of congenital anomalies in Argentina; *J Commun Genet*; January 2017;8(1):1–7.
34. Tracey S, Kuper H, Macleod D, Foster A, Lavy C; Birth prevalence of congenital talipes equinovarus in low- and middle-income countries: A systematic review and meta-analysis; *Trop Med Int Health*; March 2017;22(3):269–285.
35. Van den Eeden SK, Karagas MR, Daling JR, Vaughan TL; A case-control study of maternal smoking and congenital malformations; *Paediatr Perinat Epidemiol*; April 1990;4(2):147–155.
36. World Health Organization; *Tobacco or Health: A Global Status Report Book.* 1997, xi and 495 pp. ref. ISBN: 92156184X

37. Werler MM; Teratogen update: Smoking and reproductive outcomes; *Teratology*; 1997;55:382–388.
38. Honein MA, Paulozzi LJ, Moore CA; Family history, maternal smoking, and clubfoot: An indication of a gene-environment interaction; *Am J Epidemiol*; 2000;152(7):658–665.
39. Woods SE, Raju U; Maternal smoking and the risk of congenital birth defects: A cohort study; *J Am Board Fam Med*; September–October 2001;14(5):330–334.
40. Saha SP, Bhalla DK, Whayne TF, Gairola CG; Cigarette smoke and adverse health effects: An overview of research trends and future needs; *Int J Angiol*; Autumn 2007;16(3):77–83.
41. Dickinson KC, Meyer RE, Kotch J; Maternal smoking and the risk for clubfoot in infants; *J. Birth Defects Res A Clin Mol Teratol*; February 2008;82(2):86–91.
42. Werler MM, Yazdy MM, Kasser JR, Mahan ST, Meyer RE, Anderka M, Druschel CM, Mitchell AA; Maternal cigarette, alcohol, and coffee consumption in relation to risk of clubfoot; *Paediatr Perinat Epidemiol*; January 2015;29(1):3–10. A systematic review based on 173,687 malformed cases and 11.7 million controls; *Hum Reprod Update* (2011) 17(5):589–604.
43. Sommers A, Blanton SH, Weymouth K, Alvarez C, Richards S, Barnes D, Mitchell L, Hecht JT; Smoking, the xenobiotic pathway and clubfoot; birth defects; *Res A Clin Mol Teratol*; January 2011;91(1):20–28.
44. Hackshaw A, Rodeck C, Boniface S; Maternal smoking in pregnancy and birth defects; *Hum Reprod Update*; September–October 2011;17(5):589–604.
45. A Report of the Surgeon General. Atlanta, GA U.S. Department of Health and Human Services: The Health Consequences of Smoking: 50 Years of Progress. National Center for Chronic Disease Prevention and Health Promotion, Office on Smoking and Health, 2014. Printed with corrections, January 2014. DOI: https://doi.org/10.1093/humupd/dmr022
46. Viteri OA, Soto EE, Bahado-Singh RO, Christensen CW, Chauhan SP, Sibai BM; Fetal anomalies and long-term effects associated with substance abuse in pregnancy: A literature review; *Amer J Perinatol*; 2015;32(05):405–416.
47. Samren EB, van Duijn CM, Koch S et al.; Maternal use of antiepileptic drugs and the risk of major congenital malformations: A joint European prospective study of human teratogenesis associated with maternal epilepsy; *Epilepsia*; 1997;38(9):981–990. Lippincott-Raven Publishers, Philadelphia.
48. Veroniki AA, Cogo E, Rios P et al.; Comparative safety of anti-epileptic drugs during pregnancy: A systematic review and network meta-analysis of congenital malformations & prenatal outcomes; *BMC Med*; 2017;15:95–3536.
49. Louik C, Lin AE, Werler MM, Hernández-Díaz S, Mitchell AA; First-trimester use of selective serotonin- reuptake inhibitors and the risk of birth defects; *N Engl J Med*; 2007;356:2675–2683.
50. Nørgaard M, Pedersen L, Gislum M, Erichsen R, Søgaard KK, Schønheyder HC, Sørensen HT; Maternal use of fluconazole and risk of congenital malformations: A Danish population-based cohort study; *J Antimicrob Chemother*; 2008;62:172–176.
51. Crider KS, Cleves MA, Reefhuis J, Berry RJ, Hobbs CA, Hu DJ; Antibacterial medication use during pregnancy and risk of birth defects—National Birth Defects Prevention Study; *Arch Pediatr Adolesc Med*; 2009; 163(11):978–985.
52. Allen R, O'Brien BM; Uses of misoprostol in obstetrics and gynecology; *Rev Obstet Gynecol*; Summer 2009;2(3):159–168.
53. Callen B, Borg N, Reis M; The use of central nervous system active drugs during pregnancy; *Pharmaceuticals (Basel)*; 2013;6(10):1221–1286.
54. Werler MM, Yazdy MM, Kasser JR, Mahan ST, Meyer RE, Anderka M, Druschel CM, Mitchel AA; Medication use in pregnancy in relation to the risk of isolated clubfoot in offspring; *Am J Epidemiol*; July 2014;180(1):86–93.
55. Broussard CS, Rasmussen SA, Reefhuis J, Friedman JM, Jann MW, Riehle-Colarusso T, Honein MA; National birth defects prevention study: Maternal treatment

with opioid analgesics and risk for birth defects; *Am J Obstetr Gynaecol*; April 2011;204(4):314e.1–314e.11.
56. Yazdy MM, Desai RJ, Brogly SB; Prescription opioids in pregnancy and birth outcomes: A review of the literature; *J Pediatr Genet*; June 2015;4(2):56–70.
57. Mitchell AA; Research challenges for drug-induced birth defects; *Clin Pharmacol Ther*; 2016;100:26–28.
58. Picciano MF; Is homocysteine a biomarker for identifying women at risk of complications and adverse pregnancy outcomes? *Am J Clin Nutr*; April 2000;71(4):857–858.
59. Vollset SE, Refsum H, Irgens LM, Emblem BM, Tverdal A, Gjessing HK, Monsen ALB, Ueland PM; Plasma total homocysteine, pregnancy complications, and adverse pregnancy outcomes: The Hordaland Homocysteine Study1,2,3E; *Am J Clin Nutr*; April 2000;71(4):962–968.
60. Karakurt L, Yilmaz E, Serin E, Bektaş B, Çikim G, Gürsu F; Plasma total homocysteine level in mothers of children with clubfoot; *J Pediatr Orthop*; September–October 2003;23(5):658–660.
61. Sharp L, Miedzybrodzka Z, Cardy AH, Inglis J, Madrigal L, Barker S, Chesney D, Clark C, Maffulli N; The C677 T polymorphism in the methylenetetrahydrofolate reductase gene (MTHFR), maternal use of folic acid supplements, and risk of isolated clubfoot: A case-parent-triad analysis; *Am J Epidemiol*; 2006;164(9):852–861.
62. Molloy AM, Kirke PN, Brody LC, Scott JM, Mills JL; Effects of folate and vitamin B12 deficiencies during pregnancy on fetal, infant, and child development; *Food Nutr Bull*; June 2008;29(2 Suppl):101–111.
63. Czeizel AE, Bártfai Z, Bánhidy F; Primary prevention of neural-tube defects and some other congenital abnormalities by folic acid and multivitamins: History, missed opportunity and tasks; *Rev Article-Ther Adv Drug Safety*; July 28, 2011;2(4):2011.
64. Czeizel AE, Dudás I, Vereczkey A, Bánhidy F; Folate deficiency and folic acid supplementation: The prevention of neural-tube defects and congenital heart defects; *Nutrients*; November 2013;5(11):4760–4775.
65. Kaska L, Kobiela J, Abacjew-Chmylko A, Chmylko L, Wojanowska-Pindel M, Kobiela P, Walerzak Makarewicz W, Proczko-Markuszewska M, Stefaniak T; International scholarly research notices-obesity; *Review Article Nutr Pregnancy after Bariatric Surg*; 2013;2013:6.
66. Gernand AD, Schulze KJ, Stewart C, West KP, Jr., Christian P; Micronutrient deficiencies in pregnancy worldwide: Health effects and prevention; *Nat Rev Endocrinol*; May 2016;12(5):274–289.
67. Gildestad T, Øyen N, Klungsøyr K, Nilsen RM, Daltveit AK, Vollset SE; Maternal use of folic acid supplements and infant risk of neural tube defects in Norway; *Scandanavian J Public Health*; August 2016;44(6):619–626.
68. Moore LL, Singer MR, Bradlee ML, Rothman KJ, Milunsky A; A prospective study of the risk of congenital defects associated with maternal obesity and diabetes mellitus; *Epidemiology*; November 2000;11(6):689–694.
69. Allen VM, Halifax NSB, Armson A, Halifax NS; Teratogenicity associated with pre-existing and gestational diabetes; *J Obstetr Gynaecol Canada*; November 2007;927–934.
70. Yazdy MM, Liu S, Mitchell AA, Werler MM; Maternal dietary glycemic intake and the risk of neural tube defects; *Am J Epidemiol*; 2010;171(4):407–414.
71. Cooper WO, Hermandez-Diaz S, Arbogast PG, Dudley JA, Dyer S, Gideon PS, Hall K, Ray WA; Major congenital malformations after first-trimester exposure to ACE inhibitors; *N Engl J Med*; June 2006;354(23):2443–2451.
72. Al-Maawali A, Walfisch A, Koren G; Taking angiotensin-converting enzyme inhibitors during pregnancy. Is it safe? *Can Fam Physician*; January 2012;58(1):49–51.
73. Edwards MJ; Review: Hyperthermia and fever during pregnancy. Birth defects research; *Part A Clinical and Molecular Teratology*; July 2006;76(7):507–516.
74. Luteijn JM, Brown MJ, Dolk H; Influenza and congenital anomalies: A systematic review and meta-analysis; *Hum Reprod*; 2014;29(4):809–823.

75. Rasmussen SA, Jamieson DJ, Honein MA, Petersen LR; Zika virus and birth defects—Reviewing the evidence for causality; *N Engl J Med*; 2016;374:1981–1987.
76. van der Linden V, Filho ELR, Lins OG, 12 others; Congenital Zika syndrome with arthrogryposis: Retrospective case series study; *Br Med J*; 2016;354:i3899.
77. Nagel HT, Vandenbussche FP, Keirse MJ, Oepkes D, Oosterwijk JC, Beverstock G, Kanhai HH; Amniocentesis before 14 completed weeks as an alternative to transabdominal chorionic villus sampling: A controlled trial with infant follow-up; *Prenat Diagn*; May 1998;18(5):465–475.
78. Farrell SA, Summers AM, Dallaire L, Singer J, Wilson JM; Club foot, an adverse outcome of early amniocentesis: Disruption or deformation? *J Med Genet*; 1999;36(11):843–846.
79. Ercole C, Shojai R, Desbriere R, Chau C, Florence B, Piéchon L, Boubli L; Prenatal screening invasive diagnostic approaches; *Childs Nerv Syst*; 2003;19:444.
80. Moh W, Graham JM Jr., Wadhawan I, Sanchez-Lara PA; Extrinsic factors influencing fetal deformations and intrauterine growth restriction; *J Pregnancy*; 2012;2012:11.
81. Wasserman CR, Shaw GM, Selvin S, Gould JB, Syme SL; Socioeconomic status, neighborhood social conditions, and neural tube defects; *Am J Public Health*; November 1998;88(11):1674–1680.
82. Castilla EE, Lopez-Camelo JS, Campaña H; Altitude as a risk factor for congenital anomalies; *Am J Med Genet*; 3 September 1999;86(1):9–14.
83. Vrijheid M, Dolk H, Stone D, Abramsky L, Alberman E, Scott JES; Socioeconomic inequalities in risk of congenital anomaly; *Arch Dis Child*; 2000;82:349–352.
84. Carmichael SL, Shaw GM, Neri E et al.; Physical activity and risk of neural tube defects; *Matern Child Health J*; 2002;6:151.
85. Li Z, Zhang L, Ye R, Pei L, Liu J, Zheng X, Ren A; Indoor air pollution from coal combustion and the risk of neural tube defects in a rural population in Shanxi province, China; *Am J Epidemiol*; 15 August 2011;174(4):451–458.
86. Chen X-K, Wen SW, Fleming N, Yang Q, Walker MC; Teenage pregnancy and congenital anomalies: Which system is vulnerable? *Hum Reprod*; 2007;22(6):1730–1735.
87. Mattison DH; Environmental exposures and development; *Curr Opin Paediatr*; April 2010;22(2):208–218.
88. Lupo PJ, Symanski E, Waller DK, Chan W, Langlois PH, Canfield MA, Mitchell LE; Maternal exposure to ambient levels of benzene and neural tube defects among offspring: Texas, 1999–2004; *Env Health Perspect*; March 2011;119(3):397–402.
89. Coppola G, Costantini A, Tedone R, Pasquale S, Elia L, Foschino Barbaro M, d'Addetta I; The impact of the baby's congenital malformation on the mother's psychological well-being: An empirical contribution on the clubfoot; *J Pediatr Orthop*; July/August 2012;32(5):521–526.
90. Jaikrishan G, Sudheer KR, Andrews VJ, Koya PKM, Madhusoodhanan M, Jagadeesan CK, Seshadri M; Study of stillbirth and major congenital anomaly among newborns in the high-level natural radiation areas of Kerala, India; *J Commun Genet*; January 2013;4(1):21–31. Also quoted: World Health Organization (1959) Effects of radiation on human heredity: investigations of areas of high natural radiation. WHO Technical Report Series No. 166, Geneva
91. Lassi ZS, Imam AM, Dean SV, Bhutta ZA; Preconception care: Caffeine, smoking, alcohol, drugs and other environmental chemical/radiation exposure; *Reprod Health*; 2014;11(Suppl 3):6.
92. Padula AM, Yang W, Carmichael SL, Tager IB, Lurmann F, Katharine Hammond S, Sha GM; Air pollution, neighbourhood socioeconomic factors and neural tube defects in the San Joaquin Valley of California; *Paediatr Perinat Epidemiol*; November 2015;29(6):536–545.
93. Zhao D-H, Rao W-W, Zhao L, Yang X, Liu J-L, Wu Z-K, Du Q, Yang X-Y; Are incidence and severity of clubfoot related to the season of birth; *World J Pediatr*; August 2016;12(3):360–363.
94. Ching GHS, Chung CS, Nemechek RW; Genetic and epidemiological studies of

clubfoot in Hawaii: Ascertainment and incidence; *Am J Hum Genet*; November 1969;21(6):566–580.
95. Phatak SV, Tule V, Phatak MS, Kolwadkar PK; Antenatal sonographic diagnosis of Patau syndrome (trisomy 13): A case report; *Indian J Radiol Imaging*; 2004;14:165–167.
96. Alvarado DM, Aferol H, McCall K, Huanq JB, Techy M, Buchan J, Cady J, Gonzales PR, Dobbs MB, Gurnett CA; Familial isolated clubfoot is associated with recurrent chromosome 17q23.1q23.2 microduplications containing TBX4; *Am J Hum Genet*; 9 July 2010;87(1):154–160.
97. Gripp KW, Hopkins E, Johnston JJ, Krause K, Dobyns W, Biesecker LG; Long term survival in TARP syndrome and confirmation of *RBM10* as the disease causing gene; *Am J Med Genet A*; October 2011;155(10):2516–2520.
98. McClure P, Booy D, Katarancic J, Eberson C; Orthopedic manifestations of moebius syndrome: Case series and survey study; *Int J Pediatr*; 2016;2016:6.
99. Miller PR, Kuo KN, Lubicky JP; Clubfoot deformity in Down's syndrome; *Orthopedics*; 1995;18(5):449–452.
100. Cereda A, Carey JC; The trisomy 18 syndrome; *Orphanet J Rare Dis*; 2012;7:81. https://doi.org/10.1186/1750-1172-7-81.
101. Baty BJ, Blackburn BL, Carey JC; Natural History of trisomy 18 and trisomy 13: I. Growth, physical assessment, medical histories, survival, and recurrence risk; *Am J Med Gen*; 1994;49:175–188.
102. Bosch-Banyeras JM, Zuasnabar A, Puig A, Catala M, Cuatrecasas JM; Poland-Moebius syndrome associated with dextrocardia; *J Med Genet*; February 1984;21(1):70–71.
103. Muir L, Laliotis N, Kutty S, Klenerman L; Absence of the dorsalis pedis pulse in the parents of children with club foot; *Bone Joint J*; January 1995;B:114–116.
104. Edelson JG, Husseini N; The pulseless club foot; *Bone Joint J(Br)*; 1984;700–702.
105. Miedzybrodzka Z; Congenital talipes equinovarus (clubfoot): A disorder of the foot but not the hand; *J Anat*; 2003;202:37–42.
106. Choulakian MY, Williamsp HB; Surgical correction of congenital constriction band syndrome in children: Replacing Z-plasty with direct closure; *Can J Plast Surg*; 2008 Winter; 16(4):221–223.
107. Koskimies E, Syvänen J, Nietosvaara Y, Mäkitie O, Pakkasjärvi N; Congenital constriction band syndrome with limb defects; *J Pediatr Orthop*; January 2015;35(1):100–103.
108. Chang CH, Huang SC; Clubfoot deformity in congenital constriction band syndrome: Manifestations and treatment; *J Formos Med Assoc*; May 1998;97(5):328–334.
109. Gomez VR; Clubfeet in congenital annular constricting bands; *Clin Orthop Relat Res*; February 1996;323:155–162.
110. Moosa M, Wani M, Wani I, Bashir A, Hussain A, Mir B, Halwai M; Congenital constriction ring syndrome associated with club foot and contralateral absence of part of tibia and fibula: A case report; *Int J Orthop Surg*; 2008;14(2).
111. Aunington NJ, Kumar SJ, Guille JT; Clubfeet associated with congenital constriction bands of the ipsilateral lower extremity; *J Pediatr Orthop*; 1995;15(5):599–603.

3

Review of literature

3.1 HISTORICAL PERSPECTIVE

Dobb et al.[1] published a classical historical review regarding clubfoot treatment. Initially, treatment consisted of serial manipulations and immobilization, followed by subcutaneous tendoachilles tenotomy, and next came aseptic surgical techniques, and then, again, manipulations and immobilization. They reported the historical perspective:

Clubfoot was first depicted in ancient tomb paintings and the first treatment was described in India as early as 1000 BCE. The first written description of clubfoot was given by Hippocrates in about 400 BCE. He advocated starting manipulations as early after birth as possible, which involved repeated manipulations and strong bandaging for maintenance. On correction, special shoes were worn to prevent recurrence. The Middle Ages were the era of barber surgeons and bone setters. Then came the repeated stretching technique of Arcaeus in 1658 with his two mechanical devices to maintain correction. In the mid-eighteenth century, Cheselden used repeated stretching and tape for maintenance. Then, in 1803, came Scarpa's historical *Memoir on Congenital Club-foot of Children*, which gave the description of clubfoot, considering the talus to be typical, but the forefoot dislocating inward from the head of talus. His treatment involved strong manipulation and maintenance with a complicated mechanical device known as Scarpa's shoe. It did not succeed in others' hands and hence was not widely accepted. In 1806, Timothy Sheldrake published *Distortions of the Legs and Feet of Children*. He advocated starting the manipulations within the first two months of birth, and he believed the deformity was due equally to muscles and ligaments. The later the start of treatment, the more difficult is the cure. Then the subcutaneous Achilles tenotomy was developed. Delpech, in 1823, was the first to do subcutaneous Achilles tenotomy in two patients. Both got infected, and he stopped performing this procedure. Then, Stormier successfully completed a subcutaneous Achilles tenotomy in 1831 and continued to practice it in Hanover; he also performed it on W.J. Little, a young orthopedic surgeon from England with clubfoot and taught this technique to him, who continued to do it successfully for many years in England. Little, in 1839, thought that the deformity was due to strong intrauterine muscular contractions. In the United States, subcutaneous tenotomy for clubfoot was first performed by Rogers in 1834 and Dickson in 1835. In 1838, Guerin was the first to use a plaster cast. With the exception of tenotomies, the era of aseptic surgical techniques and anesthesia was introduced by Lister in 1867. In 1873, Esmarch introduced the rubber bandage tourniquet, and the introduction of the pneumatic tourniquet by Cushing in 1904 really revolutionized limb surgery. These evolutions also led to good and more radical clubfoot surgeries. Ponseti developed his method of manipulation and plaster casting after a thorough knowledge of movements of tarsal joints from a publication of Farabeuf in 1872, who described these joints as being polyaxial, with all axes moving simultaneously with movements. He advocated that treatment must be started shortly after birth and the right regimen must be observed to get the desired results. The foot is fully abducted and not everted. Equinus is corrected last and, if needed, Achilles tenotomy is performed (85%). Tibialis anterior transfer is done if there is recurrence. Dobb et al.[1] also assert that what is definitely missing in the literature is long-term follow-up of the quality of life of Ponseti's treated cases.

Carroll[2] wrote about clubfoot in the twentieth century and its likely future in the twenty-first century. In regard to its ethnic prevalence, it has been reported from 0.6 to 6.8 per thousand live births, with occurrence in males twice as common as in females. In the early 1900s, Hugh Owen Thomas treated clubfoot by forced manipulation with the Thomas wrench. Hippocrates, in 400 BCE treated it with gentle manipulation and bandages, while Joseph Hiram Kite in the 1930s used plaster casts instead of bandages to maintain correction. During the late 1940s, Ignatio Ponseti described his technique of plaster casting based on correction of the subtalar joint abnormal orientation. In clubfoot, the soft tissues are more resistant to pressure than the bones. Later on, with the concept of more resistant soft tissues as compared to bones, soft tissue releases came in, with safer pediatric anesthesia. In the 1960s, 1970s, and 1980s, more aggressive surgeries including complete subtalar releases were developed. With the advent of better imaging, computers, better understanding of pathoanatomy, and long-term follow-up information showing undercorrection, overcorrection, pain, stiffness, etc., aggressive surgical enthusiasm dampened. Toward the end of the twentieth century, Ponseti's technique again gained momentum. Now again, surgeons are looking toward the limitations of Ponseti's method. Finally, in the twenty-first century, the author is imagining what may happen in the future in prevention and treatment of clubfoot with various advances in epidemiology, molecular biology, biomechanics, biomaterials, surgery, and evidence-based medicine.

Gjonej et al.[3] corroborating the historical report of Hippocrates around 400 BCE as given by Dobbs et al. (2007), mentioned Arcanys (1658), describing his technique with mechanical devices and the forcible manipulation of Scarpa with his mechanical device with a shoe for maintenance, which never became popular. In 1823, Delpech was the first to describe tendoachilles tenotomy, which got infected, but improved over time. After that, there were many good manipulative treatments by Hugh Owen Thomas, Sir Robert Jones, Dennis Brown, Michael Hoke, Kite, Ponseti, Huson, and others. However, the main methods were of Kite (1939), Ponseti (1950), and the French method. The difference between the Kite and Ponseti methods are (i) the point of counter pressure in the Ponseti method is the talar neck and, in the Kite method, it is the calcaneo-cuboid joint; (ii) the first cast in the Ponseti method is in supination and, in Kite's method, it is pronation; and (iii) it is tenotomy of the tendoachilles in Ponseti's method, not so in Kite's method. However, the Ponseti method is more effective. Michael Hoke (1874–1944) was the first to start casting. In the Ponseti method, treatment is started within the first few days, with weekly casting for two months, then Achilles tenotomy, if required; after that, patients follow a strict regimen of stretching exercises and long-term bracing for four years.

Francis and Addis[4] working in Africa, have published a review article on treatment of neglected clubfoot, which is a common problem in low income countries, with very little literature available on their treatment. A neglected clubfoot is one which has been inadequately or never treated and deformity is severe and rigid. The bones become deformed with weight bearing for long periods with axial loading instead of typical plantigrade weight bearing with thick callosity, bursa, fissures, infection, breaking down, and so forth. Treatment before the walking age by the Ponseti technique can bring back the typical appearance. As the age advances, in neglected clubfoot, the spectrum of severity varies depending upon the severity and rigidity. Treatment of neglected clubfoot is largely surgical, and no single surgical procedure can correct all clubfeet, and there are many procedures available. The choice of method depends on age, severity, and rigidity varying from various soft tissue with or without osseous procedures. They described many procedures from the literature for correcting every type of clubfoot **and asserted that** Ponseti's technique of manipulation and casting is effective in children up to two years of age but they commented that Lourenco and Morcuende[5] have reported its use in a small series of 24 neglected clubfeet of older children 1.2–9 years of age with percutaneous tenotomy in all and a second posterior surgical release required in eight of the feet. The second option is soft tissue release, the standard posterior, medial, and posterior soft tissue release surgical procedure. For dynamic supination, lateral transfer of tibialis anterior to the third cuneiform. Then, there are lateral column shortening osteotomies, through the calcaneum or the calcaneo-cuboid joint to shorten the longer lateral column by wedge resections, Dilwyn Evans, or Lichtblau procedures. Calcaneo-cuboid fusion by the Evans' procedure leads to stiff foot. Combined closing wedge of cuboid and opening wedge cuneiform osteotomies (McHale and Lenhart) have also been described, which are more appropriate for patients more than eight or nine years old. Then, there are the corrective midfoot osteotomies for correcting the angular and rotational deformities at midfoot, that is, rigid pes cavus, rigid metatarsus varus (inversion and adduction). The triple arthrodesis is used for correcting major deformities. In the developed world, triple arthrodesis is primarily used as a salvage procedure for pain after previous surgeries. In developing countries, it is relevant for correcting severe and rigid deformities. Conventionally, triple arthrodesis should not be done before skeletal maturity, that is, 10–12 years of age, to avoid growth retardation during the growing age. However, Penny, working in Africa, has done it in children as young as six years old, and he feels it is only a cosmetic handicap. Talectomy has been often used in neglected clubfoot, but he quoted Penny who preferred triple arthrodesis because talectomy leaves an incongruous joint with a functional handicap.

3.2 PONSETI'S TECHNIQUE AND ITS PITFALLS

Ponseti and Smoley[6] in the reprint of their classic article of 1963 published in *The Journal of Bone and Joint Surgery* have themselves reported their results of treatment in 67 patients with 94 severe clubfoot deformities. The age of start of treatment was one week to six months after birth, with the average being one month, and with most being within the first month of birth. In 74 more severely deformed feet (79%), a heel cord section was done. They have asserted in the discussion, "Complete and permanent correction of a severe and rigid club foot is often difficult. Recurrence of the heel varus deformity and adduction of the fore part of the foot are common even after complete correction. Denis Browne splints on shoes worn full time for the first two or three months after correction, and part time thereafter until the child is from three to five years of age, are useful to prevent recurrences in many cases. However, only half of the recurrences could be blamed on the neglect of follow-up treatment." They found that 53 feet (56% of cases) had their first recurrence from 10 months to five years of follow-up. Even a majority of radiologically corrected cases had residual deformity. Regarding the 44% of good results, they found, "In the forty-one feet permanently corrected with the first treatment, the deformity tended to be less rigid, the leg muscles better developed, and the length of Denis Browne splint treatment longer than in the feet with recurrent deformities. Also, the family of patients without recurrence tended to be more cooperative. About half of the recurrences occurred from two to four months after the Denis Browne splints were discarded, usually on the family's own initiative. The recurrences could be blamed on the neglect of follow-up treatment with these splints. In other patients the recurrence was associated with a severer initial deformity and apparently poorly developed leg muscles; these recurrences seemed to be related to the severity of the primary aberration which caused the deformity." Many of them were treated, by second heel cord section and another surgical procedure. Even in these first-recurrence cases, they reported second-time recurrence in 17 feet (18%) from 18 months to 5 years of follow-up. They were treated by either resection of the tendoachilles or other surgical procedures. Out of these 17 feet, 9 feet had a third recurrence at 3–8 years of follow-up. They were all treated surgically. Yet again, one foot had a fourth recurrence, treated surgically. In summarizing their results, they found that their final results in severe deformities in young children one week to six months of age (average one month), with four recurrences were 71% good, 28% with slight residual deformity, and one failure. Therefore, it can be safely concluded that Ponseti's technique will give the best results in mild and moderate deformities and if the treatment is started within the first week of birth or up to one month of age, followed by a prolonged corrective splintage for 3–5 years, which often gets neglected. Even otherwise, with proper splintage, recurrences can occur for unknown reasons.

Huang et al.[7] operated between 1957 and 1994 on 1,521 clubfeet in 1,088 children from 3 months to 12 years of age. Out of these, in order to determine their long-term results of surgery, they reviewed only 111 patients with 159 feet, with operations between 6 months to 12 years of age by à la carte posteromedial release. The inclusion criteria were physical presentation of all patients for clinical and radiological assessment, at least 6 years after surgery, and all patients at least 13 years of age. They obtained about 92% excellent or good results. They have quoted Tarraf and Carroll[8] reporting residual deformities of adduction and supination of the forefoot as the most common persistent deformity in 95% requiring repeat surgery after soft tissue correction. Tarraf and Carroll also reported that these deformities became more evident with growth.

Azarpira et al.[9] commented on the factors responsible for recurrence with Ponseti's treatment. They reviewed the results of 196 clubfeet in 115 children with a male:female ratio of 2.6:1, a mean age at start of treatment of 5.4 days after birth (1–60 days), an average number of casts of 4.2, and follow up of 11–60 months. Thirty-nine feet had recurrence (30%). More recurrences with high statistical significance were observed with nonidiopathic clubfeet, noncompliance with bracing, low educational level, more number of casts, and with longer follow-up period. The Ponseti method is highly laborious with a very strict regimen. More failure will be present if these principles are neglected.

Zhao et al.[10] reported from a comprehensive review of well-considered inclusion criteria from 19 eligible articles out of 519 recorded reports of the Ponseti method of treatment. The presenting age in these studies was mostly within three months of birth. The Ponseti method is simple but requires careful attention to its details. Failure to observe details of manipulation, percutaneous Achilles tenotomy and tibialis anterior transfer when needed, type of brace, bracing protocol, and relapse management will increase the failure rate. Because of wide variations in the protocols of different reports, there have been variations in relapse rates. Although good correction has been reported in all reports in the initial phase of casting, with around 90% in all, recurrence has been very common in the maintenance phase of prolonged bracing and noncompliance. The rate of noncompliance was up to 61% and the relapse rate was up to 62%. The most common reason for noncompliance is discomfort and its long-term use. There are a large number of reports quoting high relapse rate. Even in the compliant group, a relapse rate of 16% has been reported. Four reasons have been analyzed by the authors for noncompliance: (i) variation in bracing protocol, (ii) varied definition of noncompliance, (iii) calculation of time period of daily bracing, and (iv) inadequate follow-up or tracking methods. Ponseti recommended bracing for four years, with proper positioning and long daily wear, to prevent relapse, which is difficult to achieve. Many modifications of braces have been described to increase compliance. Results can only improve if every detail of the Ponseti technique is adhered to.

Staheli and Ponseti and others[11] excerpt from their manual, describing every detail with photographs and diagrams with the rationale and the methodology through the last follow-up, will be quite pertinent to discuss this most prevalent method of clubfoot management all over the world. The protocol, reported for the first time, by Ponseti and Smoley in their classic article in 1963, is intensely laborious and time consuming, hence it is important to learn all of the details thoroughly, both for the caregivers as well as the recipients. It is being practiced in about 150 countries all over the world. It is extremely important to follow the exact protocol for success. The salient features of this technique, based on strong scientific evidence, are that it is important to understand the polyaxial kinematics of tarsal joints depending upon the multidirectional orientation of these joints, as well as the biology of soft tissues, that is, muscles, tendons, and ligaments. **It is very important to observe the following principles in order to obtain the best results.** The treatment should start in the first few weeks after birth, preferably within the first week of birth, but correction is possible through late childhood. Mostly, 6–7 weekly casts will correct the deformity; if not, the casting is faulty. If treatment is delayed, some cases will need surgery. The success rate will depend upon the degree of stiffness of the foot, the surgeon's experience, and the family's cooperation. This technique can be used in syndromic clubfoot also, but it is more difficult and less predictable. After castings, heel cord tenotomy is done in nearly all cases, and the foot is put in a cast for a further three weeks. After this, a prolonged period of abduction/external rotation bracing occurs. The method of achieving initial correction in the first cast is correction of the cavus by elevating the head of the first metatarsal, aligning it with the hindfoot. Later casts are in abduction of the forefoot, with counter pressure on the talar head inward without touching the heel, which leads to a composite three-dimensional movement of the whole foot around head of the talus. Plaster casting avoids pressure on bones by good molding, as well as for maintenance of correction. Casting is above the knee and given in two parts, below the knee first and then extending it to the upper thigh. Many complications can occur with improper casting technique because of the many detailed steps that are involved; the complications include rocker bottom foot, crowded toes, flat heel pad, and pressure sores. There may be many mistakes in multiple manipulations, casting, and molding steps, each one being important. Then there may be errors in heel cord tenotomy or improper braces with so many types available or neglecting the prolonged bracing protocol. **There will be recurrence in more than 80% of cases if the bracing protocol is neglected.** Illiteracy, poverty, lack of training and family support due to culture barriers and lack of communication in remote areas are also important reasons for failures. There is a lack of diligent follow-up to detect early relapses, which are most often due to noncompliance with the bracing protocol. Relapses may be of equinus due to more rapid tibial growth than growth of gastrocsoleus on account of a fibrotic tendon and atrophic muscle. Relapse can also be due to varus relapse or dynamic supination due to an overactive tibialis anterior muscle.

Goriainov et al.[12] reported a Pirani severity score as a predictor of incidence of relapse with the Ponseti treatment. All of the 80 patients included in this report were children, with average age at presentation as 23.2 days, ranging from 2 to 152 days. They found statistically significant higher relapse rate in more severe/rigid deformities with higher Pirani score with 21% relapses in 80 feet.

Bhaskar and Rasal[13] highlighted the pitfalls of the Ponseti technique in 40 treated children who started casting at the mean age of nine days, with heel cord section in all, and they got excellent results in 28 children. The problems of the Ponseti technique have been undercorrection due to faulty casting on account of poor learning of the rigid technique, with a gradual learning curve, non-compliance of bracing, improper brace, and poor follow-up.

Bhaskar and Patni[14] reported that relapses are common in clubfoot treated by the Ponseti technique and will become as severe as the initial deformity if left untreated. In the literature, some have used descriptive deforming elements to describe relapse, for example, equinus, adduction, varus, cavus, or in combination. Others have used Pirani or Dimeglio scores, and still others have described the relapse as major or minor, without definitive classification given. The authors treated 206 children with 362 feet by the Ponseti technique and identified 43 children with 78 foot relapses; this included 48 children with 86 relapses from other institutions who were referred for treatment and thus have reported 91 relapsed children with 164 feet with a mean age at presentation for casting as 10.71 days (range 7–22 days). There were 73 bilateral (Pirani score 5.6) and 18 unilateral feet (Pirani score 5.5). Percutaneous Achilles tenotomy was done in 65 bilateral cases (130 feet, 89%) and 12 unilateral (66%). They have classified these relapses into five patterns at a mean follow up of 4.5 years (range 3–5 years). Grade 1A is decreased dorsiflexion from 15° to neutral, grade 1B is dynamic adduction or supination forefoot, grade 2A is rigid equinus, grade 2B is rigid adduction/supination forefoot, and grade 3 is a combination of two or more deformities. In regard to distribution of these relapses in the bilateral group, 28% had a grade 1A relapse, 34% had a grade 1B, 16% had a grade 2A, 9.7% had a grade 2B, and the remaining 12.3% had a combination of these.

Zionts and Dietz[15] commented that Ponseti is popular, but the successful outcome is quite challenging in preventing relapses and the most common cause of relapse is failure to adhere to the long regimen of bracing after correction, besides socioeconomic and cultural issues, which need the utmost attention.

MacNeille et al.[16] reported a mini open tendoachilles lengthening in view of many complications due to closed heel cord cutting, considering its necessity in over 85% of cases and to avoid the complications. The complications of closed tenotomy, which have been reported in the literature, are bleeding due to injury to the peroneal artery, the posterior tibial artery, or the lesser saphenous vein; injury to the posterior tibial or sural nerve, and incomplete release. More rare complications reported many times in the literature and also quoted by these authors (Changulani et al. 2007) are congenital vascular anomalies and the absence of the anterior tibial and/or posterior tibial artery, with the peroneal artery assuming prominent arterial supply, and serious neurovascular damage by closed tenotomy. The authors conducted 63 tenotomies (41 patients) in the operating room, in children 5–48 weeks of age, with an average age of 12.5 weeks, through a 10 mm incision on the medial edge of the tendoachilles under vision, and all the complications mentioned were avoided.

Dobbs et al.[17] reviewed 134 infants with 219 clubfeet treated by the Ponseti method with percutaneous tenotomy performed in 222 feet (91%) at a mean age of 16 weeks. Four had serious bleeding, three due to injury to the peroneal artery and one due to injury to the lesser saphenous vein.

Burghardt et al.[18] commented that bleeding is frequently seen after tenotomy. They reported a case of active pseudoaneurysm in a child eight weeks old after percutaneous heel cord sectioning with a pulsating mass, incomplete correction, and without proper bracing. This was confirmed by color ultrasonography and managed by repeat casting and pressure moulding over the aneurysm for four weeks.

Miller et al.[19] reported that, despite the Ponseti method of treating clubfoot in children being considered the gold standard, the results have been variable in different institutions, and they quoted a large number of references from the literature reporting recurrences from 10% to 41%. The authors reviewed their results from comparison of two institutions, one following strict adherence to rigid steps in casting, bracing, and follow-up and the other loosely following the principles. They found that with strict followers, the recurrence rate was 2%, while loose followers had a 47% recurrence rate. **Following the strict regimen is difficult but possible and requires a single committed surgeon and supporting staff and commitment from the patient's parents, along with financial and other various forms of committed logistical support.**

Agarwal et al.[20] reported numerous problems during casting, tenotomy, and bracing in the Ponseti method for treating clubfoot during six years, and they reported moisture lesions, hematoma, dermatitis, pressure sores during casting and bracing, fractures, excessive bleeding on tenotomy, and tenderness at the tenotomy site.

Bor et al.[21] reported results of the Ponseti treatment in 117 clubfeet (74 infants) and with a minimum follow-up of five years, and found 44% had poor brace use and 32% underwent additional surgery other than tendoachilles tenotomy.

Changulani et al.[22] reported 32% recurrence after Ponseti's technique out of 96 feet, requiring additional surgical procedures with extensive surgery in 15 of them.

Zionts et al.[23] prospectively evaluated walking age of 94 clubfoot infants, who were treated by the Ponseti technique within 12 weeks of birth by a single surgeon and followed for at least two years. They found that, at 18 months, 90% of the children were walking freely without assistance. Patients with moderate deformities walked earlier than those with severe deformities. Overall, patients with clubfoot deformity started walking about two months later than typical children, and patients with very severe deformities or in which relapse occurred were further delayed in the age of walking.

Sala et al.[24] reviewed data from 36 fully compliant children for Ponseti's casting treatment with all other essential inclusion criteria. Their treatment was started at mean age of 15.2 days. There were delays of 1.5–2 months in various milestones, including ambulation and independent walking.

Haft et al.[25] reported follow up of 51 babies with 73 clubfeet for a minimum of two years after treatment by the Ponseti method, and they found that 41% were noncompliant for the bracing regimen and 57% of those had major recurrences, while in the 59% compliant group, only 11.5% had major recurrences. Thus, the noncompliant group had a five-times higher risk of major recurrence.

McElroy et al.[26] commented that the Ponseti method of casting is good and cost-effective, but that there are numerous obstacles in its implementation in Uganda, classifying these into six areas: (i) inadequate resources, (ii) distance to treatment centers, (iii) poverty, (iv) lack of family support, (v) attitude of caregivers, and (vi) implementing the treatment process effectively (correct casting, prolonged bracing, etc.).

Abdelgawad et al.[27] reported that out of 137 patients treated by the Ponseti method with a follow up of at least two years, at least two-thirds were noncompliant with bracing and had a recurrence requiring surgery, out of which one-third required extensive operations. Even in the remaining one-third who were compliant, 14% required surgery.

Faulks and Richards[28] reported their 15 years of experience with the Ponseti and French functional techniques and reported 95% initial correction with both methods, but relapses occurred with both: 37% with Ponseti and 29% with the French technique. However, posteromedial release could be avoided with both methods at 4.3 years average follow-up, but more children treated by the French technique walked with hyperextended knees and equinus gait, and more walked with calcaneus gait when treated by the Ponseti method.

Faldini et al.[29] reported their results of treatment in 88 clubfeet: 52 newborns, 12 nonambulating children 4–12 months of age, and 24 ambulating children. All newborns and nonambulating children were treated by the Ponseti casting technique with heel cord tenotomy in some, while all ambulating children were treated by open surgery medial or posteromedial release and cuboid wedge osteotomy. At 1–6 years of follow-up (average 5 years), results in newborns were excellent in 42, good in 6, and poor in 4. In nonambulating children in the older age group, 9 had excellent results and 3 had good results. In ambulating children, the results were excellent in 5, good in 16, and poor in 3 cases. Therefore, the need for surgery was higher in delayed-treatment cases, and early treatment is better for getting good results with casting treatment.

Lourenco and Morcuende[5] retrospectively reviewed the Ponseti technique used in 24 neglected clubfeet in 17 children with a mean age of 3.9 years (1.2–9 years) with mean follow-up of 3.1 years (2.1–5.6 years) and mobilization in a plaster of Paris (POP) cast for 1.5–6 months, mean 3.9 months. Percutaneous tenotomy was done in all, with 7 feet requiring a second tenotomy and 8 feet needing a posterior release for full correction of hindfoot. Results were 66.6% good with 4 feet having dynamic inversion. For these, a modified Ponseti technique was used which was more intensive and prolonged for manipulations and casting. However, for hindfoot correction, operative intervention was necessary.

Ganesan et al.[30] reviewed the literature from 2000 to 2015 from four electronic databases, namely, Medline, Cumulative Index to Nursing and Allied Health Literature (CINHAL), PubMed, and Scopus, for efficacy of the Ponseti method in the treatment of clubfoot (casting, heel cord tenotomy, and bracing) in children less than two years of age. Out of 1,095 identified articles, only 12 satisfied their inclusion and exclusion criteria. In most of them, treatment was started soon after birth. Out of 12 studies, relapses were noticed in nine, with maximum of 27.1% in one study (Hallaj et al. 2015). They quoted from many studies in the literature that 10%–30% relapses are very common with the Ponseti treatment. Relapses can be prevented only if the treatment is started soon after birth and casting with the right technique, and continued bracing for four years the way is it advised. Many of the reasons for relapses are still not clear. About 78% of relapses occur due to noncompliance of bracing, which is the most difficult part of treatment. Even in the bracing-compliant patients, 7% relapse is quoted by the authors as being reported in these studies. Other factors responsible are illiteracy and poverty. Improper casting, percutaneous tenotomy, and poor follow-up are other factors. Moreover, this report did not included children with clubfeet more than two years of age and older age groups.

Jowett et al.[31] reported a literature review of 74 full-text articles of the Ponseti treatment meeting their inclusion criteria. They found noncompliance of long-term bracing for four years to be the most common cause of relapse.

Dogan et al.[32] reported their experimental study in 15 rats, each for comparison between subcutaneous heel cord tenotomy and mini open tenotomy, the other side used as control. One rat in each group was reserved for study of histopathology. This was necessitated due to reports of incomplete division of the tendon and re-tenotomies leading to relapses requiring open surgery. After 31 days, in the grossly mini open group, they found slightly more thickening and adhesions. The gap was replaced in both groups by dull gray and thick scar tissue in the gap between the glistening tendon ends, but there was no difference in the strength on biomechanical testing in the two groups. Histologically, a typical tendon showed tightly packed parallel collagen fibers with few cells. In the mini open group, irregularity in the parallel pattern of collagen fibers with nonspecific collagen tissue and infiltration by mononuclear inflammatory cells was observed. In the percutaneous group, these changes were more marked than in the mini open group. The authors commented on two distinct advantages of the mini open technique: (i) assured complete tenotomy as is a must in the Ponseti method and (ii) complete avoidance of neurovascular complications seen with the percutaneous procedure. Mini open is safe and sure, especially in fatty infants when the tendon is not easily palpable, in small infants, when vascular compromise is suspected clinically or after color Doppler, or for an inexperienced surgeon initially. However, mini open requires general anesthesia, but percutaneous only requires local anesthesia.

3.3 OTHER CONTEMPORARY TECHNIQUES

McKay[33–35] in Section I of his new concept regarding clubfoot treatment, described the morbid anatomy in detail. He believed that internal rotation of the foot and failure to correct it is due to rotation of subtalar complex pivoting at the interosseous ligament, causing the calcaneum to rotate inward and the talus outward. In 1983, in Section II, he described his new concept of treating clubfoot by correcting this abnormal subtalar rotation described in Section I by reversing the rotation of the talo-calcaneal complex. In Section III, he evaluated 102 clubfeet treated by this technique over a six-year period, and he found the results to be good but needed long-term follow-up data. In addition, the foot abduction brace used in small children of pre-walking age had to be replaced by Foot Ankle Orthosis (FAO). The authors have also commented on the small size of the series.

Bensahel et al.[36] as pioneers of the functional method of clubfoot treatment, the so-called French technique, in describing the history of this technique, wrote that this technique has been erroneously called the French technique. The original French technique for clubfoot was very crude and used painful stretching, rigid taping, and splinting, which came into vogue at a large children's hospital (BUCH) in Paris, famous for using physiotherapy as a supplement to surgery for orthopedic patients, including clubfoot patients. When Professor Bensahel took over around 1970, he started his historic gentle stretching and splinting in clubfoot in newborns, which was based on sound abnormal pathoanatomy correction. In resistant cases, it was supplemented with à la carte posteromedial release, and they experienced success in the majority of cases at 96%. This was presented in 1975 in Chicago at the Tachdjian Clubfoot Course. They asserted that this technique should actually be called Bensahel's functional method of conservative treatment of clubfoot.

Turco[37] described the details of his popular early one-stage posteromedial release in resistant idiopathic congenital clubfeet in failed conservative treatment cases or in cases which recurred after previous soft tissue release. The author devised this procedure after due deliberations and realizing its necessity. He quoted many authors reporting high recurrence rate (Brockman 1930, Bertelsen 1957, Fripp and Shaw 1967, Ponseti and Smoley 1963, Salter 1965, Wynne Davis 1964, and Beatson and Pearson 1966). He also quoted Kuhlman and Bell (1957), who reported 154 operations on 53 patients of resistant clubfoot with only 31% satisfactory results and Dangelmajer (1961) reporting 60% requiring soft tissue or bone surgery out of 200 cases. Turco himself reported incomplete corrections and recurrent deformities in over 50% of cases eventually requiring one or more surgical procedures. With that background, he developed this technique of one-stage surgery. He first studied the pathoanatomy and skiagrams and then based his surgical technique of correction. Describing his surgical technique in detail, it is carried out through a single medial incision from the first metatarsal base to the tendoachilles behind the medial malleolus. As the first step to facilitate surgery in a small deformed foot, five structures are then identified: tibialis posterior tendon, the flexor digitorum longus, the neurovascular bundle, the flexor hallucis longus, and the Achilles tendon. The tibialis posterior is divided just above the medial malleolus, and the distal part of the tendon is cut at the navicular at the end of dissection and removed. Other releases are the posterior release, medial release, and partial subtalar release by tendoachilles Z plasty, posterior capsulotomy of the ankle and the subtaloid joint, dividing superficial fibers of the deltoid ligament, dividing the Henry's knot, and freeing the sheaths of flexor hallucis and flexor digitorum tendons, dividing the spring ligament and the interosseous talo-calcanean ligament from the medial side, reducing talo-navicular dislocation, and fixing with K-wire in the corrected position. In postoperative care, the POP cast is changed at three weeks and again at six weeks with stitch removal and then continued for a total of four months; a Dennis Brown splint is used for one year; and walking shoes for two years. In this preliminary report, he used this procedure in 58 feet in 41 patients up to six years of age. He does not recommend this in older children, with follow-up varying from two to seven years. He commented that evaluation of results is difficult due to so many variables. The author graded his results on clinical and radiological correction. Out of 31 feet with follow-up for two or more years, results were excellent in 15 feet, good in 12, fair in 3, and poor in 1 foot.

Turco[38] consolidated his opinion about his posteromedial release in yet another report in 1979 with 240 operated resistant clubfeet in 176 patients. The end results in 149 feet with follow-up for 2–15 years were excellent or good in 83.8%, fair in 10.7%, and poor in 5.3%. The best results obtained were in children operated on between one and two years of age. Out of 240 clubfeet, 58% were under two years of age and 82.5% were within four years of age. All older children (36%) in his series had one or more prior surgeries. The author categorically states that a completely normal foot cannot be achieved; there will be some residual deformity, such as calf atrophy, unequal lengths of feet in unilateral cases, limitation of movement, pes planus, forefoot adduction or in-toeing, radiological undercorrection in a typical-looking foot. Results evaluated were based on appearance, function, and radiology. Results have been reported in 149 feet with follow-up for more than two years (for 5–15 years in 51% of cases). Results were 84% excellent/good and 16% fare/poor. In conclusion, he asserts that the best results are obtained if the operation is done at 1–2 years of age. Previous surgery acts as a spoiler of results. For older children, he recommends triple arthrodesis at skeletal maturity.

Lichtblau[39] described combined medial and lateral release, a modified soft tissue release combined with excision of the distal part of the calcaneum, instead of excision of the calcaneo-cuboid joint and arthrodesis and to preserve the motion at the calcaneo-cuboid joint, the excision of the distal end of the calcaneum will gradually result in reforming of fibrocartilage, preserving movement at this joint. The author has found this to be very useful in recurrent or residual deformities after earlier surgeries with dense scars and severe deformities with rigidity and uninhibited lateral tarsal growth. Long-term effects of these in regard to arthritis of joints have not yet been reported. The author justifies this procedure over Evan's calcaneo-cuboid fusion with corrective wedge resection, arguing that fusion will lead to more growth on the medial side than the lateral, resulting in valgus, especially in a younger child, as well as loss of motion with a stiff foot.

Tayton and Thompson[40] in their 1979 report, described in detail the operation of soft tissue release and calcaneo-cuboid fusion, published by Dillwyn Evans in 1961 along with the long-term review of their series of 118 clubfeet treated by this technique. Like Dillwyn Evans, the authors deliberately delayed this operation until about six years of age, when all risk of relapse would be gone. All of them were resistant feet, and the average age of patients at review was 17 years and were operated by Dillwyn Evan's "collateral operation," the name preferred by Evan, although the operation internationally bears his name. This operative technique consists of four stages, the first three stages being extensive soft tissue release realigning the hindfoot. Finally, in the fourth stage, the calcaneo-cuboid wedge is excised, shortening the lateral border, and held with two staples after correcting the deformity. Stage one is plantar fasciotomy, stage two is medial release, and stage three is posterior release by Z plasty of tendoachilles and opening of the talocalcanean joint. After surgery, a plaster cast is kept for four months and the patient can bear no weight for the first six weeks. Results were assessed on the basis of eight questions for functional results and 10 points for clinical assessment. In regard to the functional assessment, 47% were good, 31% were fair, and 22% were poor. In regard to the clinical assessment, using the Wynne–Davies scoring system, 85% of the feet were clinically acceptable and using the scoring system of Main et al., 56% of the feet were satisfactory. Complications seen included shortening by 1.9 centimeters on average, more appreciated in unilateral feet; circulatory disturbance (cold feet) in 4%; stiffness of severe nature in 50% of feet; and slight degree of stiffness in 43% of feet. Pseudarthrosis of the calcaneo-cuboid joint was present in 13% of feet, a repeat collateral operation was necessary in 19% of feet, with a second repeat in 4%, and 7% were a total failure requiring triple arthrodesis. The authors considered this operation, on the whole, a good procedure with 78% acceptable functional results and 56%–85% clinically acceptable results, depending upon the method used, as above. If radiological correction is considered, only 37% had acceptable results, which has been seen by others also with a surprising amount of hidden deformity, with only 37% with full anatomical correction. Results compare favorably well with other series of this surgery. Four other observations are specifically mentioned by the authors: firstly, a high incidence of limited motion at the ankle and subtaloid joints; secondly, undercorrection of varus of the navicular in 33% of cases; thirdly, poorer results in girls than boys; and fourthly, the observation of Evans that this operation is likely to succeed below the age of four years has not been confirmed by the authors. Finally, they concluded that long-term results of the collateral operation is good for very resistant feet.

Simons[41] in part I of his report, described complete subtalar release, an extensive soft tissue release procedure for clubfeet that are not corrected by nonsurgical methods. He described his demanding technique in full detail of all four sides of subtalar release in four parts and numerous other soft tissue and anterior calcanean wedge resection, including intraoperative triple K-wire fixation under radiographic control. He also wrote that the main disadvantage of this procedure is the tendency to overcorrection.

Simons[42] in part II of his report on this procedure compared the results with less extensive procedures. In group I, 21 feet had posteromedial and lateral release, and in group II, 26 feet had complete subtalar release. He found group II to have better clinical correction, 72% as compared with 50% in group I. However, in group II, radiologically good correction was only 64%. Yet another finding was central radiolucencies seen in the calcaneum, talus, and metatarsal heads in 60% of group II which could be avascularity or not, and needs investigation with long term follow-up. The follow up period of four years in this series had no adverse effect.

Hassan et al.[43] treated 18 children (30 feet) aged 3–11 years (mean age 5.6 years) by complete subtalar release between 2000 and 2006 for recurrent or neglected clubfoot and reported good results.

3.4 ILIZAROV AND ALLIED TECHNIQUES

Jordan et al.[44] reported on the Ilizarov technique for clubfoot correction along with its modifications being very often used in this deformity. However, as we all know, it evolved as a revolutionary procedure in research for limb lengthening and deformity correction. Its history started in the nineteenth century with surgeons struggling to treat the sequelae of war injuries. They quoted Langenbeck (1869), Hopkins and Penrose (1889), and von Eiselberg (1897) making initial attempts at limb lengthening. The modern era of limb lengthening in early 1900 by the Italian orthopedic surgeon Codivilla presenting his work of limb lengthening by osteotomy and gradual traction at the American Orthopaedic Association meeting in 1905. They further quoted Abbot and Crego reporting their improved technique in the 1930s. European and American orthopedic surgeons were developing their own techniques. Although many methods of good lengthening were available, they remained localized due to poor dissemination of information. With Wagner (1963) advancing his technique in the west, Ilizarov was working in Kurgen (Siberia) developing his biological principle of distraction osteogenesis for limb lengthening.

In part 2 of this series, Goldstein et al.[45] reviewed the principals of distraction osteogenesis and discussed their indications, instrumentation, and surgical technique. Among the important contributors in this field, the name of Dr. Gavril Ilizarov stands tall.

Malizos et al.[46] retrospectively reviewed 13 feet (12 patients) with relapsed clubfoot deformity after previous surgery. They were treated with soft tissue surgical procedures. Out of these, seven were supplemented with an Ilizarov frame (mean age 7–8 years) where complete intraoperative correction was not possible. The Ilizarov frame was applied for 9–13 weeks, and there were two excellent, three good, and two fair results at four years of follow-up. They also comment that there are only a few reports of small case series with a similar approach in relapsed clubfeet, with varying results from 15% to 100% and with recurrence rates of 5%–61%. All of the published reports, including the present one, have their limitations in too many variables with respect to age, severity of deformity and treatment methods, and evaluating results. No two series are similar in all respects. On the whole, this is a good method in selected cases in children.

Saghieh et al.[47] reported their experience of treatment with ring fixators with differential lengthening and other maneuvering in nine patients between three and nine years of age with relapsed clubfeet after at least one open posteromedial release; all but one patient had two previous surgeries. The frame was removed after 75–130 days. Follow-up was 6 months to 7.5 years with a mean of 3.5 years. There were several complications, for example, pin track infections in all patients with healing with antibiotic, anterior subluxation of the talus treated by gradual posterior translation, severe flexion contractures of toes, fracture of the first metatarsal, and moderate-to-severe pain during the treatment. Evaluation was done on appearance, function, and radiological correction. There were three excellent, four good, and two fair results. Out of these, two relapsed at the last follow-up. The authors comment that their distraction treatment is not significantly better in relapsed clubfeet than surgical options, and it was a small series and had inadequate follow up for any firm conclusion.

Manjappa[48] treated 15 old resistant/recurrent clubfeet with a mean patient age of 5 years and 10 months, with 14 satisfactory results and one unsatisfactory result. The author also comments that treatment options are many with nearly the same results. There are so many variables that no two studies can be compared, but Joshi's external skeletal system (JESS) is simple and more comfortable for patients.

Suresh et al.[49] presented their results in 44 clubfeet in 26 children, from 10 months to 6 years of age (average 2.8 years), treated by JESS external fixator during two years, January 1998 to December 1999. Cases included neglected clubfeet, dropouts of plaster casting treatment, relapses after surgery, common in India. After achieving correction, the fixator is continued for another 2–3 months and then removed, putting the limb in plaster for another three months. At two years of follow-up, results obtained were 77% excellent, 14% good, and 9% poor. Common complications were 50% pin track infections, healing in due course, and pin loosening requiring removal. They further commented that the Ilizarov fixator, being bulky, will be difficult to manage in small children younger than six years of age with small feet. For such cases, the JESS fixator which was invented in the early 1990s is especially useful for small feet. Other advantages of JESS over Ilizarov are: easier application, lightweight, easy learning curve, lower inventory, and low cost. Motivated and compliant parents are pivotal to this technique, besides the judiciously performed prolonged differential distraction, for best results. Otherwise, it may be catastrophic in a small developing foot.

Oganesyan et al.[50] evaluated their results in 65 adults with 83 equino-cavo-varus deformities, due to trauma with ischemic and neutrophic changes, poliomyelitis, Charcot-Marie-tooth neuromuscular dystrophy, and untreated clubfeet, all considered unsuitable for surgery. They were all treated with the Volkov–Oganesyan–Povarov hinged distraction apparatus. Ages of patients varied from 16 to 65 years with an average of 26 years. Duration of applying the fixator was 3–13 weeks for correction, followed by an additional two months, a plaster cast for two months, and finally a custom made shoe insert for one year. Eight patients had pin track infection treated by antibiotics, five of them requiring removal of pins and three additional patients required removal of the whole assembly. In 59 feet, results were good, 20 showed satisfactory results, and 4 had poor results. In the poor results, arthrodesis improved the results.

Grill and Franke[51] treated 10 neglected equinovarus deformities in nine patients due to various causes by the Ilizarov distractor. There were three patients of congenital idiopathic clubfeet, the others were due to trauma, arthrogryposis, cerebral palsy, peripheral neuropathy, and one with two inches limb shortening. The ages of these patients ranged from 8 to 15 years. In severe deformities in children, the prevalent opinion is to wait until skeletal maturity or at least until 12 years of age and then do arthrodesis procedures preceded by soft tissue releases, leading to short and stiff foot, besides risk of complications such as skin necrosis, infection, pseudarthrosis, and vascular necrosis. The authors have obtained good results by this much less invasive method. These deformities are common in developing countries and remain neglected due to various socioeconomic reasons. They are resigned to their fate until they start getting pain. The authors recommend this treatment in such cases.

Makhdoom et al.[52] reported 21 patients (27 clubfeet) with resistant deformities between 8 and 20 years of age, with a mean age of 12 years, who were treated with an Ilizarov fixator along with limited soft tissue correction as percutaneous heel cord tenotomy and plantar fasciotomy. The fixator was kept for 3–5 months, a plaster cast for six weeks, and ankle foot arthrosis for an additional three months. They obtained 74% excellent/good results with plantigrade foot, while about 26% were unsatisfactory. They concluded that the short-term results are promising, but as follow-up continues longer, more recurrences can be expected.

Utukuri et al.[53] quoted by Makhdoom et al.[52] reported 70% unsatisfactory results at a follow-up of 47 months. However, the authors still consider Ilizarov a good option for these long-standing neglected deformities.

Ferreira et al.[54] reported their experience with the Ilizarov external fixator along with limited soft tissue correction (heel cord tenotomy and plantar fasciotomy) in 38 severe, stiff neglected clubfeet (30 patients) with mean age of 26 years (range 5–39 years), with an average follow-up of 58 months. The device was applied for an average of 16 weeks, followed by a plaster cast for six weeks and ankle-foot orthosis for six months. The results were good in 30 feet (78.9%), fair in 3 feet, and poor in 5 feet. Recurrence was observed in 59% of feet (19 feet). None of them required arthrodesis for symptomatic arthritis of the ankle or midfoot. The authors also conclude that the Ilizarov technique allows correction of all components of deformity with minimal surgery and reduced skin or neurovascular complications avoiding shortening of foot. The authors thus weigh the plus and minus points of this technique.

Refai et al.[55] reported a review of 19 relapsed clubfeet in 18 patients after Ponseti or posteromedial release, treated by an Ilizarov frame during about three years from 2005 to 2008, and they were not very satisfied with it. The age of patients varied from 4 to 15 years, follow-up varied from two to six years with a minimum of two years and frame application for an average of five weeks. Sixteen of nineteen feet were plantigrade at last follow-up. The three recurrences were in two patients, one 12 years old and other 15 years old, and both had relapsed earlier; one after posteromedial release. The authors discussed the disadvantages of the Ilizarov frame in that the frame application has to be for a long duration with continued discomfort to the patient, recurrences of deformity are found at long-term follow-up, and a higher recurrence rate in older children. They quoted several authors including Wallander et al. (1996) reporting 70% recurrence (7 out of 10 treated) and Freedman et al. (2006) reporting 11 out of 21 relapsing after the Ilizarov frame, requiring revision surgeries. The authors feel the relapses would be much higher if this technique were used in adolescents and adults.

Emara et al.[56] compared two groups of patients of complex equino-cavo-varus deformities in skeletally mature patients: Group 1 of 27 patients (29 feet) treated by triple arthrodesis fixed by an Ilizarov external fixator and group 2 of 29 patients (30 feet) clinically corrected by an Ilizarov fixator first and the Ilizarov replaced by percutaneous screws. Both groups were compared in regard to results and complications. In group 2, duration of treatment, as well as pin track infection rate, was significantly less compared with group 1.

Paley,[57] an expert in deformity correction and limb lengthening, presented his experience in 25 very complex foot deformities, which included five clubfeet. He treated these by various types of Ilizarov distraction osteotomies, which included supramaleolar, posterior calcanean, talo-calcaneal neck, midfoot, and metatarsal osteotomies. In clubfeet, he did all except metatarsal and talo-calcanean neck. Complications noted were pin track infection, deep infection, failure of separation or early union of osteotomy before correction, tarsal tunnel syndrome, toe contractures, various problems of wires, buckle fracture, requirement of secondary procedures, and skin break down. All these complications could be treated without ill effects, but lead to longer duration of treatment. Other disadvantages of this treatment in foot deformities are prolonged and painful treatment, a plantigrade but stiff foot with subnormal function.

Patwardhan and Doshi[58] described a mini external fixator (UMEX, universal mini external fixator) used in clubfoot in children, which is claimed to be an improvement over JESS. It is designed on the same principles as JESS, that is, histeogenesis of all tissues when they are put on gradual stretch. The difference is in the design of the clamp for better stability and fixation with more efficient correction, and it is used in all types of clubfeet in children. Use of a mini fixator is based on clubfoot having three components of deformity in the forefoot, hindfoot, and leg, and it is essential to have skeletal hold on these three blocks by frames with wires and connect these three blocks with distracters and clamps. It is essential to uncouple the distracters from the three blocks weekly and manipulate the foot to achieve manual derotation and then connect the distracters again. This is repeated every week until correction is achieved and then maintained for another two months for consolidation. Medial distraction is carried out four times a day, 0.25 mm each time and lateral distraction 0.25 mm twice a day. After removing the fixator, a brace is given.

Lee et al.[59] reported their experience of treating rigid equino-cavo-varus foot deformities caused by neurologic disorders by the Ilizarov technique. Such cases are difficult to correct and relapses are common. They treated 29 neurological equino-cavo-varus feet (26 patients), mean age of 18.7 years, due to lower motor or upper motor neuron diseases. Nine feet were treated by distraction histogenesis with limited soft tissue release and 20 needed additional osteotomy and/or tendon transfer/lengthening. Minimum follow up was 12 months (range 12–155 months, mean 72.9 months). The frame was kept for an average 50.3 days. Plantigrade foot was obtained in 24 feet; in five feet, residual mild varus persisted, while in four feet, deformity recurred requiring surgery. The authors feel that Ilizarov is a good option for treating such cases.

Meena et al.[60] evaluated their results of JESS and Ilizarov in neglected and relapsed clubfeet in 21 patients (28 feet) in the 3–12 years age group, with mean age of less than 8 years. In the Ilizarov group of 15 feet, results were 27% excellent, 40% good, 13% fair, and 20% poor, while in the JESS group of 13 feet, results were 15% excellent, 23% good, 23% fair, and 39% poor. Average follow up was 15 months. Their conclusion was that Ilizarov gave better results in more severe cases in older age groups, while JESS was better in younger children and less severe deformities. However, the Ilizarov frame was heavy and required somewhat more skilled management.

3.5 OLDER CHILDREN AND ADULTS

Herold and Torok[61] recommended a two-stage operation with medial release, excision of abductor hallucis, dividing tibialis posterior tendon, and heel cord lengthening as the first stage and triple arthrodesis in the second stage. Supplementary operations were also done, such as derotation tibial osteotomy and metatarsal osteotomy. Cosmetic results were excellent, and functional results were also good.

Burger et al.[62] have highlighted the overcorrected clubfoot deformities presenting in adults, which were operated on in childhood and remained asymptomatic for years. Long-term results of cases treated with posteromedial release shows overcorrection, sometimes due to revision surgeries for undercorrection, minor trauma, or some other episode triggering symptoms. Key deformities include dorsally subluxated navicular, a dorsal bunion due to hyperactive tibialis anterior, ankle, and hindfoot valgus; and a flat-topped talus. The aim of treatment is to obtain a painless, stable, plantigrade, and well-aligned foot, restoring muscle imbalance when present.

Penny[63] with long experience in Africa, recommended triple arthrodesis in rigid, neglected, very severe clubfeet with marked cavus in patients over six years of age in developing countries with limited resources. He recommends it even without soft tissue release by excising more bones and, in severe cases, a specific modified Lambrinudi triple arthrodesis excising large bone wedges.

Sobel et al.[64] reported results of three adult immigrants with severe neglected clubfeet. They did posterior, medial, and plantar release with double arthrodesis of calcaneo-cuboid and talo-navicular joints with wedge resections and obtained pain-free plantigrade feet.

Brodsky[65] highlighted the problems of a high rate of residual deformities in clubfoot over the long term, with limited studies about functional deterioration later in life. There are also untreated cases of adults with clubfoot coming for treatment due to various problems arising with age, besides the neurogenic or traumatic clubfoot. There may be overcorrection or undercorrection of deformity, with undercorrection being much more common than overcorrection. Symptoms can appear in both. Pain is a common symptom which is persistent or recurrent due to bony or soft tissue causes. Each adult patient has to be considered as different. They will essentially require arthrodesis procedures and osteotomy of the first metatarsal to correct its rigid plantar-flexion, preceded by soft tissue release.

Yadav[66] carried out extensive soft tissue release with dorsolateral wedge resection in patients from 8 to 11 years old and triple arthrodesis after 11 years of age. He treated 45 feet in 27 patients, 8–28 years of age, with 25 feet in patients 8–11 years of age and 20 feet in patients over 11 years of age. In adults, he removed more bone, leading to more shortening. The follow-up period was six months to eight years. Results were graded on clinical and functional correction. Thirty-nine out of 45 (87%) had acceptable results, with 18% still having residual equinus, and 11% had residual adduction.

Zhou et al.[67] reported their experience in a prospective study of midfoot osteotomy in pes cavus deformity, characterized by an abnormally high medial arch with change of foot shape and possibly accompanied by concomitant forefoot and hindfoot deformities. The condition may be classified as neuromuscular, congenital, idiopathic, or traumatic and is seen commonly, the most common among these being neuromuscular disorders. For severe deformities, surgical intervention is needed. Midfoot osteotomy, first described by Cole in 1940, is known to be a good treatment. The authors reviewed 17 patients 12–36 years of age (mean age of 16.8 years) and operated on between 2008 and 2012. Midfoot osteotomy was done with dorsal wedge resection from parts of navicular, cuneiforms, and cuboid, and joint-sparing internal fixation by three cannulated screws was done between the Lisfranc and Cyma lines. When required, K-wires were used for fixing the flexed toes in extension. Assessment of results was based on improvement in appearance and function. Additional soft tissue surgical procedures were required in some of the cases. Screws were removed after 3–6 months, and K-wires of toes were removed after six weeks. Osteotomy healed within a mean period of 7.8 weeks (range 6–12 weeks), and mean follow-up was 25.3 months (range 10–50 months). Patients were allowed partial weight bearing in a plaster cast after four weeks. Oteotomies healed in 6–12 weeks (mean 7.8 weeks). The results, assessed on the American Foot and Ankle Society scoring system, were 94.1% satisfactory or satisfied with minor reservations in regard to improvement in shape and function with mobility of joints, but, objectively, 88.2% were satisfied. The authors have used cannulated screws for better fixation and early resumption of exercises and bearing weight, but this is challenging and choosing the exact size of screws, neither too short to be inadequate nor too long to cross the navicular and cuboid, is difficult. Therefore, it has to be done under X-ray control. The usual methods of fixing the osteotomy by other authors have been K-wires and staples. Moreover, in regard to the results, these were only short-term results after about two years. To know the real efficacy, long-term follow-up is required. The authors have also quoted many reports of this midfoot osteotomy and are not very happy with their results: Levitt et al. 1973 reported 30% pseudoarthrodesis, Naudi et al. 2009 found 74.2% of cases of arthritis of subtalar and tarsometatarsal joints at long-term follow-up and even dysfunction of the ankle joint, more so in cases with severe cavus. Therefore, the present authors excluded severe cavus deformities from their study.

Groner and DiDomenico[68] presented an overview of various midfoot osteotomies along with other procedures for the correction of pes cavus commonly associated with neuromuscular diseases, trauma, congenital clubfoot, and others. The condition may be classified as neuromuscular, congenital, idiopathic, or traumatic. In a review of 77 cases by Brewerton (1977), numerous congenital and acquired neuromuscular causes were found in 75%, idiopathic clubfoot in 14%, and idiopathic pes cavus in 11% of cases. Further, this review revealed various diseases leading to pes cavus are Charcot-Marie-Tooth; meningomyelocele; poliomyelitis; diseases of the spinal cord such as tumors, syringomyelia, spinal muscular atrophy, and poliomyelitis; other neuromuscular conditions like muscular dystrophy, cerebral palsy, Friedreich's ataxia, Roussy-Levy syndrome, Dejerine-Sottas syndrome, and spina bifida; and traumatic cases due to severe burns, malunion of fractures, compartment syndrome, and crush injuries. Congenital disorders, such as syphilis, lymphedema, arthrogryposis, and paralytic clubfoot, have also been reported. Due to a decrease in the weight-bearing surface of the foot, symptoms appear and increase over time. Treatment is sought for fatigue, metatarsalgia, and increasing pain on walking; painful callosities under the metatarsal head/heads; and trophic ulcers, as well as for cosmetic reasons. Primary disease should be treated first before pes cavus. The authors did radiological assessment for planning the treatment, measuring several angles to find out the apex of the deformity. They are calcanean inclination angle (typical is less than 30°), Meary's angle of long axis of the talus and first metatarsal (typical is less than 5°), and calcaneo-metatarsal angle between long axis of calcaneum and first metatarsal (typical is less than 140°). Some special tests, depending upon the etiology, will also be required, such as electromyography and others. In long standing severe deformities, callosities form under metatarsal heads. Cavus may be classified into flexible and rigid cavus and also into anterior cavus, when the major deformity is at tarsometatarsal joints (Lisfranc joints) or it may be posterior at the midtarsal joints (Chopart joints). It can be combined cavus, both anterior and posterior. It may be confined to the first metatarsal head or medial cavus, also known as local cavus. It may be present at all tarsometatarsal joints when it is called global or full cavus. Various radiological angles are important to know the amount of deformity. Meary's angle is talo-first metatarsal in lateral view and typical is 0°–5°. Hibb's angle is the angle of axis of the first metatarsal with calcaneum in lateral view and it is 150° or more. Then, there is the calcanean inclination angle with weight-bearing surface, which is usually 25°–30°, and more than this is pes cavus. Claw toes may also be associated with cavus. It is important to assess the apex of deformity in order to correct the entire deformity by soft tissue releases, including various well-described tendon transfers and soft tissue releases followed by osseous procedures. Lesser deformities may be corrected by soft tissue procedures alone, but osseous procedures will also be needed for rigid deformities. Correction of foot deformity follows after the treatment of treatable primary diseases. Treatment for this common condition is surgical, but conservative measures do have their role, including physiotherapy, special shoes, or orthosis after surgery. Conservative measures are also indicated when patients are reluctant for surgery due to minor symptoms and it is possible to manage without surgery. Indications for surgery are pain, severe deformity, and ankle instability. The goals of surgery are to balance muscle forces, correct deformities, and provide a mobile plantigrade foot. Various osteotomies in rigid deformities preceded by requisite soft tissue procedures described by the authors are first metatarsal dorsal flexary wedge osteotomy and plate fixation for local cavus of first metatarsal. The Lapidus procedure involves arthrodesis of the first metatarsal and medial cuneiform joint with appropriate wedge resection and fixing with screws with or without a plate or even multiple metatarsal osteotomies in full cavus through the three-incision approach. Calcanean osteotomy is done for hindfoot cavus. Calcanean osteotomies are of various types: percutaneous or open, displacement, opening wedge, or Dwyer lateral closing wedge osteotomy after appropriate soft tissue procedures like Steindler's release and tendoachilles lengthening. Japas truncated dorsal closing wedge arthrodesis of the tarsometatarsal joint, essentially a Lisfranc joint arthrodesis. An essential prerequisite is to know the apex of the deformity, otherwise rocker bottom foot can result. Triple arthrodesis is a common procedure, in skeletally mature patients, for severe pes cavus with osteoarthritis of foot joints. Midfoot osteotomies are done for anterior cavus deformities: Cole's osteotomy, described by him in 1940, is a dorsal closing wedge osteotomy, with a wedge removed through a cut over the cuboid, cuneiforms and navicular. This osteotomy was in fact described by Saunders five years earlier and Cole popularized it. This is indicated in skeletally mature, rigid anterior cavus with apex at midfoot and contraindicated in cavus otherwise. Talo-navicular and calcaneo-cuboid joints are spared in this. Width and direction of the wedge can vary depending on any multiplanar deformity. This can be done by one, two, or three incisions, but the author does it by two incisions. Fixation of osteotomy can be done with K-wires, staples, or screws. Screw fixation has the risk of crossing the posterior joints, defeating the purpose of joint sparing, and should be meticulous. The present authors use screws due to stable fixation. Japas midfoot osteotomy, a V-shaped osteotomy, was described to improve Cole's procedure by avoiding shortening of the foot. The apex of osteotomy is in the navicular and arms extending forward through the cuboid and medial cuneiform through a single dorsal incision. This is indicated in the anterior cavus in the skeletally mature foot. Steinmann pins are used for fixing after correction. However, its disadvantages are delayed/nonunion and an uncomfortable dorsal hump. The authors feel Cole's procedure is better and easier with fewer complications. Midtarsal dome osteotomy (Wilcox and Weiner) is indicated when the apex of deformity is at midfoot. With a transverse incision over midfoot, a one-centimeter wide wedge osteotomy is done with a curved osteotome through the cuneiforms, cuboid, and base of the fifth metatarsal. The shape osteotomy allows three-dimensional correction by fixing with Steinmann pins. Plantar fascial stripping is a prerequisite to it. However, its execution is difficult. Many authors have used an Ilizarov fixator with midfoot osteotomy through a small transverse incision to have advantage of both techniques and eliminate disadvantages; besides, it allows dynamic bone regeneration by distraction osteogenesis and achieving correction in three dimensions and is thus a viable option. The authors themselves have done a subperiosteal midfoot osteotomy with a Gigli saw through four stab incisions under X-ray control at the apex of the deformity. Finally, they have concluded that surgical correction is a challenging task. No single procedure can correct every cavus, and midfoot osteotomy is a part of it. It is important to fix the apex of the deformity.

3.6 TALECTOMY

Letts and Davidson[69] presented results of seven bilateral clubfeet treated by talectomy. Age at surgery varied from 1 year and 10 months to 15 years and 7 months, with a mean of 5 years and 7 months. Three were arthrogrypotics, three meningomyelocele, and one muscular dystrophy, with an average follow-up of 5 years and 6 months (ranging from 3 years to 12.5 years). Three feet had good results, seven had fair results, and four had poor results. The authors recommended the procedure in such cases in spite of the limitations.

El-sherbini and Omran[70] presented their results in 19 rigid equinovarus feet (Demiglio grade 4) in 13 patients treated in a period of about 10 years from 2001 to 2012. Nine were arthrogrypotics, one each was due to sacral agenesis, spastic cerebral palsy, neglected congenital talipes equinovarus, and post-traumatic contracture. Their ages ranged from 3 to 26 years, with mean of 7.7 years and follow-up was 2–11 years. Other bony procedures such as excision navicular, calcaneal osteotomy, or calcaneo-cuboid fusion were done when required. All feet improved to Demiglio grade 2, and 16 feet were plantigrade. Calcaneum has to be placed exactly in the ankle mortis for satisfactory results. This is a good salvage procedure.

Usuelli et al.[71] commented that talectomy is an extreme salvage procedure generally reserved for adults. However, they used it recently in a 12-year-old with severe rigid clubfoot in Zambia as a single step short-term treatment. He walked with plantigrade foot at six months with no pain and 20° dorsiflexion/plantarflexion. They also recommend it in infants and small children in developing and poor countries instead of Ponseti's multistep long-term treatment, in which multiple visits and long-term bracing with follow-up is not possible. The authors feel that this should be reserved for older children.

Louis et al.[72] presented their results of 15 talectomies in 10 patients of arthrogryposis with clubfeet (five bilateral); nine of these patients already recurred after soft tissue operations and thus only one had primary talectomy at 2–9 years of age and followed for 3–14 years. In nine, plantigrade foot could be achieved, but with residual varus, however, the patient could walk with standard shoes. They concluded that this is a good salvage procedure, and in 46.7% spontaneous tibiocalcanean fusion occurred.

Solund et al.[73] performed 17 talectomies in 10 children of arthrogryposis with 17 clubfeet, nine of whom already had an average of three soft tissue surgeries with recurrence. At a mean follow-up of 14 years, results were satisfactory in 14 out of 17 feet. They recommend talectomy before walking age in arthrogryposis multiplex congenita.

Dias and Stem[74] performed 28 talectomies in 18 patients of myelomeningocele and arthrogryposis with 24 already operated with soft tissue release in patients 1–9 years of age. At an average follow-up of four years, 23 patients had good results. Forefoot problems persist in many, which is managed by additional surgery. Talectomy was considered a good salvage procedure.

Johnson et al.[75] provided surgical principles of talectomy for use in severe, rigid, and resistant clubfoot. They are associated with a high recurrence rate, and multiple surgeries are often needed for a satisfactory result. Talectomy has been used both as the primary or salvage procedure to treat such deformities. The authors have discussed operative technique, indications, advantages, and common complications associated with the procedure, and have also given a case report of a bilateral case in a four-year-old.

3.7 RESIDUAL DEFORMITIES

Innumerable publications have been appearing in the literature with a high incidence of residual deformities after various forms of conservative and surgical methods of treatment of resistant clubfoot, including Ponseti, Ilizarov, and others reporting as high as 95% residual deformities.

Loza et al.[76] reported results of double column osteotomy, that is, closing wedge cuboid and opening wedge medial cuneiform along with soft tissue release, to correct the residual adduction, cavus, and supination deformities in relapsed clubfoot. The wedge of bone removed from the cuboid was fitted in the medial and plantar gap of medial cuneiform open wedge defect, fixing with two K-wires. They treated 20 residual deformities in 15 children, 3–7 years of age, with an average follow up of 2.3 years. They obtained 80% excellent/good and 20% fair/poor results, which were statistically significant. This surgery is not suitable in children under three years of age with immature cuneiform ossification.

Tarraf and Carroll[8] reviewed records and X-rays of 125 children with 159 clubfeet after 210 surgeries to find residual deformities. They found that forefoot adduction and supination were the most common residual deformities present in 95% of the feet, resulting from undercorrection at the primary operation. They may not be apparent soon after surgery, but appear with growth, later requiring additional treatment. These appear to result from not releasing the calcaneo-cuboid joint and plantar fascia and not recognizing these on the radiographs.

Otremski et al.[77] reviewed their 44 clubfeet operated by Turco's one-stage posteromedial release carried out between six months and two years of age with a long term follow up of 8–11 years and found 21 (48%) having persistent deformity, and even in the other 23 feet having a typical-looking foot, 11 had radiological undercorrection. The residual deformity was due either to metatarsus varus or persisting talo-navicular subluxation.

Elgeidi and Abulsaad[78] reviewed 35 resistant bean-shaped clubfeet (27 children aged 4–9 years) due to earlier surgeries and repeated surgical treatment by double tarsal wedge osteotomy (closing wedge cuboid and opening wedge medial cuneiform) and transcuneiform osteotomy between 2008 and 2012, all with significant residual deformities of forefoot adduction and inversion with a stiff bean-shaped foot. All complicated clubfeet with multiple surgeries and syndromic cases were excluded. Posteromedial with lateral release was done in more severe cases and only posteromedial release in less severe cases. At 2–6.5 years of follow-up, results were satisfactory.

Lehman et al.[79] reported their results in revision surgeries in 40 feet (32 patients) operated on during 1979 to 1987 in a variety of relapsed or residual deformities in different childhood age groups of 1–12 years (average 5 years and 4 months), with the majority less than five years of age. The authors have quoted numerous references from the literature citing relapses or residues in 30%–50% after manipulations and casting treatment and 13%–50% poor results after one or more surgeries, all requiring additional surgeries. Surgical procedures were various types of soft tissue clubfoot release alone or with plantar or the Dillwyn Evans operation, or capsulotomies. Of the 40 feet, they have reported 9 months to 7 years of follow-up results in 29 feet only with their assessment protocol. They had 8 excellent, 11 good, 8 fair, and 2 poor results. The authors have also commented that even the best results cannot be treated as typical even after two or three surgeries because calf hypoplasia and a smaller foot, even more so than before revision surgery, will remain.

McHale and Lenhart[80] treated seven residual deformities after earlier surgeries with a bean-shaped foot by closing wedge cuboid and opening wedge medial cuneiform with good results.

Lourenco et al.[81] reported that the forefoot is the most common residual deformity after clubfoot surgery and moderate and severe forms require reoperation. The authors operated on 39 such feet by closing wedge cuboid and opening wedge medial cuneiform with good results at 4.8 years of follow-up, and they recommend this for children at least four years of age or later, when cuneiform ossification is good.

Lee et al.[82] reported that forefoot adduction is a very common residual deformity after surgery of clubfoot in children, and they found 18 such feet (35%) out of 51 operated on by posteromedial release confirmed by radiological assessment of talo-first metatarsal and talo-calcanean angles. They were operated by cuboid-cuneiform osteotomy, and there was significant improvement.

Mahadev et al.[83] commented that residual deformities after surgeries in children or even after Ponseti management in resistant clubfeet occur commonly. They do need treatment due to deformity, shoe fitting, and limitation of activities of daily living with bean-shaped foot and scarring on the medial side. The authors have managed these by a limited lateral incision with a lateral closed wedge cuboid osteotomy and transcuneiform midfoot osteotomy under image intensifier. They did this in 12 patients (14 feet) of 4–5 years of age and with follow-up for 2–3.2 years, with good results clinically as well as radiologically. The authors also commented that, in older children with rigid deformities but proper bony development, opening wedge osteotomy of medial cuneiform will offer better chances for correcting the deformity.

Hassan and Roger[84] in their comprehensive review article, commented about various names given to medial deviation of the forefoot occurring purely at the Lisfranc joint. They opined that metatarsus adductus is located at the Lisfranc joint in a purely transverse plane and the hindfoot is usually positioned under the ankle. But, in the literature, it has been called by various names by different authors for about one hundred years, that is, metatarsus adductus, metatarsus varus, metatarsus adductovarus, pes adductus, metatarsus supinatus, forefoot adductus, and hooked forefoot, and they are all synonyms. However, there are other aspects to it and they quoted Berg (1986) who described metatarsus varus combined with midfoot and hindfoot deformity along with radiographic study in 124 feet in four categories: simple metatarsus adductus (51 feet), complex metatarsus adductus when it is combined with lateral translation of midfoot (42 feet), simple skewed foot when hindfoot is in valgus (16 feet), and complex skewed foot when midfoot is laterally translated and hindfoot is in valgus (15 feet). In clubfoot, besides equinus and hindfoot varus, metatarsus adductus is the third component of clubfoot. These authors also quoted Kite (1950) as describing metatarsus varus as a combination of adduction at the Lisfranc joint along with inversion (internal rotation) of the forefoot in relation to the hindfoot, but adduction is much more prominent. Kite reasoned it out due to muscle imbalance resulting from overpower of tibialis anterior posterior as compared to peronei. They have also quoted various others to describe a foot deformity with forefoot adduction and hindfoot valgus as skewed foot, serpentine foot, Z-shaped, or S-shaped foot. For treatment of this deformity, all focused on metatarsal deformity as well as heel valgus, and double osteotomy of medial cuneiform and cuboid corrects both effectively. Haasan and Rogers have also commented that recurrent forefoot adduction is commonly seen after treatment of clubfoot in children after three years of age with Tarraf and Carroll quoting the highest incidence with 81.1%, even after first revision surgery and 47.5% after second revision surgery in a series of 159 clubfeet.

Green and Lloyd-Roberts[85] considered that, in resistant feet in infants, if limited posterior release or more extensive posteromedial release in severe cases are carried out after initial casting treatment, earlier and better functioning feet can be obtained even if some deformity remained. They treated 70 feet with this regimen, the majority within 12 weeks of age and the rest all within 26 weeks of age. Although they got only 59% excellent/good and 41% poor results (residual equinus and or varus), they were happy with the function. Many of the poor results were improved by secondary soft tissue and osseous surgeries. They reasserted forcefully to continue pursuing this technique in spite of 41% initial poor cosmetic results requiring secondary operations.

Uglow and Clark[86] reported relapse rate after two-stage surgery to avoid wound healing problems. During 1988 to 1995, the authors included 91 feet in 68 children with a mean age of 8.9 months in this study with strict inclusion criteria. They carried out a plantar medial and posterolateral extensive releases of various short and long muscles, ligaments, capsules, and so forth through separate incisions at two-weeks interval. They were preoperatively grouped into grades 2, 3, and 4 according to Dimegilo grading and grade 1 (mild and pliable) was not included. Grade 2 included 26 feet (28.6%), grade 3 included 54 feet (59.3%), and only 11 feet (12.1%) were grade 4. Residual deformities remaining after this procedure were considered relapses. There were no relapses in grade 2, 20.4% relapsed in grade 3, and the highest relapse rate was in grade 4 with 65.4%. In other words, the total relapse rate was about 86% and was statistically significant according to Cochrane–Armitage trend test, increasing with increasing severity. Mean age at relapse was 3.03 years.

Legaspi et al.[87] reviewed 24 feet in 15 patients of talectomy for recurrent equinovarus deformity; 21 with arthrogryposis multiplex, two with meningomyelocele, and one idiopathic variety, with a mean follow-up of 20 years. These deformities are well known to show resistance even after multiple surgeries. After talectomy, relapse of deformity in the hindfoot was seen in 67% at a mean follow-up of 10 years. Painful tibiocalcanean arthritis was seen in 33% of cases, requiring fusion in some. There is posterior displacement of the heel in these cases. Seven showed spontaneous tibiocalcanean fusion. Moreover, talectomy did not correct the forefoot deformity, which required additional procedures, and this has been supported by many other reports. The authors have concluded that talectomy is useful, but should be carried out with caution due to future long-term complications.

Dobb et al.[88] reported long-term (25–32 years) follow-up after extensive soft tissues release in 73 patients (45 patients) in children 12–15 months of age and failed to correct with serial casting, selected by comprehensive inclusive criteria. They were divided into two groups; in one group, more extensive surgery was done than the other. They concluded that they had poor foot function and there was correlation between the extent of soft tissue release and the degree of foot-function impairment. Repeated soft tissue surgeries can result in stiff, painful severe arthritic feet with impaired function.

Depuy and Drennan[89] observed that residual varus deformities, clinical as well as radiological, were common after posteromedial release, and they compared children of three age groups operated on at an average age of 4.4 months, 9.1 months, and 16.1 months, having similar parameters of deformities, surgery, and postoperative care and found residual deformities in 7%, 28%, and 35% of cases, respectively, with the early group faring better.

3.8 EARLY SURGERY

Kuo and Smith[90] commented on late residual deformities after clubfoot surgeries, with dynamic and stiff supination, forefoot adduction, in-toeing gait, overcorrection, rotator dorsal subluxation of the talo-navicular joint, avascular talus with collapse, and dorsal bunion. They reviewed 134 clubfeet in 95 children operated on between 1988 and 1991. They found that children operated on at earlier than six months of age had poorer results than older children. Additional surgeries were done in 21 feet (15.7%), and the most common procedure was tibialis anterior transfer. All do not require surgery and restoration of function is of primary importance, and surgery is done only when necessary.

Ryoppy and Sairanen[91] claimed that the first published report of neonatal surgery in clubfoot is from their hospital in 1959 and quoted Somppi and Sulamaa (1971). They continued, improved upon it and reported 94 operated clubfeet soon after birth, with the mean age being 12 days, and obtained 90% excellent/good results with primary surgery and 99% after secondary treatments at a minimum of two years of follow-up. They carried out tailor-made releases depending upon the severity of the deformity. The more severe the deformity, the more radical the release. The authors have also discussed many problems during surgery and after surgery and opined that it has to be learned patiently. The authors have quoted many reports regarding dissatisfaction due to their unfavorable results with neonatal surgery in clubfoot. The advantages quoted by the authors are mainly much less time needed for completing the treatment and being cost-effective with fewer hassles. However, the authors have reservations about recommending its general use because of the expertise needed for neonatal anesthesia, the steep learning curve, and the highly meticulous surgery with strict asepsis to avoid infection.

Reimann and Anderson[92] carried out surgery on children within the first three months of birth, who had severe deformities not corrected by manipulation treatment. All mild/moderate cases were corrected by conservative treatment started soon after birth. All others were operated on and this included 140 cases (40.3%) cases and posteromedial release was carried out, more extensive in more severe cases.

3.9 VARIOUS ASSESSMENT PROTOCOLS

Andriesse et al.[93] published an assessment protocol, Clubfoot Assessment Protocol (CAP). Various instruments of assessing various variables of structure and function in clubfoot exist but none seem to be entirely reliable. The authors devised 22 items of structure and function in clubfoot for assessing the inter- and intra-observer variations and found their results to be 82% and 89.5%, respectively. The authors feel that the CAP system is more reliable than others, as it is more multidimensional. However, this system also has its limitations in regard to the variables of age and interobserver-expected variations.

Dimeglio et al.[94] devised a scoring system on a scale of 0–20 for assessing various components of deformity, as well as after treatment to assess its efficacy. Four grades of clubfeet can be described: (a) Benign feet so-called "soft-soft feet," grade I, similar to postural feet, with a score of 5 to 1 (they must be excluded from statistics as they falsely increase good results); (b) moderate feet, so-called "soft > stiff feet," grade II (reducible but partly resistant, score of 5–10); (c) severe feet, so-called "stiff > soft feet," grade III (resistant but partly reducible, score of 10–15); and (d) very severe, pseudoarthrogryposic feet, so-called "stiff-stiff feet," grade IV (score of 15–20 points).

Dyer and Davis[95] described the simple scoring system of Pirani et al. in assessing the severity in 77 clubfeet before and after treatment in babies and its predictive value with the Ponseti treatment. The scoring system is based on six signs of contracture and each is scored on three grades: no abnormality is 0, moderate abnormality is 0.5, and severe abnormality is 1. Of the six signs, three relate to hindfoot and three to midfoot. Hindfoot signs are posterior crease, emptiness of heel, and rigidity of equinus. The midfoot signs are severity of medial crease, lateral border curvature, and position of the lateral side of the head of the talus. Therefore, each foot can have a hindfoot and a midfoot score of 0–3 and a total of 0–6. The authors found the Pirani score to be useful for assessing and predicting the need for percutaneous tenotomy in the Ponseti treatment. A foot with a 2.5–3 hindfoot score has a 72% chance of tenotomy; however, a low score does not eliminate chances of the requirement for a tenotomy.

Andrew et al.[96] reported the assessment of reliability of four classification systems and assessment protocols commonly used for clubfoot and described by Catterall, Diméglio et al., Harrold and Walker, and Ponseti and Smoley. This was carried out by four observers, independently, of 18 clubfeet at different stages for the first six months after birth, for a total of 190 examinations. In conclusion, they found that the Dimeglio system had greater reliability than the others, showing moderate to substantial results, but no system is entirely satisfactory. The authors further outlined the prerequisites of an ideal system: (i) it should be reliable and reproducible for this peculiar three-dimensional deformity, as well as simple to practice; (ii) it should give separate information for forefoot, midfoot, and hindfoot because the severity may differ at each level; (iii) it should be informative about flexibility and rigidity of the deformity; (iv) it should be applicable equally before, during, or after treatment at all ages; (v) it should be informative about the method of treatment to be adopted with reference to different elements of the deformity; (vi) it should predict the prognosis; and finally, (vii) it should be usable to compare the results. They feel that there is a need to develop better protocols.

Goriainov et al.[12] carried out a retrospective study from 2002 to 2006 to evaluate the reliability of the Pirani clubfoot scoring system to assess at first examination and then to assess and estimate the later relapse. Inclusion criteria were same surgeon with same protocol of stretching and casting until correction, then heel cord tenotomy, and then foot abduction bracing. Each foot was assessed on two subscores: Midfoot Contracture Score (MFCS) and Hindfoot Contracture Score (HFCS); each can be 0–3 and the total is the Total Pirani Score (TPS), which could be 0–6. Therefore, any higher Pirani score would be a relapse. The authors concluded that higher Pirani scores were statistically significant predictors of relapse and compared to MFCS, the HFCS and TPS were more valuable to diagnose relapse. A more vigilant follow-up would be essential to diagnose and treat early relapse.

Fan et al.[97] investigated interobserver reliability of the Pirani and Dimeglio scoring systems in 173 idiopathic clubfeet of different severities and number of casts needed. The correlation of both was poor in mild and very severe deformities (requiring 2 or 7–8 casts, respectively) of deformity. The two were different; while the Dimeglio system evaluated reducibility of deformity, the Pirani system evaluated morphology of deformity. They commented about the need for a more objective and reliable evaluation system.

Gao et al.[98] also investigated, in Aukland, New Zealand, all clubfeet treated from 2007 to 2011 and the reliability of the Pirani and Dimeglio scoring systems in predicting the number of casts required. Patients required 2–10 casts from start to initiation of brace, but both scoring systems had a poor correlation, in spite of these being used widely all over the world. Their prognostic value, therefore, remains questionable.

Hussain[99] in a letter to the editor, commented about two articles published regarding the Pirani scoring system vis-à-vis the Ponseti casting treatment. Regarding a Dyer and Davis article entitled, "The role of the Pirani scoring system in the management of club foot by the Ponseti method," he argued and highlighted the absence of a good universal scoring system for classification and evaluating treatment of clubfoot. Complete correction of all elements of deformity, as well as restoration of function has to be evaluated. There should be two systems, one for evaluating deformity and the other for evaluating function. The Pirani system cannot assess both effectively, and both are highly important for any patient. However, it can roughly predict whether a fewer or greater number of casts will be required. Regarding the other article by Shack and Eastwood, "Early results of a physiotherapist-delivered Ponseti service for the management of idiopathic congenital talipes equinovarus foot deformity," he claimed also lack of evidence for comparison. They have concluded that each author has his own selection criteria to justify their findings. There is a definite need to have a universal CAP (Clubfoot Assessment Protocol).

3.10 IMAGING TECHNIQUES: SKIAGRAMS, ULTRASONOGRAPHY, CT, AND MRI

3.10.1 Skiagrams

Beatson and Pearson[100] described a simple radiological technique, easily done as an outpatient procedure. They did it in 200 typical feet and 147 resistant clubfeet with three types of surgeries and compared before and after the operation, correlating with clinical assessment. Radiographs are taken as antero-posterior view radiographs with the foot in a 30° of plantar flexion, with the tube directed cranially 30° from the perpendicular and lateral view with 30° plantar-flexion. Measurements are then taken of the angular relationships between the long axes of the calcaneum and the talus. The mean of the two is called the talo-calcanean index. In the lateral view, the range in clubfeet was from minus 5° to 40° and in typical feet, it was from 15° to 55°, with a large overlap. In the antero-posterior view, the range in clubfeet was from 0° to 55° and in typical feet, it was from 10° to 50°. However, indices in clubfeet were calculated as 0° to 55° and typical as 40° to 85°, with much less overlap. The authors, therefore, concluded that a talo-calcanean index of 40° is to be taken as typical and a good method of differentiating typical from atypical. Results are from three types of surgeries: medial soft tissue release, Dillwyn Evans procedure, and tibialis anterior lateral transfer. In the post-treatment assessment, there is a definite improvement in the angles, but complete correction is not present. In conclusion, they advocated the procedure for routine use.

Sambandam and Gul[101] reported a technique of stress radiographs for clubfoot for initial and post-treatment assessment for better insight, because of misinformation due to positioning in X-rays in relaxed attitude of the foot. They designed a radiolucent splint for fixing the stressed foot before X-rays for better assessment of deformity pre- or post-treatment in regard to angles and axes. They used it in 21 severe clubfeet that underwent posteromedial subtalar release (PMSTR), taking two sets of radiographs, one with manual positioning and the other with this splint. They found a significant difference in the values of the two sets in the midfoot and the forefoot radiological parameters. In the hindfoot, it was not useful, but in the forefoot and the midfoot residual deformities, which are common, it is quite informative. Assessment of residual deformity improved significantly with the use of this technique and the authors advocated its routine use. It becomes a simulated weight-bearing X-ray in pediatric patients, where weight bearing is not possible. The authors also mentioned its limitation of a small number of patients.

Prasad et al.[102] used 12 radiological parameters in weight-bearing anteroposterior (AP) and lateral positions, pre- and post-soft tissue release surgery in 50 clubfeet, to assess the radiological correction vis-à-vis clinical correction. The twelve parameters were: in AP views, (1) talo-calcaneal angle, (2) talo-first metatarsal angle, (3) calcaneo-fifth metatarsal angle, and (4) talo-navicular subluxation; and in the lateral view, (5) talo-calcaneal angle, (6) tibio-talar angle, (7) tibio-calcaneal angle, (8) talo-first metatarsal angle, (9) calcaneo-fifth metatarsal angle, (10) first-fifth metatarsal angle, (11) talar dome flattening, and (12) the talo-calcaneal index (TCI), which is a mean of the AP and lateral TCA. Clinical criteria were based on the Laaveg and Ponseti scoring systems, and 58% were grouped as very good and good and the other 42% as satisfactory and poor results. The authors found a statistically significant correlation with clinical in AP-TCA and a good rating in lateral-TCA, with a conflicting view quoted by the authors by others in the literature. However, TCI has been found to be a better index, which is also reported by many authors, including Beatson and Pearson, specifically, although there is no complete correction of angles and correlation with clinical correction. The authors recommended routine use of these radiological parameters at follow-up in surgically treated cases to assess the results. Use of a wide range instead of single parameter would be better for assessment of postoperative results.

Simons[103] described a radiographic diagnosis of talo-navicular subluxation before ossification of navicular occurs. There are seven basic combinations of deformities that occur in clubfoot. X-rays before operation diagnose which of the combinations are present in a particular clubfoot. Furthermore, X-rays during operation determine whether or not all the deformities have been corrected and whether or not any further procedures are required. The author describes that there are four basic deformities, and therefore 16 combinations are theoretically possible, but only seven have been seen to be enough. There are two reasons for this: firstly, talo-navicular subluxation is always seen in combination with hindfoot varus, eliminating several deformity combinations, and secondly, equinus is the most difficult to correct by conservative treatment, and many other deformities get corrected before it. In other words, when other deformities are present, equinus will always be there in combination with these.

Kang and Park[104] evaluated the clinical value of lateral tibio-calcaneal angle (LtiC) on lateral radiograph with foot and ankle in full dorsiflexion instead of physical examination ankle dorsiflexion angle (ADF) only, to find out the need for percutaneous Achilles tenotomy after Ponseti casting in 125 clubfeet after proper selection criteria, excluding Dimiglio grade 1 cases and taking only those cases with a minimum follow-up of two years treated during 2006 to 2012. It was found that patients having a LTiC angle of >80° had more incidence of relapse when tenotomy was not done, even when the ADF angle was favorable and more than 15°, which was due to pseudocorrection at the midfoot breakage. They concluded that the LTiC angle of plain X-ray is a more objective finding and prognostic indicator for a need of percutaneous tenotomy as compared to the ADF angle of physical examination.

Radler et al.[105] conducted a study of the Ponseti treatment with percutaneous tenotomy from two centers, treatment starting within three weeks of birth and performing AP and lateral skiagrams of the foot before and after treatment, lateral X-rays of the ankle with full dorsiflexion and anteroposterior X-rays of the foot. Lateral tibio-calcaneal ankle in lateral X-rays and talo-calcanean angles in anteroposterior and lateral X-rays were done before and after tenotomy. A significant improvement of the lateral tibio-calcaneal angle in lateral ankle radiographs of 16.9° was present, but the talo-calcanean angles were insignificant. Both centers showed nearly identical results.

3.10.2 Ultrasonography

Keret et al.[106] studied 281 ultrasound findings to correlate accuracy of prenatal findings with findings after birth and subsequent treatment given to 147 infants born with clubfoot. Clubfoot can be diagnosed in more than 60% of cases. The earliest diagnosis was made at 12 weeks and the latest at 32 weeks. In 29%, it failed to diagnose at early stage. In 86%, it was diagnosed between the twelfth and twenty-third weeks and the remaining 14% between the twenty-fourth and thirty-second weeks. The early or late detection of deformity was due to early, late, or very late onset in development of clubfoot in utero. There could be a possibility of some false negatives in early negative scans and, conversely, there may be false positives being transient positional deformity. Prenatal ultrasonic findings correlated well with physical findings after birth, but not so with the severity of deformity as the method of treatment, conservative or surgical. The authors reported accurate diagnosis in 62% of cases.

Rosselli et al.[107] highlighted the advantages of prenatal ultrasonographic diagnosis in cases of diagnosed clubfeet in 178 patients, between 2003 and 2012, for genetic counseling, early treatment, and better prognosis. Diagnosis can be made early with the advantage of genetic counseling, amniocentesis for other defects, and early start of treatment with better prognosis than others diagnosed after birth. El-Adwar and Taha[108] in Egypt commented on the limited role of conventional radiography in the infant foot as the major parts of the bones are not ossified. They, therefore, evaluated reliability of the Ponseti treatment for clubfoot correction vis-à-vis clinical and ultrasonographic findings and whether ultrasonic variables correlated with each other and with the Pirani score before and after treatment. They studied 17 infants with 24 clubfeet, using the Pirani score and various ultrasonic parameters (medial malleolus navicular distance, navicular alignment in relation to the talar head, medial soft tissue thickness, talar length, and calcaneo-cuboid distance) before and after Ponseti casting treatment, starting at a mean of 30 days and reexamination at a mean of 6.3 months with a follow-up of a mean of 14.3 months. There were four recurrences, and ultrasound was found to be useful to alert the surgeon to this.

Bhargava et al.[109] compared various (about twelve) parameters of sonography in different positions of clubfoot with radiographic studies to evaluate their relative superiority before and after the Ponseti treatment, sonography being a noninvasive, radiation-free imaging technique. The study was carried out in 31 unilateral clubfeet, comparing with typical feet. All sonographic parameters correlated well with the severity of deformity, but radiography did not do so. On comparing both methods, sonography was better as compared with radiography in regard to correction of various components of the deformity, in addition to being noninvasive.

Chawla et al.[110] evaluated ultrasonography in 82 clubfeet in 54 children, correlating its various parameters with the Pirani six-point scoring system before and after Ponseti casting treatment and found this to be a simple, cost-effective, noninvasive, useful, and promising investigation. Ultrasonographic parameters used were: medial malleolar to navicular distance (MMN) measured on medial view, calcaneo-cuboid distance (CCD) and calcaneo-cuboid angle (CCA) on lateral view, talar length (TAL) on dorsal view, and tibio-calcaneal distance on posterior view. They found statistically significant correlation with the Pirani score by measuring the Pearson correlation coefficient.

3.10.3 CT scanning

Farsetti et al.[111] studied the computed tomography of two groups of congenital clubfoot patients treated with two distinct protocols. Forty-seven clubfeet were treated according to the traditional protocol of their hospital and 61 were treated according to the Ponseti technique. The normal feet of the unilateral deformities served as controls. All patients were followed to skeletal maturity. Declination angle of the neck of the talus, torsion angle of the ankle, declination angle of the neck of the talus, and the calcaneo-cuboid angle were studied at maturity by CT images. Authors found that the Ponseti manipulative technique provided better anatomical results in comparison to their traditional technique.

Windisch et al.[112] dissected seven idiopathic clubfeet and two normal feet of aborted fetuses in this study, with special emphasis on the shape of the cartilage and bones. A 3D micro-CT system, generating a series of X-ray attenuation measurements, was used to produce computed reconstructed 3D data sets of each of the separated bones. Based on these micro-CT data scans, a high-definition 3D color printing system was used to make a four times enlarged clubfoot model, exactly representing all the bony malformations. This model showing the complex pathoanatomy of this disease was designed for use in workshops of orthopaedic surgeons and physiotherapists, for training.

Johnston et al.[113] assessed the bony pathoanatomy of clubfoot by a 3D reconstruction of transverse CT images in 27 feet at ages 3–10 years. Interosseous deformity of the bones was determined by principal axes to quantify, while intraosseous deformity was estimated by visual inspection of the reconstructed images. Midfoot adduction and rotation were analyzed on the AP view of the forefoot, while hindfoot prono-supination was analyzed on the AP view of the ankle in posterior part. This technique allows visualization of deformities which normally cannot be analyzed on plain radiographs, and also shows that a variety of interosseous relationships make up the clinical entity known as clubfoot. Abnormal talar pronation ("intorsion") was an unexpected finding of this 3D analysis.

Ippolito et al.[114] studied the measurement of talo-calcanean angle (Kite's angle) for assessing clubfoot correction in 48 treated clubfeet by manipulation and above knee casting and postero medial release if necessary and 38 normal feet at the end of skeletal maturity. They used standing AP radiographs and 3D CT scan reconstructions. They concluded that plain radiography as misleading in 75% of cases and recommended other imaging techniques as CT for better correctional assessment results

3.10.4 MRI

Cahuzac et al.[115] evaluated magnetic resonance imaging (MRI) in 12 infants, all under 16 months of age, of unilateral clubfoot. They calculated, objectively in three dimensions, the volumes of cartilage and osseous structures by multiplanar reconstructions, as well as their axes in talus and calcaneum and compared them with the typical. The volume was 20% less in ossific center of calcaneum in clubfoot than typical, but reduction of volume of the talus was double that of the calcaneum. Long axes of ossific nucleus of the talus in clubfoot and typical compared with cartilaginous anlage were both medial, but inclination angle is more in clubfoot than the unaffected side. However, in calcaneum, they were similar in both the unaffected foot and the clubfoot. Cartilage anlage axes in clubfoot and the typical foot in the talus were both medially rotated compared with bony structure, but with a smaller angle in the clubfoot. They have concluded that plain radiography gives a single-dimension view, while this is a three-dimensional quantification of medial rotation of the talus. Therefore, a preoperative measurement of position of the talus will be useful preoperatively.

Kamegaya et al.[116] studied *in vivo* talo-navicular alignment by MRI imaging of the cartilage anlage and not of the ossific nucleus in the transverse plane in 26 clubfoot patients (36 feet) with mean age of 9 months. Talar neck angle (TNA) was greater in clubfeet than in typical feet, and the difference in the mean angle was statistically significant, with clubfeet as $44.0° \pm 8.1°$ and typical as $30.8° \pm 5.5°$, $p < 0.001$. There is a statistically significant difference between surgically treated and conservatively treated patients with angles more in the surgical group. With regard to anatomical relationship between midpoint of the navicular and long axis of the head, in the operative group, medial shift of the navicular was present in 18 feet and none had lateral shift; but in the conservative group, 12 showed medial and 6 showed lateral shift. All nine typical feet had lateral shift of the navicular. To conclude, in MRI, TNA was more in clubfoot than typical, and more so in the surgical group than the conservative group, thus helping in knowing the pathoanatomy in clubfoot and helping in the choice of treatment.

Richard and Dempsey[117] studied the MRI changes in chondro-osseous anatomy and the joint relationships in tibiotalar, talo-navicular, and talocalcaneal joint relationships after treatment in six infants by the French functional method of treatment in clubfoot, pretreatment and three months after treatment. It was found that equinus looking clinically improved was still present at the calcaneum and was associated with rocker bottom indicated by dorsal displacement of the cuboid on the calcaneum. However, varus deformity did improve.

Duce et al.[118] studied the volume of muscle, subcutaneous fat, tibia, fibula, and arteries in the lower legs in six clubfeet and five controls of adolescents and adults and found anatomical differences. All clubfeet had soft tissue surgeries. Three-dimensional T^1 weighted image and three-dimensional magnetic resonance angiography (MRA) were done. Segmentation software for volumetric, anatomical, and image analysis and Kolmogorov–Smirnov tests were performed. Volume of affected legs, muscles, and bones in lower parts in the unilateral clubfoot was significantly reduced as compared with the control in unilateral cases, while muscular fat content increased. No difference in location of vasculature was observed, but hypoplasis was seen. It appears that this is due to development rather than due to the result of previous surgeries.

O'Connor et al.[119] reported that radiography definitely had a predictive value in talo-navicular alignment in the majority, but MR predicted TN relationships in all cases, while radiography was inconclusive. It is proposed that MR should always be done when radiography is indeterminate or when there is disparity between the clinical and radiographic assessment.

Wang et al.[120] studied seven infants with 11 clubfeet by three-dimensional gradient-echo of MR sequences with multiplanar reconstructions to demonstrate complex deformities in clubfeet. By this method, talo-navicular dislocation was demonstrated in 9 out of 11 feet. They concluded that the non-ossified parts can be seen also in MRI, while three-dimensional T1-W and T2-W scans can give continuous data so that thin-slice, high-resolution multiplanar reconstructions (MPRs) can be done. MPR is a powerful tool for facilitating measurements in various bones, which will give important information for grading the severity of the disease. Therefore, this should be used wherever possible.

3.11 CONCLUSIONS

3.11.1 Historical

Dobb et al.[1] reviewed the history of clubfoot dating back to 1000 BCE and then proceeding ahead to 400 BCE, the era of Hippocrates, starting manipulative treatment, bandaging, and special shoes. Those basic principles are practiced even today, but with modern modifications. After that, with the advent of anesthesia, surgical treatments started, which progressed to many techniques with numerous medications. The author commented about what is missing in the literature, that is, long-term follow-up of Ponseti's treated cases with their quality of life. Carroll[2] wrote about clubfoot in the twentieth century and its likely future in the twenty-first century. In the early 1900s, it was the era of splintage, then around 1940, Ponseti's casting started, then in the 1960s, 1970s, and 1980s in more rigid deformities and with the advent of anesthesia, surgical releases became popular, and toward the end of 2000, again Ponseti's technique gained momentum. Now again, surgeons are looking toward the limitations of the Ponseti method. Further, things are likely to change in the future with advances in epidemiology, molecular biology, biomechanics, biomaterials, and surgery. Francis Nyiiro, MD, CURE Hospital, Addis Ababa, Ethiopia Nyiiro[4] (www.ptolemy.ca/members/archives/2011/Clubfoot/index.html), wrote about his and others' African experience of treatment of neglected clubfoot, which is common there that surgical options like triple arthrodesis, talectomy, midfoot osteotomies in older age groups are more often done, but for small children, Ponseti's technique is practiced.

3.11.2 Ponseti's technique pearls and its pitfalls

Ponseti and Smoley[6] in their classic article themselves asserted that permanent correction of a severe and rigid clubfoot is often difficult. Recurrence of the heel varus deformity and adduction of the fore part of the foot are common even after complete correction and even up to four recurrences have been performed. However, only half of the recurrences could be blamed on the neglect of follow-up treatment. It can be safely concluded from this article that Ponseti's technique will give the best results, in mild and moderate deformities, if the treatment is started within the first week of birth or up to one month of age, followed with a prolonged corrective splintage for 3–5 years, which often gets neglected. Even otherwise, with proper splintage, recurrences can occur for unknown reasons. Azarpira et al.[9] commented that the real Ponseti method is highly laborious with a very strict regimen. More failure will be present if these principles are neglected. Zhao et al.[10] analyzed the reasons for common failures from 19 eligible articles out of 519 recorded reports of the Ponseti method of treatment and found recurrences to be very common in the maintenance phase of prolonged bracing and noncompliance. The rate of noncompliance was up to 61% and the relapse rate was up to 62%. The most common reason for noncompliance is discomfort and its long-term use. Results can improve only if every detail of the Ponseti technique is adhered to. Staheli and Ponseti[11] in their manual commented that "the protocol is intensely laborious and time consuming, hence important to learn all details intelligently, both for the care givers as well as recipients. There will be recurrence in more than 80% of cases, if bracing protocol is neglected." Illiteracy, poverty, lack of training and family support, transport in remote areas, and lack of diligent follow-up are important reasons for failures. Relapses may be due to more tibial growth than gastrocsoleus on account of fibrotic tendon and atrophic muscle and dynamic supination. Goriainov et al.[12] found statistically significant higher relapse rate in more severe/rigid deformities. Bhaskar and Rasal,[13] McElroy et al.,[26] Zionts and Dietz[15] and Jowett et al.[31] highlighted the pitfalls of the Ponseti technique: faulty casting due to poor learning of the rigid technique, noncompliance/ improper bracing, and poor follow-up. Bhaskar and Patni[14] reported a high relapse rate of 36.7% and even described a 5-pattern classification of relapses. Dobbs et al.,[17] Burghardt et al.[18] and MacNeille et al.[16] highlighted the bleeding and nerve injury complications of heel cord tenotomy. Miller et al.[19] commented that following a strict regimen with Ponseti's technique is difficult and possible only with a single committed surgeon, supporting staff and patient's parents with financial and other logistic support. Agarwal et al.[20] reported numerous problems and complications with the Ponseti method. Faldini et al.[29] commented that need for surgery was higher in delayed treatment cases, and early treatment is better for getting good results with casting treatment. Ganesan et al.[30] reviewed the literature from 2000 to 2015 from four electronic databases from 12 eligible articles and quoted that 10 to 30% relapses are very common with Ponseti treatment. Bor et al.,[21] Changulani et al.[22] and Haft et al.[25] also reported a high relapse rate with the Ponseti technique. Zionts et al.[23] and Sala et al.[24] reported good results with Ponseti with fully compliant patients.

3.11.3 Other contemporary techniques

There are a number of surgical techniques reported in the literature: the old classic McKay[33-35] and evidence based correction, Bensahel et al.,[36] so called French casting technique, Turco,[37] description of posteromedial release and its report of 1979, which is very popular even now, Lichtblau[39] combined medial and lateral modified release avoiding calcaneo-cuboid fusion; Tayton and Thompson,[40] Dillwyn Evan's fusion; Simons[41] complete subtalar release; Ilizarov's technique and its modifications performed by Jordan et al.,[44] Malizos et al.,[46] Saghieh et al.,[47] Manjappa,[48] Grill and Franke,[51] Makhdoom et al.,[52] Ferreira et al.,[54] Refai et al.,[55] Oganesyan et al.,[50] described their individual experience with their hinged distraction system; then the JESS technique by Suresh et al.,[49] Emara et al.,[56] did triple arthrodesis but fixed with Ilizarov frame. Paley[57] also described his experience with Ilizarov in clubfoot. Patwardhan and Doshi[58] described a mini external fixator (UMEX i.e., Universal Mini External Fixator). Lee et al.[59] reported their experience of treating rigid clubfeet due to neurologic disorders by the Ilizarov technique. Meena et al.[60] evaluated their results of JESS and Ilizarov in neglected and relapsed clubfeet. All had good experience using their own methods. They all have their place, but with proper experience with the technique and in properly selected cases.

3.11.4 Ilizarov and allied techniques

Ilizarov and other allied techniques work on differential distraction in clubfoot and are good in properly selected cases. Goldstein et al.[45] reviewed the principles of distraction osteogenesis and discussed their indications, instrumentation, and surgical technique. Among the important contributors in this field, the name of Dr. Gavril Ilizarov stands tall. Malizos et al.[46] commented after treating 13 relapsed clubfeet along with review of other reports that there are varying good results from 15% to 100% and with recurrence rates of 5%–61%. They also have their limitations in too many variables with respect to age, severity of deformity and treatment methods, and evaluating results. No two series are similar in all respects. On the whole they recommended the techniques. Saghieh et al.[47] commented that distraction treatment is not significantly better in relapsed clubfeet than surgical options, and it was a small series and had inadequate follow up for any firm conclusion. Manjappa[48] treated 15 old resistant/recurrent clubfeet and commented that with so many variables, no two studies can be compared, but Joshi's external skeletal system (JESS) is simple and more comfortable for patients. Suresh et al.[49] presented their results in 44 clubfeet treated by JESS fixators and found it to be better than Ilizarov's, being lighter, low cost, and easier to apply. Oganesyan et al.[50] evaluated their results in 65 adults with 83 equino-cavovarus deformities due to other causes, other than congenital clubfoot with their modified apparatus and got good results in 65 feet. Grill and Franke[51] treated 10 neglected equinovarus deformities in nine patients due to various causes by the Ilizarov distractor. The authors recommend this treatment in such cases. Makhdoom et al.[52] reported 21 patients (27 clubfeet) with resistant deformities between 8 and 20 years of age. They obtained 74% excellent/good results with plantigrade foot and concluded that the short-term results are promising, but with long term follow-up more recurrences occur. Utukuri et al.[53] quoted by Makhdoom et al.[52] reported 70% unsatisfactory results at a follow-up of 47 months. Ferreira et al.[54] reported their experience with the Ilizarov external fixator along with limited soft tissue correction (heel cord tenotomy and plantar fasciotomy) in 38 severe, stiff neglected clubfeet and reported recurrence in 59% of feet (19 feet). Refai et al.[55] reported a review of 19 relapsed clubfeet in 18 patients after Ponseti or posteromedial release, treated by an Ilizarov frame. They discussed the disadvantages of the Ilizarov frame as: a frame application for a long duration with continued patient discomfort, recurrences at long-term follow-up, and a higher rate in older children. They quoted several authors, with Wallander et al. 1996 reporting 70% recurrence and Freedman et al. 2006 reporting 52% relapsing after the Ilizarov frame, requiring revision surgeries. The authors feel the relapses would be much more if this technique were used in adolescents and adults. Patwardhan and Doshi[58] described a mini external fixator (UMEX, universal mini external fixator) used in clubfoot in children, which is claimed to be an improvement over JESS. Lee et al.[59] reported their experience of treating rigid clubfeet due to neurologic disorders by the Ilizarov technique and feel that it is good for treating such cases.

Meena et al.[60] evaluated their results of JESS and Ilizarov in 21 neglected and relapsed clubfeet patients. Their conclusion was that Ilizarov gave better results in more severe cases in older age groups, while JESS was better in younger children.

3.11.5 Older children and adults

Many authors have described their experience in this group of patients: Herold and Torok[61] described a 2 stage triple arthrodesis with good results; Burger et al.[62] treated overcorrected feet in adults by arthrodesis. Penny,[63] with long experience in Africa, also recommended triple arthrodesis. Sobel et al.[64] and Brodsky,[65] Yadav[66] also recommended triple arthrodesis in adults. Zhou et al.,[67] Groner and DiDomenico[68] used joint-sparing midfoot osteotomies with good results.

3.11.6 Talectomy

Letts and Davidson,[69] El-sherbini and Omran[70], Usuelli et al.,[71] Louis et al.,[72] Solund et al.,[73] Dias and Stem[74] and Johnson et al.[75] used talectomy as a salvage procedure, for straightening out the foot from the gross deformed position with incongruous articular surfaces.

3.11.7 Residual deformities

There is a very high incidence of residual deformities as a result of treatment by various conservative and surgical treatments, as high as 95% in some reports, which are treated by many techniques. Loza et al.[76] reported results of double column osteotomy, i.e., closing wedge cuboid and opening wedge medial cuneiform osteotomy along with soft tissue release. Elgeidi and Abulsaad[78] treated this surgically by double tarsal wedge osteotomy (closing the wedge cuboid and opening the wedge medial cuneiform). Lehman et al.,[79] McHale and Lenhart,[80] Lourenco et al.,[81] Lee et al.,[82] Mahadev et al.,[83] Hassan and Roger,[84] Green and Lloyd-Robert,[85] Uglow and Clark,[86] Legaspi et al.,[87] Dobb et al.,[88] and Depuy and Drennan[89] treated these cases by various types of revision surgeries including soft tissue and osseous procedures.

3.11.8 Early surgery

Kuo and Smith,[90] Ryoppy and Sairanen,[91] Reimann and Anderson[92] performed surgeries in neonates and early infancy with a high relapse rate.

3.11.9 Various assessment protocols

There are various types of assessment protocols, but none of them is entirely satisfactory. Andriesse et al.[93] published the CAP, and this system had its limitations in regard to the variables of age and interobserver-expected variations.

Dimeglio et al.[94] devised a scoring system on a scale of 0–20. Dyer and Davis[95] described the simple scoring system of Pirani et al. The scoring system is based on six signs of contracture and each is scored on three grades. Andrew et al.[96] reported the reliability of four classification systems and assessment protocols commonly used for clubfoot, described by Catterall, Dimeglio et al., Harrold and Walker, and Ponseti and Smoley. The authors further outlined many prerequisites of an ideal system. They feel that there is a need to develop better protocols. Gao et al.[98] and Fan et al.[97] investigated interobserver reliability of the Pirani and Dimeglio scoring systems. The correlation of both was poor. Hussain[99] commenting about the usefulness of the Pirani system in the Ponseti technique and that there is a definite need to have a universal CAP.

3.11.10 Imaging techniques: Skiagrams, ultrasonography, CT, and MRI

Beatson and Pearson[100] described a simple and outpatient radiological technique, talo-calcanean angle and index, quite practicable in preoperative and postoperative assessment. Sambandam and Gul[101] reported a technique of stress radiograph that is quite informative in the common forefoot and midfoot residual deformities. Prasad et al.[102] used twelve radiological parameters and claimed that use of a wide range instead of a single parameter would be better for assessment of postoperative results. Simons[103] described a radiographic diagnosis of talo-navicular subluxation before ossification of navicular occurs. Kang and Park[104] concluded that LTiC angle of a plain X-ray is a more objective finding and prognostic indicator for a need of percutaneous tenotomy as compared to the ADF angle of physical examination. Keret et al.[106] correlated prenatal ultrasound findings with findings after birth and reported accurate diagnosis in 62% of cases. Rosselli et al.[107] highlighted the advantages of prenatal ultrasonographic diagnosis in genetic counseling, amniocentesis for other defects, and early start of treatment for better prognosis than others diagnosed after birth. El-Adwar and Taha Kotb[108] in Egypt stressed ultrasound being more reliable than conventional radiography in the infant foot due to no ossification of many bones. Bhargava et al.[109] compared radiography and sonography and found sonography was better as compared with radiography. Chawla et al.[110] evaluated ultrasonography, correlating its various parameters with the Pirani six-point scoring system, and found it is statistically significant. Farsetti et al.[111] the Ponseti manipulative technique provided better anatomical results in CT in comparison to their traditional technique. Windisch et al.[112] devised a model showing the complex pathoanatomy of this disease for use in workshops of orthopaedic surgeons and physiotherapists, for training and found it to be useful. Johnston et al.[113] concluded that visualization of deformities which normally cannot be analyzed on plain radiographs, like a variety of interosseous relationships in clubfoot, were unexpected findings of this 3D analysis. Ippolito et al.[114] used standing AP radiographs and 3D CT scan reconstructions and concluded that plain radiography as misleading in 75% of cases and recommended other imaging techniques as CT for better correctional assessment results.

Cahuzac et al.[115] evaluated MRIs to be better at giving a three-dimensional quantification of medial rotation of the talus as compared with plain X-rays giving a single-dimension view.

Kamegaya et al.[116] concluded that, in MRI, the talar neck angle was bigger in clubfoot than typical and more so in the surgical group than the conservative group, thus helping in knowing the pathoanatomy in clubfoot and helping in choice of treatment. Richard and Dempsey[117] also found that clinically improved equinus after treatment was still present in MRI because MRI shows even the cartilage. O'Connor et al.[119] also found MRI is more sensitive showing talo-navicular relationship in all cases and proposed that MRI should always be done when radiography is indeterminate. Wang et al.[120] concluded that we can also see the non-ossified parts in MRI, while three-dimensional T1-W and T2-W scans can give continuous data.

The references have also been divided into corresponding sections for ease of referencing.

REFERENCES

1. Dobb MB, Morcuende JA, Gurnett CA, Ponseti IV; Treatment of idiopathic clubfoot: An historical review; *The Iowa Orthop J*; 2000;20:59–64.
2. Carroll NC; Clubfoot in the twentieth century: Where we were and where we may be going in the twenty-first century; *J Paediatr Orthop Part B*; January 2012;21(1): 1–6.
3. Gjonej A, Gjonej R, Selman E; Clubfoot since ancient time up to now; *Journal of Osteoarthritis Open Access J Ost Arth*; 2016;1:1–3.
4. Francis N, Addis A; Review article: Treatment of neglected clubfoot; *Surgery in Africa- Monthly Review*; http://www.Ptolemy.ca/members/archives/2011/clubfoot/indexx.html.
5. Lourenco AF, Morcuende JA; Correction of neglected idiopathic club foot by the Ponseti method; *J Bone Joint Surg*; 2007(B);89(3):378–381.
6. Ponseti IV, Smoley EN; The classic congenital club foot: The results of treatment; *Clin Orthop Relat Res*; 2009;467:1133–1145.
7. Huang YT, Lei W, Zhao L, Wang J; The treatment of congenital club foot by operation to correct deformity and achieve dynamic muscle balance; *J Bone Joint Surg*; 1999;81-B(5):859–862.
8. Tarraf YN and Carroll NC; Analysis of the components of residual deformity in clubfeet presenting for reoperation; *J Paediatr Orthop*; 1992;2(12):207.
9. Azarpira MR, Emami MJ, Vosoughi AR, Rahbari K; Factors associated with recurrence of clubfoot treated by the Ponseti method; *World J Clin Cases*; 2016;4(10):318–322.
10. Zhao D, Li H, Zhao Li, Liu J, Wu Z, Jin F; Results of clubfoot management using the Ponseti method: Do the details matter? A systematic review; *Clin Orthop Relat Res*; 2014;472(4):1329–1338.
11. Staheli L, Ignacio P et al. *Clubfoot: Ponseti Management Manual*; 2009; Third edition. 32 pages, 8.5" × 11", Four-Color, English & Others, ISBN-13 978-1- 60189-002-3
12. Goriainov V, Judd J; Uglow M; Does the Pirani score predict relapse in Clubfoot?; *J Child Orthop*; 2010;4(5):439–444.
13. Bhaskar A, Rasal S; Results of treatment of clubfoot by Ponseti's technique in 40 cases: Pitfalls and problems in the Indian scenario; *Indian J Orthop*; 2006;40:196–199.

14. Bhaskar A, Patni P; Classification of relapse pattern in clubfoot treated with Ponseti technique; *Ind J Orthop*; July–August 2013;47(4):370–376.
15. Zionts LE, Dietz FR; Bracing following correction of idiopathic clubfoot using the Ponseti method; *J Am Acad Orthop Surg*; 2010;18(8):486–493.
16. MacNeille R, Hennrikus W, Stapinski B, Leonard G; A mini-open technique for Achilles tenotomy in infants with clubfoot; *J Child Orthop*; 2006;10(1):19–23.
17. Dobbs MB, Gordon JE, Walton T, Schoenecker PL; Bleeding complications following percutaneous tendoachilles tenotomy in the treatment of clubfoot deformity; *J Paediatr Orthop*; 2004;24(4):353–357.
18. Burghardt RD, Herzenberg JE, Ranade A; Pseudoaneurysm after Ponseti percutaneous Achilles tenotomy: A case report; *J Pediatr Orthop*; 2008;28:366–369.
19. Miller NH, Carry PM, Mark BJ, Engelman GH, Georgopoulos G, Graham S, Dobbs MB; Does strict adherence to the Ponseti method improve isolated clubfoot treatment outcomes? A two-institution review; *Clin Orthop Relat Res*; 2016;474(1):237–243.
20. Agarwal A, Kumar A, Shaharyar A, Mishra M; The problems encountered in a CTEV clinic. Can better casting & bracing be accomplished? *Foot and Ankle Specialist*; 2016;6(9):513–521.
21. Bor N, Coplan JA, Herzenberg JE; Ponseti treatment for idiopathic clubfoot: Minimum 5-year followup; *Clin Orthop Relat Res*; 2009;467:1263–1270.
22. Changulani M, Garg NK, Rajagopal TS, Bass A, Nayagam SN, Sampath J, Bruce CE; Treatment of idiopathic club foot using the Ponseti method: Initial experience; *J Bone Joint Surg Br*; 2006;88:1385–1387.
23. Zionts LE, Packer DF, Cooper S, Ebramzadeh E, Sangiorgio S; Walking age of infants with idiopathic clubfoot treated using the Ponseti method; *J Bone Joint Surg Am*; October 2014;96(19):e164.
24. Sala DA, Chu A, Lehman WB, Van Bosse HJ. Achievement of gross motor milestones in children with idiopathic clubfoot treated with the Ponseti method; *J Paediatr Orthop*; January 2013;33(1):55–58.
25. Haft GF, Walker CG, Crawford HA; Early clubfoot recurrence after use of the Ponseti method in a New Zealand population; *J Bone Joint Surg Am*; 2007;89(3):487–493.
26. McElroy T, Konde-Lule J, Neema S, Gitta S. Understanding the barriers to clubfoot treatment adherence in Uganda: A rapid ethnographic study; *Disability and Rehabilitation*; 2007;29:11–12.
27. Abdelgawad AA, Lehman WB, van Bosse HJ, Scher DM, Sala DA; Treatment of idiopathic clubfoot using the Ponseti method: Minimum 2-year follow-up; *J Paediatr Orthop B*; March 2007;16(2):98–105.
28. Faulks S, Richards BS; Clubfoot treatment: Ponseti and French functional methods are equally effective; *Clin Orthop Relat Res*; 2009;467(5):1278–1282.
29. Faldini C, Traina F, Nanni M, Sanzarello I, Borghi R, Perna F; Congenital idiopathic talipes equinovarus before and after walking age: Observations and strategy of treatment from a series of 88 cases; *J Orthopaed Traumatol*; 2016;17:81–87.
30. Ganesan, LA, Al-Jumaily A, Balasankar SK, Naik GR; Ponseti method in the management of clubfoot under 2 years of age: A systematic review; *Pub Lib of Sc*; 2017;2(6):e0178200.
31. Jowett CR, Morcuende JA, Ramachandran M; Management of congenital talipes equinovarus using the Ponseti method: A systematic review; *J Bone Joint Surg (B)*; 2011;93(9):1160–1164.
32. Dogan A, Uzumcugil O, Sarisozen B, Ozdemir B, Emre Akman Y, Bozdaq E, Sunbuloglu E, Bozkurt E; A comparison of percutaneous and mini-open techniques of Achilles tenotomy: An experimental study in rats; *J Child Orthop*; 2009;3(6):485–491.
33. McKay DW; New concept of an approach to clubfoot treatment: Section I—principles and morbid anatomy; *J Pediatr Orthop*; 1982;2(0):347–356.
34. McKay DW; New concept and approach to clubfoot treatment: Section II—correction of the clubfoot; *J Pediatr Orthop*; 1983a;3(1):10–21.
35. McKay DW; New concept and approach to clubfoot treatment: Section III—evaluation & results; *J Pediatr Orthop*; 1983b;3:141–148.

36. Bensahel H, Bienayme B, Jehanno P; History of the functional method for conservative treatment of clubfoot; *J Child Orthop*; 2007;1(3):175–176.
37. Turco VJ; Surgical correction of the resistant club foot. One-stage posteromedial release with internal fixation: A preliminary report; *J Bone Joint Surg Am*; April 1971;53(3):477–487.
38. Turco VJ; Resistant congenital club foot—one-stage posteromedial release with internal fixation. A follow-up report of a fifteen-year experience; *J Bone Joint Surg Am*; September 1979;61-A(6):805–814. PMID:479227.
39. Lichtblau S; A medial & lateral release operation for clubfoot; *J Bone Joint Surg*; 1973;55-A(7):1977–1984.
40. Tayton K and Thompson P; Relapsing clubfeet late results of delayed operation; *J Bone Joint Surg*; 1979;61B(4):474–480. Also quoted: Evans D. Relapsed club foot. *J Bone Joint Surg* 1961,43-B:722–733.
41. Simons GW; Complete subtalar release in Clubfeet. Part I: A preliminary report; *J. Bone Joint Surg*; 1985;67-A(7):1044–1055.
42. Simons GW; Complete subtalar release in clubfeet. Part II: Comparison with less extensive procedures; *J Bone Joint Surg*; 1985;67-A(7):1056–1065.
43. Hassan et al.; Complete subtalar release; *Foot and Ankle Surg*; 2010;(16):38–44.
44. Jordan CJ, Goldstein RY, McLaurin TM, Grant A; The evolution of the Ilizarov technique Part 1: The history of limb lengthening; *Bulletin of the Hospital for Joint Diseases*; 2013;71(1):89–95.
45. Goldstein RY, Jordan CJ, McLaurin TM, Grant A; The evolution of the Ilizarov technique Part 2: The principles of distraction osteosynthesis; *Bulletin of the Hospital for Joint Diseases*; 2013;71(1):96–103.
46. Malizos KN, Gougoulias NE, Dailiana ZH, Rigopoulos N, Moraitis T; Relapsed clubfoot correction with soft-tissue release and selective application of Ilizarov technique; *Strategies Trauma Limb Reconstr*; 2006;3(3):109–117.
47. Saghieh S, Bashoura A, Beriawi G, Afeiche N, Elkattah R. The correction of the relapsed club foot by closed distraction; *Strategies Trauma Limb Reconstruct*; 2010;5(3):127–135.
48. Manjappa CN; Joshi's external stabilization system(JESS) application for correction of resistant clubfoot; *The Internet J Orthop Surg*; 2009;18(1).
49. Suresh S, Ahmed A, Sharma VK; Role of Joshi's external stabilisation system fixator in the management of idiopathic clubfoot; *J Orthop Surg (Hong Kong)*; 2003;11:194–201.
50. Oganesyan OV, Istomina IS, Kuzmin VI; Treatment of equinocavovarus deformity in adults with the use of a hinged distraction++ apparatus; *J Bone Joint Surg Am*; April 1996;78(4):546–556.
51. Grill F, Franke J; The Ilizarov distractor for the correction of relapsed or neglected clubfoot; *J Bone Joint Surg*; 1987;69-B(4):593–597.
52. Makhdoom A, Pir Qureshi AA, Jokhio MF, Siddique KA; Resistant clubfoot deformities managed by Ilizarov distraction histogenesis; *Indian J Orthop*; 2012;46(3):326–332.
53. Utukuri MM, Ramachandran M, Hartley J, Hill RA; Patient-based outcomes after Ilizarov surgery in resistant clubfeet; *J Pediatr Orthop B*; 2006;15:278–284.
54. Ferreira RC, Casto MT, Frizzo GG; Correction of neglected clubfoot using the Ilizarov external fixator; *Foot & Ankle Internat*; 2006;27(4):266–273.
55. Refai MA, Song SH, Song HR; Does short-term application of an Ilizarov frame with transfixion pins correct relapsed clubfoot in children? *Cli Orthop Retat Res*; 2012;470(7):1992–1999.
56. Emara K, El Moatasem el H, El Shazly O; Correction of complex equino cavo varus foot deformity in skeletally mature patients by Ilizarov external fixation versus staged external-internal fixation; *Foot Ankle Surg*; 2011;17(4):287–293.
57. Paley D; The correction of complex foot deformities using Ilizarov distraction osteotomies; *Clin Orthop Relat Res*; 1993;293:97–111.
58. Patwardhan S, Doshi C; Mini fixator for correction of neglected clubfoot; *Int J Paediat Orthop*; 2016;2(1):6–9.

59. Lee DY, Choi InHO, Yoo WJ, Lee SJ, Cho Tae-Joon; Application of the Ilizarov technique to the correction of neurologic equinocavovarus foot deformity; *Clin Orthop Relat Res*; 2011;469(3):860–867.
60. Meena RC, Meena DS, Patni P, Saini N, Chauhan A; Jess & Ilizarov in neglected/relapsed CTEV: A prospective comparative study; *IOSR J Dent and Med Sc*; 2014;13(9):20–26.
61. Herold HZ and Torok G; Surgical correction of neglected clubfoot in the older child and adult; *J Bone Joint Surg Am*; 1973;55(7):1385–1395.
62. Burger D, Aiyer A, Myerson MS; Evaluation and surgical management of the overcorrected clubfoot deformity in the adult patient; *Foot Ankle Clin N Am*; 2015;20(4):587–599.
63. Penny JN; The neglected clubfoot; *Tech Orthop*; 2005;20(2):153–166.
64. Sobel E, Glorgini R, Velez Z; Surgical correction of adult neglected clubfoot: Three case histories; *J Foot Ankle Surg*; 1996;35(1):27–38.
65. Brodsky JW; The adult sequelae of treated congenital clubfoot; *Foot Ankle Clin N Am*; 2010;15:287–296.
66. Yadav SS; Observations on operative management of neglected clubfoot; *Intnat Orthop (SICOT)*; 1981;5:189–192.
67. Zhou U, Zhou B, Liu J, Tan X, Tau X, Chen W, Tang K; A prospective study of midfoot osteotomy combined with adjacent joint sparing internal fixation in treatment of rigid pes cavus deformity; *J Orthop Surg Res*; 2014;9–44.
68. Groner TW, DiDomenico LA; Midfoot osteotomies for the cavus foot; *Clin Podiatr Med Surg*; 2005;22:247–264. Also Quoted: i. Cole WH. The treatment of claw foot. *Bone Joint Surg* 1940,22:895–908. ii. Japas LM. Surgical treatment of pes cavus by tarsal v-osteotomy. *J Bone Joint Surg [Am]*, 1968,50:927–944. iii. Wilcox PG, Weiner DS. The Akron midtarsal dome osteotomy in the treatment of rigid pes cavus. *J Pediatr Orthop*, 1985,5(3):333–338.
69. Letts M, Davidson D; The role of bilateral talectomy in the management of bilateral rigid clubfeet; *Am J Orthop (Belle Mead NJ)*; February 1999;28(2):106–110.
70. El-sherbini MH, Omran AA; Midterm follow-up of talectomy for severe rigid equinovarus feet; *J Foot Ankle Surg*; 2015;54(6):1093–1098.
71. Usuelli FG, Lastroni G, Grassi M, Malerba, F; Talectomy in a neglected clubfoot in Zambia: A low cost one step option in a developing country; *J Foot Ankle Surg AP*; January–June 2014;1(1):32–33.
72. Louis CS, David J, Leong JCY; Talectomy for club foot in arthrogryposis; *J Bone Joint Surg*; November 1984;66-B(5).
73. Solund K, Sonne-Holm S, Kjolbye JE; Talectomy for equinovarus deformity in arthrogryposis. A 13 (2-20) year review of 17 feet.; *Acta Orthop Scand*; August 1991;62(4):372–374.
74. Dias LS, Stem LS; Talectomy in the treatment of resistant talipes equinovarus deformity in myelomeningocele and arthrogryposis; *J Pediatr Orthop*; January–February 1987;7(1):39–41.
75. Johnson GR, Han P, Giacopelli JA; Role of talectomy in the treatment of rigid talipes equinovarus deformities; *J Am Podiatr Med Assoc*; April 1995;85(4):189–197.
76. Loza ME, Bishay SNG, El Barbary HM, Zaki Hanna AAA, Taraf YNE; Double column osteotomy for correction of residual adduction deformity in idiopathic clubfoot; *Ann R Coll Surg Eng*; 2010;2(8):673–679.
77. Otremski I, Salama R, Khermosh O, Wientroub S; Residual adduction of the forefoot a review of the Turco procedure for congenital club foot; *J Bone Joint Surg Br*; 1987;69-B(5):832–834.
78. Elgeidi A and Abulsaad M; Combined double tarsal wedge osteotomy and transcuneiform osteotomy for correction of resistant clubfoot deformity (the "bean-shaped" foot); *J Child Orthop*; 2014;8(5);399–404.
79. Lehman WB, Atar D, Grant AD, Strongwater AM; Re-do clubfoot: Surgical approach and long-term results; *Bull NY Acad Med*; November-December 1990;66(6):601–616.
80. McHale KA, Lenhart M; Treatment of residual clubfoot deformity—the 'bean—shaped' foot-by opening wedge medial cuneiform osteotomy and closing wedge

cuboid osteotomy: Clinical review and cadaver correlations; *J Pediatr Orthop*; 1991;11:374–381.
81. Lourenco AF, Dias LS, Zoellick DM, Sodre H; Treatment of residual adduction deformity in clubfoot: The double osteotomy; *J Paediatr Orthop*; 2001;21(6):713–718.
82. Lee DK, Benard M, Grumbine N, Pokrassa M, Weinstein S; Forefoot adductus correction in clubfoot deformity with cuboid cuneiform osteotomy: A retrospective analysis; *J Am Podiatr Med Assoc*; 2007;97:126–133.
83. Mahadev A, Munajat I, Mansor A, Hui JHP; Combined lateral and transcuneiform without medial osteotomy for residual clubfoot for children; *Clin Orthop Rel Res*; 2009;467(5):1319–1325.
84. Hassan N, Roger J; Management of metatarsus adductus, bean-shaped foot, residual clubfoot adduction and Z-shaped foot in children, with conservative treatment and double column osteotomy of the first cuneiform and the cuboid; *Ann Orthop Rheumatol*; 2015;3(3):1050.
85. Green ADL, Lloyd-Roberts GC; The results of early posterior release in resistant clubfoot; *J Bone Joint Surg*; 1985;67-B:588–593.
86. Uglow MG, Clarke NMP; Relapse in staged surgery for congenital talipes Equinovarus; *J Bone Joint Surg*; 2000;82-B(5):739–743.
87. Legaspi J, LI YH, Chow W, Leong JC; Talectomy in patients with recurrent deformity in club foot. A long-term follow-up study; *L Bone Joint Surg (Br)*; 2001;83(3):384–387.
88. Dobb MB, Nunley R, Shoenecker PL; Long term follow up of patients with clubfeet treated with extensive soft tissue release; *J Bone Joint Surg*; 2006;88A(5):986–996.
89. Depuy J, Drennan JC; Correction of idiopathic clubfoot: A comparison of early versus delayed posteromedial release; *J Pediatr Orthop*; 1989;9:44–48.
90. Kuo KN, Smith PA; Correcting residual deformity following clubfoot releases; *Clin Orthop Relat Res*; 2009;467(5):1326–1333.
91. Ryoppy S, Sairanen H; Neonatal operative treatment of club foot—A preliminary report; *J Bont Joint Surg*; 1983;65-B(3).
92. Reimann I, Becker-Andersen H; Early surgical treatment of congenital clubfoot; *Clin Orthop Rel Resarch*; July–August 1974;102:200–206.
93. Andriesse H, Hagglund G, Gunbritt J. The clubfoot assessment protocol (CAP); description and reliability of a structured multi-level instrument for follow-up. *BMC Musculoskeleta Disord* 2005;6:40.
94. Dimeglio A, Bensahel H, Souchel P, Mazeau P, Bonnet F; Classification of clubfoot; *J Paediatr Orthop B*; 1995.
95. Dyer PJ, Davis N; The role of the Pirani scoring system in the management of club foot by the Ponseti method; *J Bone Joint Surg*; 2006;88-B(8):1082–1084.
96. Andrew M. Wainwright AM, Tanya A, Benson MK, Tim N; Theologis: The classification of congenital talipes equinovarus; *J Bone Joint Surg*; 2002;84-B(7):1020–1024.
97. Fan H, Liu Y, Zhao Li, Chu C, An Y, Wang T and Li w; the correlation of pirani and dimeglio scoring systems for ponseti management at different levels of deformity severity. *NPJ*; Scientific reports 2017, No.7, article No.14578(2017). doi: 10.1038/s41598-017- 14977-7
98. Gao R, Tomlinson M, Walker C; Correlation of Pirani and Dimeglio scores with number of Ponseti casts required for clubfoot correction; *J Paediatr Orthop*; 2014;34(6):639–642.
99. Hussain FN; The role of the Pirani scoring system in the management of club foot by the Ponseti method. Correspondence; *J Bone Joint Surg [Br]*; 2007;89-B:561–563.
100. Beatson TR and Pearson JR; A method of assessing correction in clubfeet; *J Bone Joint Surg*; 1966;48-B(1):49–50.
101. Sambandam SN, Gul A; Stress radiography in the assessment of residual deformity in clubfoot following postero-medial release; *Int Orthop*; June 2006;30(3):210–214.
102. Prasad P, Sen RK, Gill SS, Wardak E, Saini R; Clinico-radiological assessment and their correlation in clubfeet treated with posteromedial soft-tissue release; *Int Orthop*; 2009;33(I):225–229.
103. Simons GW; Analytical radiography of clubfeet; *J Bone Joint Surg*; 1977;59-B(4):485–489.

104. Kang S, Park S-S; Lateral tibiocalcaneal angle as a determinant for percutaneous Achilles tenotomy for idiopathic clubfeet; *J Bone Joint Surg*; 2015;97-A(15):1246–1254.
105. Radler C, Michael MH, Suda R, Burghardt R, Herzenberg JE, Ganger R, Grill F; Radiographic evaluation of idiopathic clubfeet undergoing Ponseti treatment; *J Bone Joint Surg Am*; 2007;89:1177–1183.
106. Keret D, Ezra E, Lokiec F, Hayek, S, Segev E, Wientroub S; Efficacy of prenatal ultrasonography in confirmed club foot; *J Bone Joint Surg*; 2002;84-B(7):1015–1019.
107. Rosselli P, Nossa S, Huerfano E, Betancur G, Guzman Y, Castellanos C, Morcuendo J; Prenatal ultrasound diagnosis of congenital talipes equinovarus in Bogota (Colombia) between 2003 and 2012; *Iowa Orthop J*; 2015;35:156–159.
108. El-Adwar KI, Taha Kotb H; The role of ultrasound in clubfoot treatment: Correlation with the Pirani score and assessment of the Ponseti method; *Clin Orthop Relat Res*; September 2010;468(9):2495–2506.
109. Bhargava SK, Tandon A, Prakash M, Arora SS, Bhatt S, Bhargava S; Radiography and sonography of clubfoot: A comparative study; *Indian J Orthop*; 2012;46:229–235.
110. Chawla S, Gupta M, Pandey V, Jain A, Manoj K; Clinico-sonographical evaluation of idiopathic clubfoot and its correction by Ponseti method–A prospective study; *The Foot*; 2017;33:7–13.
111. Farsetti P, De Maio F, Russolillo L, Ippolito E: CT study on the effect of different treatment protocols for clubfoot pathology. *Clin Orthop Relat Res.* May 2009; 467(5):1243–1249.
112. Windisch G, Salaberger D, Rosmarin W, Kastner J, Ulrich E G, Haldi-Brändle V, Anderhuber F. A model for clubfoot based on micro-CT data. *J Anat*; June 2007; 210(6):761–766.
113. Johnston CE 2nd, Hobatho MC, Baker KJ, Baunin C; Three-dimensional analysis of clubfoot deformity by computed tomography. *Journal of Pediatric Orthopedics*. Part B [01 Jan 1995, 4(1):39–48]
114. Ippolito E, Fraracci L, Farsetti P and De Maio F; Validity of the anteroposterior talocalcaneal angle to assess congenital clubfoot correction; *American Journal of Roentgenology* 2004;182:5;1279–1282.
115. Cahuzac, JP, Baunin C, Luu S, Estivalezes E, Sales de Gauzy J, Hobatho, MC; Assessment of hindfoot deformity by three-dimensional MRI in infant club foot; *J-P J Bone Joint Surg*; 1999;81-B(1):97–101.
116. Kamegaya M, Shinohara Y, Kuniyoshi K, Moriya H; MRI study of talonavicular alignment in club foot; *J Bone Joint Surg [Br]*; 2001;83-B:726–730.
117. Richard BS, Dempsey M; Magnetic resonance imaging of the congenital clubfoot treated with the French functional (physical therapy) method; *J. Paediatr Orthjopp*; March 2007;(2):214–19.
118. Duce SL, D'Alessandro M, Du Y, Jagpal B, Gilbert FJ et al.; 3D MRI analysis of the lower legs of treated idiopathic congenital talipes equinovarus (Clubfoot); *PLOS ONE*; 2013;8(1):e54100.
119. O'Connor PJ, Bos CF, Bloem JL; Tarsal navicular relations in club foot: Is there a role for magnetic resonance imaging? *Skeletal Radiol*; August 1998;27(8):440–444.
120. Wang C, Petursdottir S, Leifsdottir I, Rehnberg L, Ahlstrom H; MRI multiplanar reconstruction in the assessment of congenital talipes equinovarus. *Pediatr Radiol*; 1999;29:262–267.

the equinus component of clubfoot deformity. The posterior talo-fibular ligament also assumes importance in its role in equinus deformity.

In front of the ankle, there are four tendons anteriorly, from the medial to lateral side, tibialis anterior and extensor hallucis longus, anterior tibial vessels and the deep peroneal nerve, and then extensor digitorum longus and peroneus tertius further lateral. Behind the ankle, on the medial side, there are the tibialis posterior and flexor digitorum longus tendons behind the medial malleolus, acting as a pulley for them. The flexor hallucis longus tendon, separated by posterior tibial vessels and nerves, is further behind the tibia and passes in a groove behind the talus and then passes down into the foot in the groove of the sustentaculum tali in the sole at Henry's knot, joined by the flexor digitorum longus. On the lateral side the peronei pass behind the lateral malleolus, acting as a pulley for them. There are two extensor retinacula, superior and inferior, which are only thickened deep fasciae, preventing bowstringing of the tendons. The superior retinaculum is just above the ankle joint, attached to the lower 2.5 cm of the tibia and fibula. The saphenus nerve, long saphenus vein, and superficial peroneal nerve cross superficial to it under the skin. The inferior extensor retinaculum is y-shaped, starting at its attachment on the calcacaneum in front of the depression at the interosseous talocalcanean ligament, and is medially divided in two layers. One passes behind the peroneus tertius and extensor digitorum longus tendons and the other in front, dividing into two diverging limbs in a Y shape going medially. One goes superiorly and is attached to the medial malleolus, superficial to extensor tendon, but enclosing the tibialis anterior tendon in two layers; the other goes inferiorly, superficial to the extensor tendons and is attached to the plantar aponeurosis.

The most free, prominent, essential, and important movement of the foot is plantar and dorsiflexion occurring at the ankle, this being a hinge joint. The axis of this joint passes through the two malleoli and the body of the talus, and movements occur in the sagittal plane at a right angle to the axis of movement like any other hinge. Moving motors, that is, the muscle–tendon complexes performing plantar flexion, are behind this axis and those performing dorsiflexion are in front of this axis. The range of dorsiflexion is about 20° and plantar flexion is 30°–50° from the neutral position. At the end of dorsiflexion movement, the talus gets locked in the ankle joint mortis, with no possibility of further dorsiflexion at the ankle joint, because the wider anterior part of the body of the talus comes in close contact with the narrow posterior part of the ankle mortis. However, in plantar flexion, which is more free, the narrow posterior part of the talus comes in front in the wider part of the ankle mortis, permitting some side-to-side and rotatory movements, which assumes importance in clubfoot deformity.

4.1.2 The foot

There are 26 bones in the foot: 14 in the toes, 5 metatarsals forming the forefoot, and 7 tarsals: 3 cuneiforms, the navicular and cuboid forming the midfoot, and the talus and calcaneum forming the hindfoot. The shape and size of each bone with their multiplanar articular surfaces is such that, in the articulated foot, all of them fit together to give an arched shape to the foot as required for its complex function. There are 33 joints: 14 in the toes, 5 tarsometatarsal joints, 8 in the midfoot, 2 in the hindfoot, and 4 in the ankle region. It will also be important to know about the bones of the foot, its ligaments, and various foot joints.

4.1.2.1 BONES OF THE FOOT

The **talus** consists of a head, neck, and body. Most of it is articular, except for the neck, a small area on the superior surface and sulcus tarsi on the undersurface (forming sinus tarsi with similar sulcus calcanei on calcaneum), narrow medially and wider laterally. The head is directed forward, slightly downward and medially. Its head is oval/round articulating with the similar concave-surfaced navicular in front. On the undersurface of the head, in front of the sulcus, it has three articular areas separated by blunt ridges: anterior is continuation of the navicular area, the middle one is for spring ligament, and posterior is for the sustenculum tali. The neck is a small constricted area, inclined medially at an angle of about 140°, giving attachment to ligaments and capsules and vascular supply; on the undersurface, it has well-marked sulcus tali. The body is cuboidal, with the dorsal surface being trochlear in shape, articulating with the lower end of the tibia, making the ankle joint. The undersurface articulates with the posterior articular surface of the calcaneum. Medial and lateral surfaces articulate with medial and lateral malleoli, respectively. The borders give attachments to capsules and the sulcus tali gives attachment to the strong interosseous talo-calcanean ligament inside the sinus tarsi, a tunnel shape with the calcaneum underneath.

The **calcaneum** is directed forward, upward, and laterally and is cuboidal in shape with six surfaces. The dorsal surface, in the middle third, has an oval articular surface for articulating with the body of the talus. In front of it is the sulcus calcanei from medial to lateral side giving attachment to the interosseous ligament, wider laterally and narrower medially. Further anterior are two articular facets on sustentaculum tali and another one in front of it for the talus. The anterior surface is cancavo–convex for the cuboid. The posterior surface has three parts: the middle part is rough, giving attachment to tendoachilles. The plantar surface is rough, marked posteriorly by calcaneal tuberosity, giving attachment to the plantar aponeurosis and flexor digitorum brevis. The lateral surface is rough with two grooves for the peronei, divided by a ridge. There are two peroneal retinacula, superior and inferior, the superior retaining the peronei behind the lateral malleolus and the inferior on the lateral surface of the calcaneum. The medial surface is concave, accommodating all the tendons, nerves, and vessels of the foot under the flexor reticulum to prevent bowstringing.

The **navicular** lies between the talar head and the three cuneiforms distally. Its distal surface is convex and articular, divided into three for articulating with the cuneiforms. The proximal surface is oval concave for articulating with the head of the talus. The medial surface is a rough projection called the tuberosity and gives attachment to the tibialis anterior. The plantar surface is concave and the dorsal is convex, and both are rough.

The **cuboid** is placed laterally, articulating with the calcaneum by its corresponding concavo-convex surface. In front, it has two articular facets for the fourth and fifth metatarsal bases. Medially, it has two articular surfaces for the navicular behind and the lateral cuneiform in front. The plantar surface has a deep groove for the peroneus longus tendon going from the lateral to the medial side.

The three **cuneiforms** are wedge-shaped, articulating with the navicular behind and the bases of the first, second, and third metatarsals in front. The medial cuneiform is the largest and the intermediate is the smallest. The dorsal surface of the medial cuneiform is narrower than the plantar; this is the reverse in the other two.

4.1.2.2 CAPSULES, LIGAMENTS, AND JOINTS OF THE FOOT

The **subtalar joint** is a complex joint having a great role in the pathology of clubfoot. It consists of three joints. There is a very small insignificant joint at its anteromedial end for the talus. There are two significant joints: one with the sustentaculum tali and the third, the most posterior and the largest, forms the so-called subtalar joint. In front of this is the curved sinus tarsi, a tunnel, narrow medially and getting wider as it moves to its lateral end. The strong interosseous talo-calcanean ligament is attached to both the talar and calcanean sulci. The talus is inclined with the calcaneum, by the longitudinal lines through their axes, at an angle of 25°–40° in anteroposterior skiagram and 35°–50° in lateral skiagram, and the mean of the two is called the talo-calcanean index, which is an important measurement in clubfoot.

The **talo-calcaneo-navicular joint** is also a complex joint with an important role in clubfoot pathology. It is formed by the head of the talus behind, the navicular in front, and the plantar-calcaneo-navicular (spring) ligament underneath, articulating with talus above. Therefore, in the typical foot, there are three articular areas at the bottom of this joint: from anterior to posterior, they are part of the navicular continuing below, the spring ligament, and the sustenculum tali. In clubfoot, there will only be two, with the spring ligament area missing. Because of the varus deformity, the navicular shifts medially and downward close to the sustenculum.

The **calcaneo-cuboid joint** is an important joint in clubfoot deformity and gets deformed increasingly with increasing age. It has concavo-convex articular surfaces of the two articulating bones, joined by a strong capsule.

The **cuneo-navicular** and **intercuneiform joints** also have a role in clubfoot deformity. There are also the **tarsometatarsal joints** and **metatarso-phalangeal joints**. The movement of intertarsal and tarsometatarsal joints is not uniplanar. It is multiplanar and coupled, occurring in three dimensions because of the peculiar orientation of their articular surfaces. The types of movements occurring at these joints are flexion-extension around the horizontal axis, adduction-abduction around the vertical axis, and inversion-eversion around the longitudinal axis. All three of these types of movements are coupled in varying degrees and occur simultaneously. This feature of movements is highly important in clubfoot and is the cause of varying degrees of deformities in clubfeet patients and why no two cases are exactly the same. Movement at the toes occurs mostly in flexion-extension in the horizontal axis, but a slight amount of adduction-abduction can also occur in the vertical axis.

4.1.2.3 MUSCLES AND TENDONS OF THE FOOT

Long muscles of the leg continue in the foot as tendons on the dorsal, plantar, medial, and lateral sides (extrinsic muscles), whereas there are intrinsic muscles of the foot that are also important. Plantar muscles are more significant and are in four layers, but there are some dorsal muscles of the foot too. There are three compartments in the leg: extensor muscles in the anterior, peronei in the lateral, and flexors in the posterior compartment.

Anterior compartment: The tibialis anterior, a powerful muscle, traverses down from the anterior aspect of the leg, under the superior extensor retinaculum, to the medial side of the foot to attach to the navicular and the base of first metatarsal and is a dorsi-flexor and inverter of the foot and is often responsible for dynamic persistence of inversion in clubfoot. The extensor digitorum longus also descends behind the retinaculum, and its four slips get attached to the bases of the middle and distal phalanges. The peroneus tertius is a small muscle, and its tendon is attached to the base of the fifth metatarsal. The extensor hallucis longus traverses from the leg to get attached to the base of the distal phalanx of the first metatarsal. They are extensors (dorsiflexors) of the ankle and toes.

Lateral compartment: **Both the peronei are lying behind the lateral malleolus groove, with** peroneus longus lying posterior to peroneus brevis tendon. They traverse down underneath the superior peroneal retinaculum longus going into the sole in the groove of the cuboid to be attached to the medial cuneiform and the adjacent base of the first metatarsal. The peroneus brevis gets attached to the base of the fifth metatarsal. They are evertors and plantar flexors.

Posterior compartment: There is a superficial and deep group of three muscles each. The superficial are gastrocnemius, soleus, and plantaris. Lower down they unite into the common tendoachilles and get attached to the posterior tuberosity of the calcaneum. The three deep muscles are the tibialis posterior, flexor digitorum longus, and flexor hallucis longus. The tibialis posterior and flexor digitorum longus tendons pass behind the medial malleolus groove under the flexor retinaculum into the sole of the foot. The tibialis posterior has nine insertions; the main portion is attached to the navicular tuberosity and the rest to all other tarsals except the talus and to the bases of the second, third, and fourth metatarsals in the sole, **which are significantly abnormal and contracted in clubfoot.** The flexor digitorum longus crosses into the sole behind the tibialis posterior tendon, and further down it comes closer to the flexor hallucis at the Henry's knot in the middle of the sole for easy recognition. The flexor hallucis longus gets attached to the base of the distal phalanx of the great toe, while the flexor digitorum longus divides into four slips to be attached to the distal phalanx of the lateral four toes. Deep fascia is present underneath the skin as plantar aponeurosis, which has a central thick and strong part and thin lateral and medial parts covering the first layer of muscles of the sole. There are four layers of short muscles of the sole, from superficial to deep: the first layer includes the flexor digitorum brevis, abductor hallucis, and abductor digiti minimi, the second layer consists of the flexor digitorum accesorius and lumbricals, the third layer contains the flexor hallucis brevis, and the fourth layer consists of plantar interossei. The dorsal short muscles are the dorsal interossei and extensor digitorum brevis. In severe clubfoot deformities, the muscles of the sole also play their role in enhancing the deformity. The abductor hallucis is especially important in clubfoot and is hypertrophied.

4.1.2.4 ARCHES OF THE FOOT

The foot has to be an elastic structure for biomechanical efficiency, in order to bear static weight on standing, weight bearing on walking, running, or jumping from height. There are the longitudinal and transverse arches in the foot. Both arches are higher medially than laterally, with the dome formed at the talo-navicular joint for its mechanical efficiency. First of all, skin and subcutaneous tissues of the sole of the foot are thick-textured and suited for weight bearing. All the tissues, right from the skin to the deepest tissues, participate to meet this functional requirement. The bony framework with multiple small bones of different shapes articulating with each other, various capsular, ligamentous structures, and plantar aponeurosis make a requisite arched, hard structure with spring action. There are various tendons from the leg, going into the foot from all sides, and short muscles of the foot contributing to the maintenance of the arches by providing a dynamic spring action during weight bearing in all functions. In severe clubfoot deformities, there is disorganization of the arched function of the foot and there is a definite functional handicap, even for normal functions with diminished earning capacity involving physical labor, in addition to the appearance along with the consequent psychological handicap. The weight bearing is on the lateral side or dorsolateral with callosity and bursa to provide the cushioning effect.

4.2 PLANES AND AXES OF MOVEMENTS

It is imperative to know that clubfoot is a three-dimensional deformity; a line is one dimensional having only length; a flat shape is two dimensional having length and breadth, like a rectangle or square; and likewise, anything three dimensional will have a depth also, for example, any solid object or body part. So the foot is a three-dimensional structure.

To define it in other words, there are antero-posterior (sagittal), side-to-side, and vertical planes. Movements occur in all three directions, parallel to these imaginary planes, in varying proportions, but the axis will be at a right angle to the plane. If one wants to describe the three planes specifically in the foot, they are the sagittal, frontal or coronal, and horizontal planes. The sagittal plane is an imaginary line running from back to front, dividing the foot into medial and lateral parts with the line passing through the second toe, and the movements of this plane, parallel to this line, are plantar and dorsiflexion around a horizontal axis at a right angle to the plane passing, from right to left, through the malleoli. The frontal or coronal plane passes from side to side and divides the foot into front and back parts; the movements of this plane are parallel to it and will be inversion and eversion around a sagittal axis. The horizontal plane is parallel to the ground, dividing the foot into dorsal and plantar parts, and the movements of this plane, parallel to it, will be adduction and abduction around a vertical axis (Table 4.1).

However, our foot, because of the shape, which is given to it by multiple bones with varied shapes and their corresponding joints articulating in different planes, has composite polyaxial movements in all the three planes at all joints in varying proportions and does not have monoaxial movements. They are coupled and of a complex nature (Figure 4.1a–f).

4.3 PATHOANATOMY OF CLUBFOOT

Idiopathic congenital clubfoot is one of the most common conditions seen in orthopedics, but it still remains an unsolved problem. There are a

Table 4.1 Planes and axes of foot movements

S. No	Plane	Axis	Movements
1.	Sagittal from back to front dividing the foot into right and left parts	Coronal from right to left	Flexion/extension
2.	Coronal from top to bottom dividing the foot into anterior and posterior parts	Sagittal from back to front	Inversion and eversion (rotational movements)
3.	Horizontal from right to left dividing the foot into dorsal and plantar parts	Vertical axis (top to bottom)	Adduction and abduction

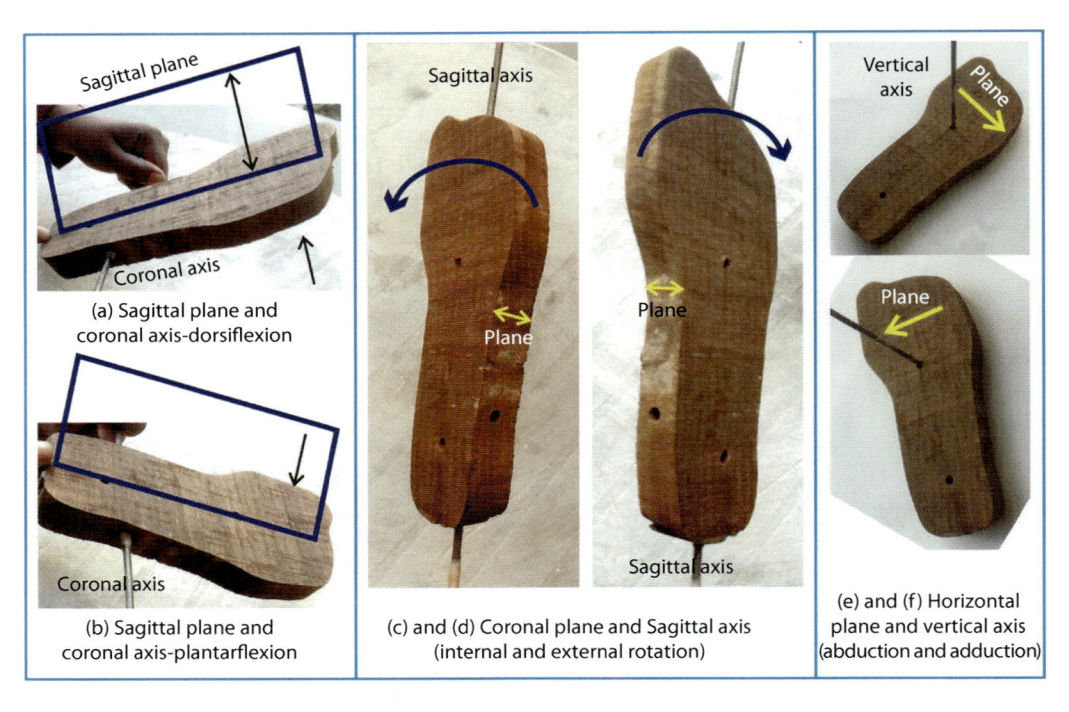

Figure 4.1 Description explaining the 3 planes and their axes of movements: **(a)** and **(b)** Movements occurring in sagittal or anteroposterior plane and around coronal or horizontal axis. **(c)** and **(d)** Movements in coronal plane but around a sagittal or anteroposterior axis. **(e)** and **(f)** Movements in horizontal plane and vertical axis.

number of reasons for that. **Firstly,** the severity of the deformity varies from very mild and easily correctable by stretching to a very severe and completely rigid foot. All grades of the deformity are seen in between the two ends of the scale. Moreover, in regard to the individual components of the deformity, they are also variable in every case. **Secondly,** the age of presentation is extremely variable, ranging from soon after birth to very late in childhood to late adulthood or even later. **Thirdly,** as the child grows, there are adaptive changes of typical growth in the bones from lying in the abnormal position due to deformity, leading to a further increase of the deformity with increasing rigidity; therefore, problems of management increase with increasing age. There are symptoms and signs due to weight bearing depending upon severity and duration the patient had been walking. **Fourthly,** in developing countries, including India, many children are not brought to a hospital at an early age due to lack of awareness, poverty, or illiteracy or they are irregular in return visits to a hospital for various reasons, making treatment more difficult. **Fifthly,** besides these, there are many more problems in long-standing cases seen from time to time affecting the deformity. They are (i) scars from one or more previous surgeries, further modifying the pathoanatomy; (ii) other deformities frequently seen with clubfoot, such as congenital genu varum/valgum or compensatory genu recurvatum in long-standing cases with equinus; (iii) many other unusual complications, which create more problems for the patients and will be discussed; and (iv) last, but not least, there may still be some complex pathoanatomical factors that are not yet completely understood or new ones still to be discovered, because **each clubfoot is different**.

Recurrence rate or incidence of undercorrected deformities has been reported to be high, ranging from 36% to 68%, by many authors (Bertelsen,[2] Singer and Fripp,[3] Turco[4] 1979). However, Huang et al.[5] quoted Tarraf and Carroll[6] reporting still higher incidence of residual adduction and supination of the forefoot as the most common persistent deformity in 95% of 159 club feet, which required repeat surgery after primary soft-tissue release. This, obviously, will be true for extreme deformities also in children, adolescents, and adults.

4.3.1 Review of literature on pathoanatomy

Congenital clubfoot, although the most common congenital defect with voluminous literature, is yet full of controversies. It is a maze and is extremely difficult to navigate. It will be interesting to trace the history of congenital clubfoot. Shands[7] has described three names to choose from as the first surgeons to perform surgery on clubfoot: William Detmold in 1938 reported it first, while Dickson in 1935 and Rogers in 1936 performed the same procedure earlier. Similarly, there are conflicting views about the basic pathology of this condition. According to one school of thought, the primary blame is on the muscle (Stewart,[8] Flinchum[9] and Fried[10]), while the other school believes bones to be primarily responsible (Bissell,[11] Irani and Sherman,[12] Waisbrod,[13] Settle[14]), mainly the talus, and still others consider it to be a composite defect of muscle as well as bones (Bechtol and Mosman,[15] Wiley[16]). Turco,[17] McKay[18,19] and Simons[20,21] laid the blame on the subtalar joint, while Goldner[22] stressed the atypical position of the talus in the ankle joint. Subluxation or dislocation of the talo-navicular joint was stressed by Turco[4] and Simons[20,21] while McKay[18,19] felt that this was not present. This confusion about the anatomical location of the defect leads one to concur with the truth in the statement of Hippocrates[23] that "there are more than one types of club foot." With my lifetime association with this deformity, **I feel that there is an extremely wide variation in the severity of this deformity at birth, and these variations further increase with age due to innumerable factors, some of them still not completely understood, which has led to different conclusions by different authors**. The story of the blind men and the elephant holds very true here, as each one analyzes the elephant from his own angle without thinking about the whole proposition.

From the above, it is clear that pathoanatomy has to be studied more diligently to solve these controversies. On reviewing the literature of anatomical dissections, it was found that only a few authors had studied the pathoanatomy on cadaveric feet. Until our dissections, only 80 dissections had been reported in the English literature with a maximum number of 16 dissections by Settle[14] and all these, too, with conflicting views. The details of 80 dissections are shown in Table 4.2, with all their dissenting views.

Stewart[8] dissected two clubfeet and performed 20 surgeries in clubfoot and commented about the pathoanatomy. The most frequent, persistent, and troublesome was inversion of the heel caused by malinsertion of tendoachilles on the medial side of the calcaneum with forward extension on its medial surface acting as a positive deforming force. Abductor hallucis was also contracted in two cases. His conclusion was that abnormal insertion of tendons was a positive deforming force.

Flinchum[9] dissected a unilateral deformed foot from a 6½-months-old and reported shortening of the deltoid ligament, the tendoachilles tendon was inserted on the medial side of the calcaneal tuberosity, the tibialis anterior tendon was inserted more on the first metatarsal base than on the navicular and was a major muscle offering resistance to correction, the mass of the peronei muscles were half the thickness and tendons longer than the unaffected side. No histological difference was noted in the muscles and nerves. Bony changes were considered to be secondary in nature. The head of the talus was prominent dorsally and was pointing toward the fifth metatarsal. No other abnormalities in bones were seen. In four surgeries on clubfeet, he found fascial extensions of tibialis anterior on medial side, as well as plantar side of the foot.

Fried[10] reported that the tibialis posterior tendon was thickened and showed fibrosis beyond medial malleolus and had hypertrophied broader attachments. Equinus deformity was due to the composite action of weaker stretched extensors and contracted overaction of triceps surae and tibialis posterior. The peronei were also stretched and weaker. He described bony changes as secondary.

Bissel[11] dissected bilateral clubfeet in a five-year-old who died of pneumonia. His tendoachilles was cut 5 months before death, which was small in length and attached more medially on calcaneum. After removing all muscles, the deformity still persisted. There was rotation of the tibia and fibula, the foot was severely rotated with the plantar surface facing medially, and the inner border of the foot touched the tibia. The deltoid ligament was short and thick. The plantar ligaments were all short and thick, especially on the medial side. The superior talo-navicular ligament was thin and lengthened. Middle and posterior parts of the lateral collateral ligament were thick, short, and cord-like, and the

Table 4.2 Showing the details of anatomical dissections in stillborn fetuses—Review of literature

Year	Author name	Work done	Abnormal findings
1818	Antonius Scarpa	3 clubfoot specimens	Insertional abnormalities
1820	Mackever	3 specimens	Insertional abnormalities
1832	Tourtual	1 specimen	Insertional abnormalities
1839	Little	4 infants	Insertional abnormalities
1851	Adams	Fetus bilateral	Talar deformity
1855	Adams William	3 specimens	Talar deformity
1879	Kocher	Premature infant unilateral	Talar neck deformity
1884	Parker and Shattock	18-month-old infant bilateral 3-month-old infant bilateral 7-month-old infant bilateral Full-term fetus bilateral	Talar deformity
1888	Bissell	5-year-old child bilateral	Talar deformity
1889	Bussel-Hagen	2 young children unilateral	Talar deformity
1893	Burell	Stillborn infant unilateral	Talar deformity
1897	Nichols	Stillborn infant bilateral	Talar deformity
1899	Shevkunenko	12 specimens	Insertional abnormalities
1920	Pfrang	1 specimen	Deformity in talus
1929	Bohm	7-month-old fetus unilateral	Talar deformity, muscle abnormalities
1950	Bechtol and Mossman	16 weeks and 6 months fetuses unilateral (2)	Malinsertion of tendons
1951	Stewart	Stillborn infant bilateral	Malinsertion of tendons
1953	Flinchum	6½-month-old fetus unilateral	Many talar neck deformity
1959	Wileys	6 equinovarus feet, full-term infants	All deformed tali
1963	Irani and Sherman	11 equinovarus feet, full-term infants	**All deformed tali**
1963	Settle	**16 clubfeet**	Talar deformity
1973	Waisbrod	6 clubfeet	**Talar deformity**
1981	Mittal et al.	**15 clubfeet, 6 unilateral and 3 bilateral**	**Skin contracture primary; deep fascia, muscles, ligaments, bones—secondary**

middle was attached well in front of the middle of the calcaneum. Even after cutting the lateral and medial ligaments, it was not possible to dorsiflex the foot more than 90°. Other features were projection of the talar head on dorsal aspect, attachment of the tarsal scaphoid to the inner malleolus, apparent absence of the typical prominence of both malleoli, the outer surface of the calcaneum convex from before backward and comparatively lengthened, its anterior articular surface facing medially and forward and larger than typical, as well as being rotated internally on its longitudinal axis. His conclusions were that the deformed shape of equinovarus is due to increased anterior length and decreased posterior part length. He also concluded that the deformed shape is primarily due to osseous changes, while tendons, ligaments, and fasciae had altered shape due to osseous changes.

Irani and Sherman[12] reported anatomical defects in 11 clubfeet. They studied detailed dissections and even cross sections. Soft tissues were completely removed to study individual bones. On cross sections, they found legs were thinner on the deformed side in full-term fetuses, with vessels and nerves being typical. On dividing the talo-navicular, plantar calcaneo-navicular, and the capsule of the subtalar joint, the deformity could be completely corrected. The typical curve on top of the talus was decreased, the lateral articular surface of talus was decreased, and its medial surface was pressed against the medial malleolus in severe deformities. The head of the talus was deviated medially. In the calcaneum, its anterior part was more uncovered, and the sinus tarsi was widened. In very severe deformities, the calcaneum was more concave on the medial side. The navicular articulated with the talus infero-medially and may touch the medial malleolus. The neck of the talus was short and the head-body angle was decreased to 115°–135° (from the normal angle of 150°–155°). The navicular was smaller in size. In conclusion, they blamed the talus as being the most deformed, and there were no primary abnormalities of vessels, nerves, muscles, and tendons. The maximum abnormality was in in the anterior part of the talus and resulted from defective cartilage anlage.

Waisbrod[13] quoted Lloyd-Roberts,[41] who stated, "This is an undeniably disheartening state of affairs which is in no way redeemed by the knowledge that little or no improvement has occurred since Brockman's review was published thirty-five years ago," and he added: "What are the features that are likely to make a club foot resist treatment, there is no ready answer?" With this in mind, he reported pathoanatomy of clubfoot in different stages of fetal development. He also quoted Muller[40] on review of literature of the last 120 years, and reported 65 dissections of clubfeet, 41 of them in fetuses. Thirty-nine of the dissected feet showed talar deformity, especially of the head and neck; the rest had insertional abnormalities. The author himself dissected eight fetuses with unilateral deformities, six from the Israel University Anatomy Department. Soft tissues were dissected and compared with typical tissue. Tali were removed, photographed, and placed in their original position. Cut sections of talus were micro-radiographed after injecting contrast. Measurements were made of the head-neck angle in the deformed. The angle ranged from 124° to 154°, whereas in control feet, it was 150°–157°. The average angle on the control sides was 153° and on the deformed sides was 134°. Three of the feet could be manipulated into plantigrade position, and it was impossible for the other five. In regard to soft tissues, the gastrosoleus was smaller on the affected side and the tendocalcaneus was thinner and insertion was typical on the calcaneum in all cases. The tibialis anterior was typical in all but one, where insertion was only on the medial cuneiform. In five cases, the tibialis posterior muscle was much smaller and the tendon too was thinner and shorter, but the navicular insertion was thickened and adherent near the medial malleolus. No talo-navicular dislocation was seen, but the talus was deformed and short with a thinner and longer neck and a pointed head with the angle of declination markedly decreased. Ossification centers were either absent or smaller and eccentric. Vascular channels in the talus were few and disorganized. The feet, which could be manipulated to the plantigrade position, had typical tali. He concluded that the most striking abnormalities were in the talus.

Settle[14] described 16 anatomical dissections in clubfeet. He dissected muscles and nerves and took their biopsies. He coated the talus with radio-opaque medium, replaced it, and took radiographs. Arthrograms were also taken in the fetuses by injecting dyes and placing lead foil in the talo-navicular joint before X-rays. His findings were as follows: the talus was 75% the size of a typical talus and the talar articular surfaces at the ankle were shallower and articulating in the plantar flexed position. The talar neck showed the main abnormality with medial and plantar deviation of its body and the navicular articulating with this deviated talar head further increasing the deformity. Talo-navicular and calcaneo-cuboid joints faced medially and plantarward and were placed one above another instead of lying side by side. Two accessory joints were noted, one between the navicular and medial malleolus and the other between the posterolateral part of the calcaneum and the lateral malleolus. In one very severe deformity, a third accessory joint was present between the sustentaculum tali and the medial malleolus. Soft tissues showed shortening on the medial side and lengthening on the lateral side. Muscles and nerve biopsies showed no abnormalities. Skiagrams were compatible with gross findings.

Bechtol and Mossman[15] described two anatomical dissections showing the neck of the talus more medially deviated with deformed head, the cuboid shifted medially half its width and articulated with the medial corner of the calcaneum, leading to navicular shifting medially with close contact with the medial malleolus. Metatarsals were normal. Biopsy of muscles in a second fetus showed many embryonic abnormal fibers throughout the muscle with slower growth and thus shortening and deformity.

Wiley[16] dissected six full-term specimens of equinovarus, one of calcaneovalgus and one metatarsus varus, obtained one to three days after death, and all were compared with controls. Severity of deformity varied from case to case. The gastrocnemius was shorter and thinner, while the tibialis posterior and the tibialis anterior, and others too, were shorter and thinner but less than typical. There were no insertional abnormalities, as seen in other reports. Regarding bony abnormalities, the talus was in equinus with its neck angled medially and the navicular articulated with it with medial displacement.

Turco[17] commented that more than 50% of clubfeet remain undercorrected after treatment from birth onward or have recurrent deformities and require further treatment including one or more surgeries. In the pathoanatomy, he stressed the knowledge of biomechanics of the talocalcaneo-navicular joint. It differs from other ball-and-socket joints in that the socket here moves around the ball with expansion and contraction with each movement, because it is partly composed of fibroelastic ligaments. Although the calcaneum does not articulate with the navicular, they move as one unit with their ligaments around the talus, with some movements at the subtalar joint. During dorsiflexion and plantar flexion, the movement occurs both at the ankle as well as at the talocalcaneo-navicular joint. Due to this, during dorsiflexion, the foot also pronates and the calcaneum everts with the navicular, and the talo-navicular socket deepens in dorsiflexion and covers more of the head of the talus. While in plantar flexion, the foot supinates and the calcaneum inverts and the navicular moves downward and medially, rotating under the talus and the posterior end of the calcaneum moving upward and laterally. Capacity of the talo-calcaneo-navicular joint decreases, exposing more of the talar head dorsally. Clubfoot can be considered as a fixed exaggeration of typical equinovarus movement with talo-navicular dislocation, and in resistant clubfoot, pathological contracture of soft tissues prevents reduction of the navicular and calcaneum on the head of the talus. The three movements, equinus, inversion, and adduction, occur simultaneously rather than in isolated movements. Therefore, talo-navicular dislocation is an integral part of this deformity which needs to be corrected.

Turco,[4] discussed and highlighted his clinical observations that the majority of failures occurred when surgery was performed early, at less than one year of age (6 out of 10 of his own cases) and also when they are operated on after 6 years of age. Surgery is best performed at 1–2 years of age. As the child grows, deformity may increase and require triple arthrodesis in children over 8 years of age. Surgery in children older than this age should be done in selected cases, when skin is pliable and all tarsal joints are good and well preserved. He has reported iatrogenic talar abnormalities during conservative treatment due to excessive pressure and more fibrosis in prolonged conservative treatment in more severe deformities. He has also stressed pes planus due to overcorrections after complete releases. In surgery of rocker-bottom footed patients, flat foot resulted more often. He also reported skew-foot deformity with valgus as well as metatarsus adductus.

The author has noted regeneration of sectioned tibialis posterior tendon during a subsequent surgery. The author has also reported variation in pathological anatomy depending upon the age, severity, and previous treatment: talo-navicular subluxation/dislocation component, shape of talar head, and variation in the soft-tissue contracture component. The author also discovered some unusual pathoanatomical findings: flexor digitorum accessorius in 6.6%, a well-developed plantaris muscle in two feet, absent tibialis posterior tendon in eight feet (3.3%), and talo-calcanean coalition was seen in eight feet. The author has also commented that there are no typical feet after surgery, but effort should always be made to achieve that.

McKay[18,19,24] with his 20 years of experience describes, in three sections, pathoanatomy of clubfoot and method of treatment. In section I of his work, he gives a detailed description of pathoanatomy and principles of correction. He believes that failure to achieve correction is due to not recognizing horizontal rotation in the subtalar complex. In section II he describes closed treatment and provides a detailed description of surgical procedures and immediate postoperative management and, especially, the technique of lengthening of flexors to prevent their sheath to prevent scarring and hinged cast to start early ankle movements. In section III he describes the results of 102 clubfeet treated based on the above principles. He further commented in the first section that maximum deformity in clubfoot is due to inward rotation of the whole foot on the talus:

at the ankle causing equinus and heel varus and at the talo-calcaneal, talo-navicular, and calcaneo-cuboid joints, whereas the talus does not move and hence it remains small. Because of navicular shifting medially and plantarward, head/neck and body angle to the talus is also reduced due to their changed direction articulating with the navicular. With increasing age, this angulation decreases more and more. So correction has to be achieved early at all these joints. After correction, early motion to preserve movements of the ankle and encourage growth are paramount to correction. He then describes the morbid anatomy of the subtalar complex, consisting of three joints: talo-calcanean, talo-navicular, and calcaneo-cuboid. The calcaneum, along with the rest of the foot, rotates horizontally inward, pivoting on the interosseous talo-calcanean ligament and it comes under the head of the talus, and its tuberosity moves closer to the lateral malleolus, and this horizontal rotation of the calcaneum is more important than equinus for proximity of the calcanean tuberosity to the lateral malleolusm, though sagittal axis rotation (equinus) is also present. The navicular has to be brought to its typical position in correction. The author also described the pathoanatomy of the calcaneo-cuboid joint, which also is malpositioned with contracture of various ligaments, causing inversion and forefoot adduction. In section II he describes his new method of correcting the abnormal subtalar rotation based on the pathoanatomy of section I. He commented that non-operative correction can succeed in only 15% of cases and that also when prolonged bracing is continued. However, he still recommends it for two reasons: firstly, the patient may fall in 15% of success category cases and secondly, even if failed, the tissues do get stretched for better surgical correction. He described his technique for manipulative treatment. He believes that failure is mainly due to not recognizing horizontal subtalar rotation. His method of correction is based on the idea that the talus is rolled back into the ankle joint and equinus horizontal rotation of the subtalar joint and malposition of the talo-navicular and calcaneo-cuboid joints are corrected to achieve full correction of deformity, provided these are done early and movement started early in treatment, so as to promote growth of the talus. He described the detailed surgical procedure to correct the above abnormalities in 102 feet.

Ghali et al. report[25] confirmed what Simons presented in 1977 at a pediatric orthopedic international seminar in San Francisco, California: that only complete subtalar release can accomplish the derotation of the calcaneum in a single operation, because the scar of surgery will make subsequent surgeries extremely difficult.

Simons[20,21] also felt that both the soft tissue and osseous abnormalities are present, with soft tissues playing a more important part, and he described his complete subtalar release procedure, an extensive surgical procedure releasing the talus completely, done with a highly meticulous surgery, a magnifying loupe, under X-ray control and fixing the reduction with K-wires, in addition to excising a dorsolateral wedge retaining the calcaneo-cuboid joint. The author also quoted McKay[18,19] who followed his concept of calcaneal rotation presented in 1977. However, the author's complete subtalar release differs from McKay's in a number of ways, in the details of releasing different structures and the method of repositioning, in using intraoperative radiographs and postoperative care. McKay used different criteria for repositioning, no intraoperative X-rays, and he used hinged casts for early motion. There were many others minor details in the various surgical steps, which differed from those of McKay.

Antonio Scarpa[39] (1752–1832), in his memoir on congenital clubfeet in 1803 and, in 1818, in *The Classic* presented a complete review of literature on clubfoot. The first description of pathoanatomy of congenital clubfoot was also given by him, which is valid even today. He concluded that the deformity was due to medial twisting of the navicular, cuboid, and the calcaneum with respect to the talus. The talus, itself, was not altered in shape, but it was oblique in shape, particularly in older children and adults. He was convinced that the muscle abnormalities were secondary to distortion of bones. It is important to know that his description of pathoanatomy is the real beginning of understanding the complex pathoanatomy of clubfoot. He also described his method of treatment by manipulations and braces incorporating steel springs.

Windisch et al.[27,28] reported their findings in a comprehensive two-part study of pathoanatomy in seven idiopathic clubfeet in aborted fetuses between the twenty-fifth and thirty-seventh week of gestation and compared with two control feet of similar gestation period. In part I they felt that anatomical dissection is a very useful tool to describe the results of morphological changes of each isolated structure, which of course is not possible during surgical approaches. In part I, they studied bones and joints, and in part II, they studied ligaments, tendons, and muscles. In part I, seven feet were classified on the degree of severity into four grades: grade 1, mild or benign (one foot); grade 2, moderate deformity (one foot); grade 3, severe deformity (two feet); and grade 4, very severe deformity (three feet). They studied the articular surfaces and shapes of bones. Shapes and angles of all bones were studied by goniometer and Vernier caliper and their relationships. Their findings were slight internal tibial torsion, greater with more severe clubfoot; talus smaller in size with neck deviated medially and downward, more with increasing severity; and the calcaneum is smaller in size and is the main abnormal bone, as found in this study, with distorted articular surfaces corresponding to other bones, with the posterior articular surface as horizontal facilitating talar translation. It is deviated in equinus and varus. The talus showed neck-body inclination angle increasing with severity from 28° to 48° (typical 22°–24°), calcanean articular surface inclined antero-laterally, and head was inclined medially and downward. The navicular is broader dorsally and flattened antero-posteriorly, articulating with the sustentaculum, as well as with the medial malleolus in very severe cases. The cuboid and the three cuneiforms in the grade 3 and 4 deformities and the metatarsal also had some abnormalities. The authors have also commented that clubfoot is a three-dimensional deformity, and to quantify the different components of abnormalities, it will be essential to have data from multiple studies. Therefore, they did it by generating the data from multiple MRI studies by a computer-guided three-dimensional reconstruction in the horizontal, vertical, and sagittal planes, and they concluded that ossification disturbance of the calcaneum to be the primary fault.

In part II,[28] they studied pathoanatomy of ligaments, tendons, and muscles. Shape of the calcaneum and other bones influenced abnormalities of muscles, ligaments, and tendons conforming to the misshapen bones. On detailed study of the stabilizing system of ligaments, tendons, and muscles, they found adaptation of these tissues to be different according to the bony architecture, confirming, thereby, the bony deformity, especially the calcaneum, as the primary defect, while all soft-tissues structures adapting to the bones in order to provide the best functioning advantage for that deformed shape. The authors have quoted many reports agreeing with this hypothesis, but some others disagree with it. The authors have quoted from the literature that the calcaneofibular ligament is the most controversial, and it is lengthened in some parts and shortened in others. The authors have tried to explain this on the basis of their adaptation to the shape and requisite function. The authors also agree that it is difficult to prove all these facts because of the nature of this complex, three-dimensional deformity.

Pinto et al.[29] carried out radiographic studies retrospectively in the lateral weight-bearing position in 14 patients with unilateral clubfoot, who were operated on by the McKay technique, after a follow-up of 2–16 years with an average of 6.53 years. The talus was compared between the unaffected and the operated foot. They assessed the deformity of talus in the dome sphericity, head, height, and length, percentage, and degree of navicular subluxation; abnormalities of the Gissane angle; and the trabecular bone pattern. Abnormalities of the dome and head were present in 92.8% and of the trabecular pattern in 100%. The talar length ratio ranged from 0.61 to 0.88 in operated and control feet (mean 0.79; SD = 0.09), while height ratio ranged from 0.57 to 0.98 (mean 0.82; SD = 0.12). The Gissane angle was more in all operated feet, and all of them showed navicular subluxation at a rate ranging from 6.43% to 59.75% (mean 26.34%; SD = 16.66%). They concluded that talar abnormalities persist in 100% of cases after surgery.

We have seen in review of literature of pathoanatomy, that there is hardly any consensus in basic pathology. Similarly, management of clubfoot has been a controversial issue in the literature. Various conservative treatments with or without minimum invasive procedures have conflicting views, and a host of operative procedures already exist in the literature. Equally so, orthopedic surgeons are constantly confronted with new surgical procedures and medications, each with its own merits and demerits, and it requires a solid judgment to determine the most appropriate procedures for your patients. However, there is a general agreement that manipulation, serial plaster casts advocated by Kite[42] and now the innovation by Ponseti, based on rationality, which is a popular manipulation and casting treatment all over the world especially during the last 25 years, still offer the best treatment for all mild and moderate deformities, provided the treatment is given as recommended by their experts until the last follow-up. Ponseti had recommended the four Rs: Right age, Right type of deformity, Right regime of casting, and Right long-term bracing schedule. However, to strictly follow these four Rs is an extremely difficult task and all are not being adhered to what had been recommended because of inherent difficulties. The fault lies both with the caregivers as well as the beneficiaries. Only the highly dedicated and committed team of caregivers and conscientious recipients can do it. This problem is also noticeable with regard to the choice of surgical procedures for resistant and recurrent deformities. There are a large percentage of cases treated in childhood, which remain uncorrected or recur or continue undercorrected due to poverty and illiteracy, or they get various complications which do need to be corrected. This is so because such deformities are more common in developing countries, including India. The reason for these issues lies, in the first instance, in the incomplete understanding of basic pathoanatomy of the deformity, Therefore, a considered decision of comprehensive study of pathoanatomy of clubfoot by anatomical dissections in stillborn fetuses was taken after long-term clinical observations of solid evidence in its favor.

4.3.2 Author's pathoanatomy study

The study of pathoanatomy by the author had a dual purpose: firstly, to clarify the controversies found in the literature, whether muscles, bones, or both muscles and bones are the primary defect. The second objective of study of pathoanatomy was to evolve a new surgical technique based on complete correction of this pathoanatomy, including skin contracture. The author had a firm conviction about the presence of skin contracture, being of primary importance in pathoanatomy, which had not drawn attention earlier and remained neglected.

It was indeed a difficult task to find an adequate number of clubfeet in stillborn fetuses for dissection. However, it was a chance discovery of 15 such feet, in the six-to-nine month gestation period, in the anatomy museum of Government Medical College Patiala, India, from 400 stillborn fetuses collected in over two decades from various parts of Punjab and neighboring states. It is worth mentioning that this was **exclusive research material** with such a big collection of deformed feet in India, **"the one and only one."** How and from where such a large number of clubfeet in the foetal collection reached the anatomy museum is a guessing game. There is a well-known saying that **"Truth Is Stranger than Fiction."** This has to be, because truth is based on facts while fiction is a creation of the human mind. Complete pathoanatomy was studied in these 15 deformed feet, nine unilateral and three bilateral. They did not have any other obvious congenital deformity such as anencephaly, spina bifida, and so forth. The abnormal anatomy was compared with the unaffected foot in the unilateral and, in bilateral, with the same number of control feet of the same gestation period. These dissections were carried out in the mid 1970s. From a review of literature, only 80 dissections had been reported, with sixteen as the largest number and most with only one or two dissections. Ours has been the second largest series, with 15, and until now I have not been able to find more. Conflicting views, as described earlier, have been expressed in these reports.

The basic anatomy and the surgical techniques, (the first-generation technique) were documented in *Indian Journal of Orthopaedics*[30] in 1981 and *International Orthopaedics (SICOT)*[31] in 1987 (Figure 4.2) respectively.

Methods: Crown-rump length of fetuses was measured for determining the gestation period. Lower limbs were amputated above knee and preserved in jars containing formalin and duly labeled from 1-A to 15-A for abnormal feet and from 1-N to 15-N for control feet. After removing the skin, muscles were dissected out. Origin direction and insertion of all the leg muscles, that is, tibialis anterior, extensor digitorum longus, extensor hallucis longus, peroneous longus, peroneous brevis, extensor hallucis longus, peroneous longus, peroneous brevis, gastro-soleus, tibialis posterior, flexor hallucis longus, and abductor hallucis, were studied. However, extensor and flexor digitorum longus were examined for their origin alone as they were divided where they split into various slips before going to their insertions into toes. After removal of the muscles, they were tagged with labels for

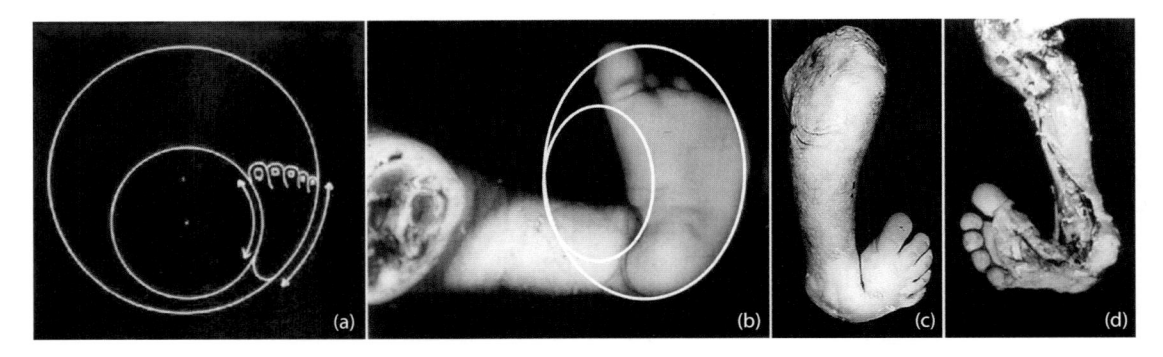

Figure 4.2 (a) and (b) Two circles provide evidence of skin contracture on a simulation diagram and actual cadaver clubfoot. (c) A cadaver clubfoot and leg seen from dorsal side. (d) Same foot after skin removal, showing clearly gross abnormalities of tibialis anterior, gastrosoleus/tendoachilles, dorsolateral hump.

identification. The tendon length, muscle length, and muscle mass of each muscle was measured with the help of a Vernier caliper and compared with the control. Then, the ligaments and joints were studied. In the ligaments, the spring ligament, the trio (deltoid ligament, conjoint posterior capsule of the ankle joint/subtaloid joints, and posterior talo-fibular ligament), besides the plantar ligaments and all other ligaments including toe joints were studied. Detailed anatomy of various joints (ankle, subtaloid, talo-calcaneo-navicular joint, calcaneo-cuboid, and others) was studied.

The angle of tibial torsion was measured by passing two pins, one proximally and the other distally, into the tibia. The tibia was fixed vertically and the ends of the pins were marked below and tibial torsion was measured by drawing parallelograms. The individual bones were dissected out and osteology of all the bones was studied. Head-body angle of the talus was measured by drawing two lines, one joining the center of the head of the talus and center of the anterior part of the body at the neck, and the second line joining the center of the anterior and posterior ends of the body. It was also done by the parallelogram principle. The talus and calcaneum were then sectioned to study their ossification centers.

4.3.2.1 AUTHOR'S OBSERVATIONS ON DETAILED MORBID ANATOMY

Muscles: The insertional abnormalities were similar in all the unilateral as well as bilateral deformed feet. Abductor hallucis was hypertrophied and smaller. Tendoachillis insertion was found to be extending on the medial side of the calcaneum in all the deformed feet. The tibialis anterior tendon was seen crossing the anterior border of the tibia in the lower part, lying on the medial surface. It was thick at its insertion, and its insertion on the plantar surface of the medical cuneiform and first metatarsal was more prominent than on their medial sides. The tibialis posterior tendon was also thicker and formed a thick fibro-tendinous mass in the sole. It was not possible to identify the nine individual insertions to various tarsals and metatarsals in the tiny feet of the fetuses. Regarding the length and mass of muscle in the extensor digitorum longus, extensor hallucis longus, and peronei, the total length of the muscle including its tendon was greater than typical and muscle mass was less in all the unilateral feet, while in bilateral cases, the findings differed a little. The gastro-soleus, tibialis anterior and posterior, flexor digitorum longus, flexor hallucis longus, and abductor hallucis were consistently shorter and thicker in all the unilateral feet, while in the bilateral feet, the findings were not so consistent (Figure 4.3a).

Figure 4.3b,c shows a dissected unilateral clubfoot compared with normal; (b) showing talo-navicular dislocation with talus in situ, (c) plantar surface of talo-navicular joint with navicular very close to sustentaculum tali and spring ligament not seen in the joint. There are two articular facets in the deformed foot on the plantar side, the one for the spring ligament is missing.

Ligaments, bones, and joints: The deltoid ligament was found to be thicker and shorter, much more in the posterior part. The spring ligament, which typically forms a large triangular area of the talo-calcaneo-navicular joint, disappeared from the joint and was found to be replaced by a thick

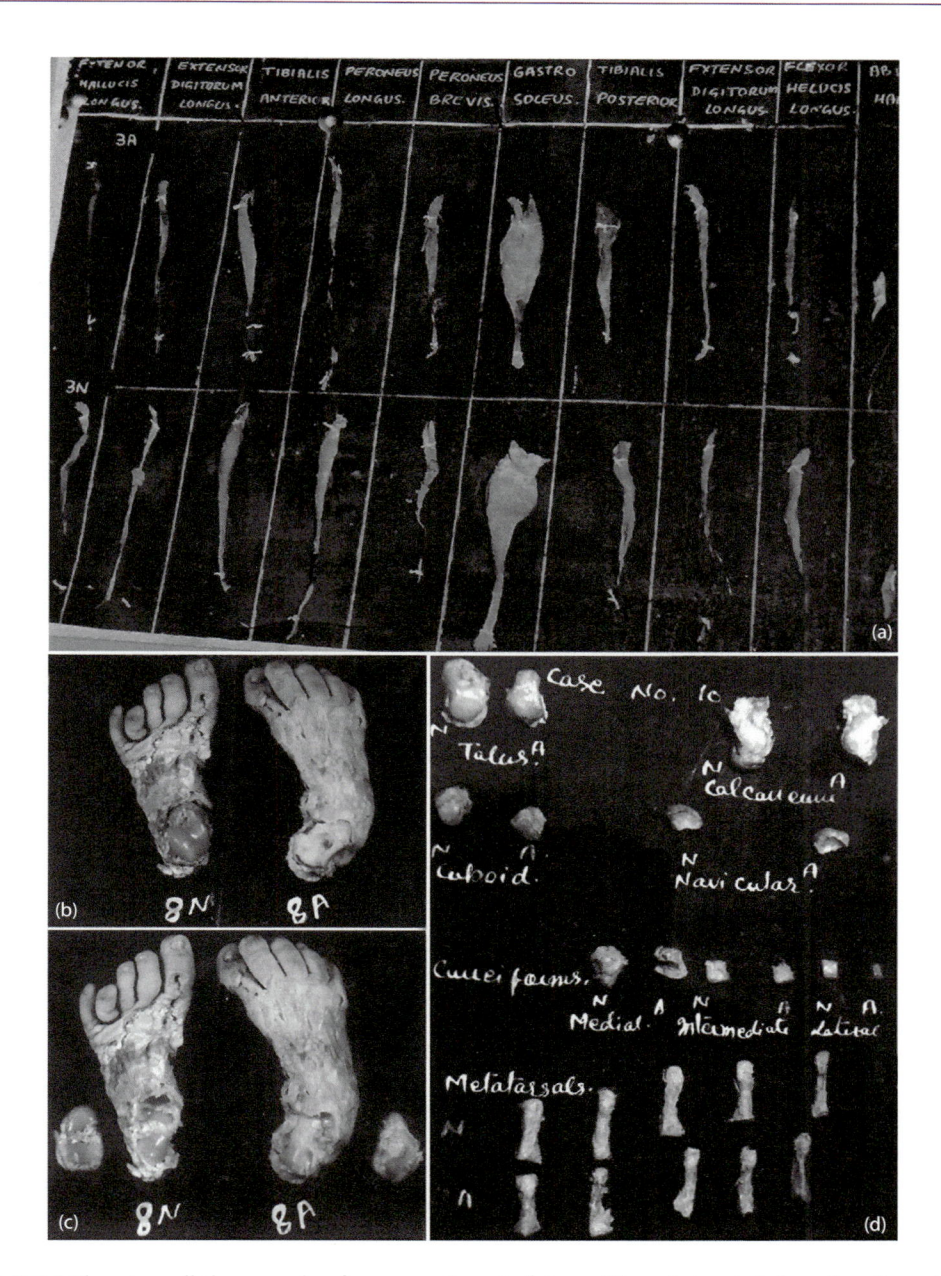

Figure 4.3 (a) Showing all the muscles from a cadaveric fetus with unilateral deformity, dissected out and labeled, compared with controls shown below each. (b) and (c) Deformed foot compared with control showing, talo-navicular dislocation with normal articular area of spring ligament underneath the head of talus missing in deformed foot. The navicular is lying adjacent to sustentaculum tali. (d) Showing differences of bones from the normal in the deformed foot in a unilateral deformity, with abnormal abbreviated as A and normal as N.

fibrous tissue mass underneath the navicular and sustentaculum tali, not visible from the superior aspect. From the superior aspect, the navicular was seen approximating the sustentaculum tali, and the spring ligament was lying entirely under these bones (Figure 4.3c). The conjoint posterior capsule of the ankle and subtaloid joint was replaced by a thick and short sheet of fibrous tissue mass, bringing the posterior distal end of the tibia closer to the calcaneum. This also extended laterally to the lateral malleolus, merging with the posterior talofibular ligament and medially up to medial malleolus, merging with the deltoid ligament. The ankle joint was in equinus position and shallower, and there was very little difference between the anterior and posterior diameters. Medial malleolus was small and lying almost in contact with the navicular in all the abnormal feet. The angle of tibial torsion was slightly less than typical in the clubfeet.

Talo-navicular joint/subtaloid joint: Head of the talus was regularly dislocated or subluxated dorsolaterally, with navicular articulating more on the medial and plantar side of the head of the talus, getting closer to the sustentaculum tali and medial malleolus. The inferior surface of the talus had two articular surfaces instead of the typical three. The one for the spring ligament was missing The articular surfaces of the subtaloid joint were distorted and smaller, and the area for the interosseous ligament was proportionately much larger (Figure 4.3c,d).

Talus: The talus, in all nine unilateral cases, was consistently smaller than the control in all its diameters, but this was not so in bilateral feet. In all the abnormal feet, the talus was abnormal in shape. Various borders dividing the different surfaces were not clearly demarcated as in typical feet, and various surfaces merged into each other. The comma-shaped medial articular surface was smaller and merged more or less with the superior surface. The superior articular surface was less convex, deformed, and shallower than the typical side. The inferior surface had two articular surfaces instead of the typical three, the one for the spring ligament was missing in the deformed foot. The articular surface for the navicular was more on the infero-medial surface than anterior. The area for interosseous ligament was larger in proportion to the inferior articular surface in the abnormal tali. The neck was small and deviated medially. The head/neck and body angle in the deformed tali varied from 108° to 145° as compared with the typical angle of 150°. The ossification center on cut section was smaller and irregular and was not yet developed in some cases.

Calcaneum: The calcaneum in all the unilateral deformed feet was smaller than typical in all its diameters. In all the abnormal feet, the posterior articular surface on the superior surface was very small and distorted. The sustentaculum tali was attenuated. In very severe deformities, the calcaneum was curved with the convexity laterally. On cut section, the ossification center was smaller than typical and irregular.

Other Bones: The cuboid and navicular were smaller in deformed feet. The navicular was smaller than typical in all its diameters in all unilateral clubfeet, and was displaced medially and downward. The three cuneiforms were smaller than typical in all the unilateral feet, but they were not consistently so in the bilateral feet. The measurements of metatarsals did not reveal any conclusive findings (Figure 4.3d).

It has been observed that the unilateral deformed feet have displayed consistently similar findings as compared with typical feet, while in the bilateral deformed feet, this was not so. The reason for this discrepancy in unilateral and bilateral deformities is that, in bilateral cases, the foot for comparison belonged to a different fetus. Bilateral feet, though not strictly comparable, however, did provide material for studying the abnormalities in clubfeet which were uniformly present.

4.3.2.2 BIOMECHANICS OF ABNORMAL MUSCLES, LIGAMENTS, AND JOINTS

The tibialis anterior tendon had directional and insertional abnormalities. It crossed the anterior border and medial surface of the tibia in lower part with its insertion on the medial cuneiform and first metatarsal more prominent on their plantar aspects, rather than their medial sides. This could be a reason for dynamic recurrence of the deformity after treatment as a result of muscular imbalance. This abnormality of direction and insertion accentuated the inversion and adduction effect of the muscle. Wiley[16] also observed the same directional abnormality of the tibialis anterior. The thinner and longer extensors of toes and peronei were weaker and thus had a lesser effect than typical to oppose equinus and inversion and thus indirectly contributed to the deformity. Hypertrophied smaller gastro-soleus, with its insertion extending on the medial side of the calcaneum, was considered a major force for causing equinus and also contributing to inversion too. Stewart[8] and Flinchum[9] reported similar abnormalities of the tendoachilles insertion. The tibialis posterior was also thick and short and a major deforming force. The abductor hallucis, although a small muscle, was short and hypertrophied and contributed to forefoot adduction, also reported by Stewart.[8]

After removing all the muscles, the foot still remains deformed but somewhat lesser, which means that the ligaments and bones also play their part in the deformity. The deltoid ligament was thick and short, especially the posterior fibers, and held the foot in equinus and inversion position. The abnormality of the deltoid and spring ligaments and the posterior capsule of the ankle joint all play a complementary role in causing and maintaining the deformity. In regard to the abnormalities of bones, the talus was the most deformed. The talus was small and deformed lying in abnormal position and played an important role in the causation and maintenance of the deformity. Its ossification center was small and irregular, suggesting a primary defect in the cartilage anlage. Waisbrod,[13] Shapiro and Glimcher[43] also commented on the irregular ossification center of this bone. The calcaneum too was smaller and abnormal in shape with a smaller and irregular ossification center, thus also playing an important role in the etiology of this condition. The other tarsal bones were also abnormal, but to a lesser extent, playing some role in the etiology.

From this detailed study of all the soft tissue and bones, it was concluded that **congenital club foot is a composite defect of the skin, fasciae, muscles, capsules, ligaments, and bones**. However, skin contracture was considered as the most important, because without correcting the skin contracture, the deeper correction is unthinkable. All the tissues developed abnormally in the embryonic stage due to certain defects in the germ plasm, which is still not clearly understood. There were gross changes in the soft tissue, as well as in the bones, especially the talus and calcaneum, which get further accentuated by adaptive changes with increasing age.

It was further concluded that the knowledge of pathoanatomy has to be applied clinically in the management of these deformities and correct the morbid anatomy as completely as possible, starting from the correction of skin contracture, followed by deeper correction and realignment of the foot to achieve the best possible results.

4.4 EVOLUTION OF SURGICAL TECHNIQUES

These were evolved in 3 phases with a distinct timeline, as a need based issue.

4.4.1 Evolution of first-generation surgical techniques on the author's pathoanatomy

Evidences of skin contracture: After having studied the pathological anatomy in dissected specimens of clubfoot in great detail and understanding its importance, it is imperative to recapitulate, once again, the important anatomical factors, with their clinical interpretations, responsible for the deformity and evolve a rational and effective surgical procedure for all severe and rigid deformities, achieving a correction, better than other procedures, which is more accepted by the patients.

4.4.1.1 SKIN CONTRACTURES

With continuous exposure to clubfoot for years together, it has been a matter of daily observation in every clubfoot, even in the newborn infants that during conservative treatment of manipulations and serial casting, skin of the foot on the postero-medial side becomes stretched and tight along with deeper tissues, while on the dorsolateral aspect it becomes wrinkled and loose. Further, the more severe and more rigid the deformity, the tighter is the skin on the postero-medial aspect. Obviously, the skin room is smaller and contracted with crowding of too many bones and soft tissues inside, like a small zipped pouch with too many objects stuffed in, or a fetus in utero, or a gymnast huddled in a small chamber, or a tortoise in its shell, or a closed fist with palmar skin contracted. A bigger bag is needed if you want to have too many objects freely mobile and systematically arranged in it. Clubfoot is a three-dimensional composite deformity, from the skin to the deeper tissues acting as a definite obstacle to good correction. Only deeper corrections were relied upon in all earlier surgical techniques. Therefore, it was also decided that during study of pathoanatomy in cadaveric clubfeet of still born fetuses, evidence for skin contracture must also be confirmed before the deeper soft tissues, bones, and joints dissections and compared with the typical. They are heterogeneous in nature. They may be primary only, present since birth, variable in degree, depending upon the severity and rigidity of deformity. They may get complicated by secondary contractures due to iatrogenic scars of previous surgeries or rarely due to direct trauma to the deformed foot or indirectly due to compartment syndrome after crush injury to the leg, leading to ischemic increase in severity of congenital deformity. There are so many clinical evidences of all varieties, which will be shown in Chapter 5. Besides the skin contracture, which is of prime importance, there are deeper abnormalities also of muscles and ligament and capsules as well as bones and joints. There is ample evidence of skin contracture as outlined below:

1. It can be seen from a two-circle diagram on a deformed foot of a stillborn fetus; the medial border of the foot is represented by the smaller circle and the lateral border by the larger circle. We will see that the medial border is clearly smaller than the lateral border of the foot. This is a one-dimensional view, and the same would be true of the other two dimensions, clubfoot being a three-dimensional deformity. A similar simulation two-circle diagram demonstrates the same (Figure 4.2a,b).
2. *Surface area*: This discrepancy can be confirmed by measuring the surface area of the posteromedial and dorsolateral aspects.
3. *Casting treatment*: We all very well know and appreciate that during conservative treatment of manipulation and casting treatment by Ponseti or others, an essential maneuver is stretching the posteromedial skin.
4. *Influence of age*: As age increases, the posteromedial side of the foot including skin grows less than the dorsolateral aspect, because the bones are lying in a deformed position, and there will be more growth toward the side of lesser resistance. Hence, the deformity increases with age and, accordingly, skin contracture will also increase.
5. *Unusual congenital contractures*: Rare congenital defects, including syndromic clubfeet, arthrogryposis multiplex congenita, associated osseous coalitions and polydactyly, constriction bands, and absent digits, have more severe primary skin contractures.
6. Heterogeneous secondary contractures due to scars of one or more previous surgeries. They may be adherent, extensive, bowstring, or keloid single or multiple scars.
7. Sometimes, there is additional hallux varus with midfoot varus as an additional skin contracture requiring correction.

These arguments leave no doubt about the reality of the presence of skin contracture, which must be remediated prior to correction of the deeper deformed structures as detailed above.

Because of the importance of pathoanatomy, it may be classified for simplification for a better understanding:

1. *Posterior contractures*: These are mainly due to a tight tendoachilles and a contracted/thick posterior capsule common to both the ankle and subtaloid joints, which is known as conjoint posterior capsule (CPC) of both ankle and subtalar joints, fixing the calcaneum to the posterior end of tibia in rigid equinus.
2. *Lateral contractures*: These are firstly due to thick, short, and wide interosseous talo-calcaneal ligament maintaining the talo-calcanean dislocation/subluxation and thereby varus deformity and secondly due to the posterior part of the lateral collateral ligament, also called posterior talo-fibular ligament, maintaining the equinus. Therefore, lateral contractures of these ligaments are responsible for preventing the correction of deformity.
3. *Varus at tarsal complex*: Besides the heel varus, it is at the midfoot due to muscular and ligamentous contractures, as well as bony abnormalities, especially of the talus. It is present at the talo-calcaneo-navicular, subtaloid, and calcaneo-cuboid joints. The muscles mainly responsible are tibialis posterior, flexor hallucis longus, flexor digitorum longus, and short flexors including the abductor hallucis. The main offending ligaments are the spring ligament, deltoid ligament, and the interosseous talo-calcanean ligament. In infancy, the deformity is mainly due to muscles and ligaments, but later, bones also get deformed. At birth, mostly the talus shows the maximum abnormality, but later, due to growth, adaptative changes occur in the other foot bones also due to overgrowth of the dorsolateral aspect, mainly the calcaneo-cuboid area, resisting correction of the deformity by soft-tissue dissection alone.
4. *Metatarsus varus*: In addition, tarsometatarsal joints are the other areas of varus deformity. This is ligamentous in the early stages, but, rarely, in older patients, adaptative changes occur in the bones.

5. *Plantar contractures*: These are also due to contracture of plantar fascia and short muscles arising from the calcaneum as well as plantar ligaments.
6. *Shortening of vessels and nerves*: They too are contracted. They must be protected by meticulous dissection and avoid sacrificing even the minor one in these mega-correction techniques. They can be lengthened only by gradual stretching and observation of circulation and sensations. There is a learning curve and it is not a quick fix technique.

These were the pathoanatomical features of dissections and clinical pathoanatomy. Based on these, the first-generation surgical technique was evolved in children and both the "pathoanatomy" and surgical technique evolved from it were published in *Indian Journal of Orthopaedics*[30] in 1981 in *International Orthopaedics (SICOT)*[31] in 1987 in the special Munich Congress issue (accepted in 1985) respectively. To give this technique a name, this was subsequently designated as the **DOLAR surgical technique**, which is an acronym of **DO**rso-**LA**teral **R**otation skin flap for correction of resistant clubfeet. This was a definite improvement for the treatment of such cases. Clubfoot, a three-dimensional deformity, definitely requires correction of skin contracture before deeper correction can be achieved. This technique is described in full detail in the Chapter 5.

4.4.2 Second-generation surgical technique

The first-generation surgical technique continued to be used in more and more patients gradually for more than two decades, leading to increasing awareness from patients to patients, in print and electronic media. Over the years, more and more resistant deformities in children, adolescents, and some adults started presenting. Many of them were residual or recurrent cases, already treated/operated by other techniques. In them, skin contracture was even more severe and was not correctible by rotation flap alone in spite of being three-dimensional. To achieve more expansion of skin contracture, Z plasty was added on the medial side to the rotation flap incision, to provide additional lengthening of skin on the medial side. Thus the DOLAR incision was converted to DOLARZ or DOLAR + Z plasty incision, giving rise to **second-generation or DOLARZ surgical technique**. With more skin expansion, better, deeper correction could be achieved, that too with a longer, flexible, and better functioning foot, without any arthrodesis procedure. Occasionally, a small insignificant gap remained at the posterior end of incision, which was covered by a small partial thickness (Thiersch) skin graft shaved off from the lower part of the leg or a small relaxing incision given proximally. Gradually, with increasing experience, in still more severe contractures in adults with bigger size foot, instead of one, even two Z-plasties and occasionally even three Z-plasties have been added to the rotation flap incision successfully. This continued further for more than a decade and was documented by Mittal[44] in an international journal. This publication was a case report with a unique pathoanatomy, that is, triple plus dislocation, a new pathoanatomy feature complicating the deformity and requiring correction with details given in Chapter 5, Case No. 14 (Figure 5.16a,b).

4.4.3 Third-generation technique with newer pathoanatomical features

Background: In spite of a voluminous maze of literature, especially after the advent of unrestricted use of the Internet for anything and everything, this still remained an unsolved problem. Millions of DALYs are wasted worldwide due to clubfoot related physico-psycho-socioeconomic handicap with tremendous GBD, which has to be dealt with at the global level. There are a large number of reasons for residual deformities, recurrences, and the obstacles in correction of deformities. The real breakthrough in the advancement of clinical research in pathoanatomy has been in the third phase during the last 7–8 years. With spreading awareness about availability of this treatment for rigid, recurrent, and severe untreated clubfeet, there has been a spurt of such cases presenting for treatment, especially in older age groups. Earlier they were sitting at home resigned to their fate. **They were not amenable to even the second-generation** DOLARZ technique. The skin cavity was extremely tight in these cases and required further expansion to avoid arthrodesis. As "necessity is the mother of invention," there has been tremendous advancement in clinical research of pathoanatomy during the last few years, and a large number of new features have been discovered, This has resulted in innovation of the third-generation surgical techniques, with many new features related to further expansion of skin as well as others for deeper corrections and not related to skin. Most of these newer pathoanatomical features have been published recently in *International Orthopaedics* (*SICOT*) February, 2018, as online-first publication (http://link.springer.com/article/10.1007/s00264-017-3741-6) and its print version in the June 2018 issue. Various newly discovered features including that **"Each Clubfoot Is Different"**, are being described below.

4.4.3.1 EACH CLUBFOOT IS DIFFERENT

We find this phrase mentioned in the literature by many authors, even as early as 400 BCE when Hippocrates made a statement and said, "there are more than one type of clubfoot." It just remained a statement without any explanation and real significance. I have worked it out, proving its truth beyond doubt, dealing with thousands of clubfeet, of all shades of deformities coming for conservative and surgical treatment during the last more than half a century. It is felt that it may be more appropriate if congenital clubfoot is designated **as clubfoot disease, including every clubfoot, even the rarest of the rare**.

The evidence is in abundance, as below:

1. There are four components of deformity; equinus, adduction, inversion, and cavus, and all are in different combinations in each case, thus every case will be different even at the time of birth.
2. Different age of presentation in every case from birth to late age further widens the difference, with deformity increasing with age.
3. Different influence of weight bearing in every case due to variation in the components of deformity as well as the time period for which the patient has walked.
4. Effect of differing modalities of treatment, conservative and one or more surgeries and heterogeneous/extensive scars.
5. Type of clubfoot, congenital or acquired, and if congenital, idiopathic, isolated, or syndromic deformities.
6. Associated congenital defects of the foot with variation in each one of them, for example, osseous coalitions, polydactyly, hallux varus, or unusual congenital skin contracture.
7. Effect of other congenital defects of the lower limbs on the deformity like genu varum, genu valgum, wind-swipe deformity of the knees, shortening, hypoplasia.
8. Delayed acquired morbidities, for example, painful dorsolateral callosity or inflamed or infected bursa, stress fracture, or painful plantar horn.
9. Other lower limb defects such as osteoarthritis of proximal joints of the ankle, knee, and spine due to longstanding abnormal weight bearing.
10. Post-treatment radiological variations other than the coalitions and multiple digits.
11. The acquired causes of clubfoot with their varied effects.

Therefore, clubfoot is a disease with a large number of variants as enumerated above and each is different. All the above arguments should leave no doubt that each patient has to be dealt with as a separate entity, requiring individual assessment, and surgical treatment will vary accordingly.

4.4.3.2 A GENERIC NAME

There are scores of confusing and diverse terms relating to the failed clubfoot deformities, for example, neglected, recurrent, relapsed, residual, resistant, recalcitrant, severe, rigid, untreated, undercorrected, metatarsus adductus, syndromic, and isolated, with or without heterogeneous surgical scars from one of more surgeries, at all ages from early childhood to late adulthood with the equal number of surgical procedures reported in the literature for their treatment but with no success. It was concluded after due deliberation, that all the above assembly of misleading names must be included under one family, because of the commonality of aim for all of them, that is, achieving a better looking and functioning correction that is more acceptable to patients. Hence, a generic unifying name of extreme deformities was given to them. Further on, they were classified into three hierarchic grades as **trimorphic extreme deformities**. Each grade is three dimensional: Grade 1, partially flexible joints, mostly seen in children; Grade 2, slightly mobile joints, mostly adolescents and adults; and Grade 3, little or no mobility, mostly adults with some degree of overlap among them.[32]

4.4.3.3 EVOLUTION OF DOLARZ-E—ADDING V-Y PLASTY TO ROTATION AND Z PLASTY (DOLARZ)

An extensive search of the literature revealed a large number of publications with very crucial and significant evidence from India and abroad, namely: Ponten,[33] Bhattacharya et al.,[34,35] Bhattacharya[36] and Cormack and Lamberty[37] mostly from plastic-surgery journals. Bhattacharya and his coworkers from India have done pioneering work in this regard, quoting others also. They deliberated that composite tissues, to cover gaps, used in plastic surgery for flaps consist of skin, subcutaneous tissue, and deep fascia with or without muscle tissue. A very good microvascular circulation exists in all these tissue planes, forming dense vascular arcades with a large number of perforators arising from all the three main lower limb vessels, namely, the posterior tibial, peroneal, and anterior tibial vessels. These perforators are musculocutaneous, fasciocutaneous, and even direct cutaneous ones, forming dense vascular networks. Deep fascia plays a significant role and is a highly vascular structure having suprafascial and subfascial vascular plexuses. Contrary to the common belief of no such optimism, there is a well-maintained microcirculation, both vascular as well as lymphatics, in this area.

Therefore, there is plenty of evidence-based proof to convince the scientific world about this nature's marvel. Based on these evidences and with confidence, the third-generation surgical technique was innovated and a meticulously executed distal-based V-Y plasty was also added to the rotation and Z plasty incision, to close the gap near the medial malleolus. This has been named DOLARZ-E, whereas E stands for extended. Besides this, additional Z-plasties were added in the medial part of the incision when required in more medial contracture. This has been termed as mega-correction, which may appear too aggressive or alarming, but is completely rational. This, three-in-one incision, all plastic surgery procedures, have been used by the author, an orthopedic surgeon, for the first time in clubfoot. To the best of my knowledge, I have not found the use of these three plastic-surgery procedures, in a single incision (three-in-one) by any plastic surgeon. However, one has to be very meticulous, remaining superficial to the deep fascia, not to damage the perforators with their microcirculation.

4.4.3.4 EQUINUS IN A NEW PERSPECTIVE

Equinus is the most important component of the clubfoot deformity. The name of the deformity, that is, equinovarus also suggests its significance. By convention, equinus is defined as plantar flexion at the ankle joint only, while plantar flexion at the intertarsal and tarsometatarsal joints (midfoot) is called cavus and still distally at the metatarsophalangeal and interphalangeal joints is called plantar flexion of a particular joint of that toe. Plantar flexion of the first tarsometatarsal joint is quite common in clubfoot and is called medial cavus, and with this, there is hyperextension of metatarsophalangeal joint of big toe or cock-up big toe, a usual accompaniment. When cavus is present at the whole of the midfoot, it is complete cavus and may be associated with hyperextension at other metatarsophalangeal joints also. So there are multiple names for a single directional deformity, that is, plantar flexion. Looking at the practical aspect, if we correct the equinus of the ankle only, equinus will still remain due to plantar flexion at all the distal joints as discussed. Our primary aim is correction of the deformity to the best possible extent. To achieve this, every plantar-flexion deformity at the foot, from ankle to toe joints, should be considered under a single name. Obviously, for complete correction of equinus, plantar flexion at all the joints from ankle to toes also need to be corrected. It was, therefore, considered to treat all plantar flexions from ankle to toe joints as part of equinus. Therefore, the other three levels of plantar flexion, that is, heel equinus (proximal foot), cavus (midfoot) and plantar flexion of toes (distal foot) were also included in equinus. This has been documented in the latest publication of the author in February 2018.[3]

Therefore, from the applied point of view, equinus has been viewed as a complex deformity comprising five hierarchic grades in increasing severity from G1 to G5. One or more or all five may be present in varying proportions in any case and are designated as EQ1–EQ5:

1. EQ1 is equinus at the ankle. This is the conventional plantar flexion at the ankle.
2. EQ2 as heel equinus, which is hidden equinus. The foot may appear plantigrade on standing with compensatory hyperextension at the knee, which is indirect evidence

of frequent residual equinus after treatment, conservative or surgical. It can be detected by many ways. If lesser degree of heel equinus is present, it will become evident only when the patient sits on his feet with knees flexed, a position of activities of daily living (ADL) in India. The other way of knowing this is passive dorsiflexion at the ankle with flexed knee, which will be less than usual; it can be seen as a decreased talo-calcanean angle (Beatson and Pearson[38]) and can even be measured.

3. EQ3 is plantar flexion at the midfoot at intertarsal and tarsometatarsal joints. It is called cavus by convention.
4. EQ4 is, by convention, called flexion deformity at the toe joints.
5. EQ5 is again at the ankle, but is an extreme version. This is unusual and presents in a long-standing deformity. In this, equinus at the ankle joint is present and there is also an oversized talus due to a long-standing equinus deformity (since birth), and the talus cannot go back into the ankle mortis on passive dorsiflexion due to talus lying anteriorly for many years.

In other words, it can be divided into the 5 grades EQ1–EQ5 and is present at four levels: EQ1 and EQ5 at the ankle; EQ2 is heel equinus at the proximal foot; EQ3 is at the midfoot, that is, intertarsal and tarsometatarsal joints; and EQ4 is at distal foot, that is, the toes. If we want to correct equinus completely, all levels of plantar flexion will have to be corrected and not only equinus of the ankle (Figure 4.4a).

4.4.3.5 HETEROGENEITY OF SCARS

This is a highly important aspect, because the author has seen innumerable varieties of scars during the last ten years or so that it will be quite pertinent to show these. Even the congenitally present primary contractures are extremely variable. Scars may vary in number (single or multiple) or quality (adherent, extensive, keloid, bowstring, etc.). All these varieties of primary contractures and secondary contractures due to scars will be shown in Chapter 5, along with their surgical treatment. They invariably require excision of the scars and varying skin expansion techniques (Figure 4.4b–i).

4.4.3.6 DEFORMITIES AT THE TOES

Sometimes in extreme deformities, as defined above, other deformities at the toes, such as (i) hallux varus (Figure 4.5a), (ii) isolated medial cavus with hyperextension of the metatarso-phalangeal (MP) joint with flexion deformity of interphalangeal (IP) joints of the great toe only, and (iii) complete midfoot cavus with hyperextension of all MP joints and flexion of IP joints at all toes, may be present. Hallux varus will have to be taken care of by an additional V-Y plasty at the great toe. We will also have to deal with the complete midfoot cavus deformity (EQ3). Flexion deformities at all interphalangeal joints of all the toes will also have to be corrected to achieve a very good looking and functioning foot (Figure 4.5b).

4.4.3.7 MUSCULAR ABNORMALITIES

Abductor hallucis is a small muscle and is hypertrophied in clubfoot, and it does play an important role in causing adduction and medial cavus. Tibialis posterior is a very powerful deforming force and its tendon has nine insertions, which can best be seen in adolescents and adults in grade 3 extreme deformities with fully developed tendons and bones. Contracture of this muscle is highly important, both in static as well as dynamic action. Its nine tentacle-like insertions pull the navicular and anterior end of the calcaneum with the rest of the bony attachments toward the medial malleolus and push the talar head dynamically during weight bearing and walking at every push off. This facilitates dorsolateral talo-navicular subluxation/dislocation with multiaxial movement at the subtalar joint due to the coupling of movements because of the direction of the articular surfaces. All the nine crowded insertions have to be divided to free the bones to spread them out, which will be shown later in the surgical techniques.

Tibialis anterior: I have seen unusual pathoanatomical features of the tibialis anterior. The first case was with its over-action, leading to a bizarre deformity in a very interesting 23-year-old male having a reversed foot gait, who had unilateral residual congenital clubfoot deformity with scars of early childhood surgery. This patient had a static and dynamic deformity aggravated by a long-standing contracted and overacting tibialis anterior, which can be seen in Figure 4.5d. The patient was walking in an almost 180° inverted

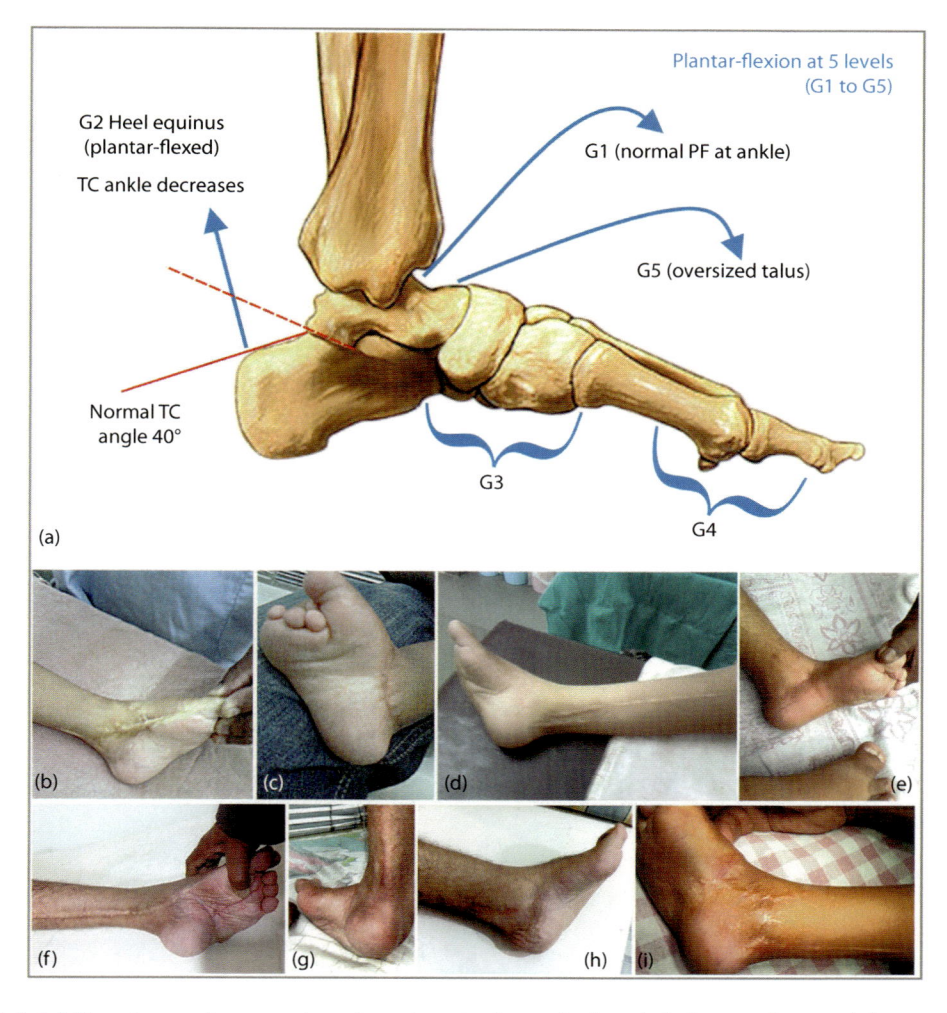

Figure 4.4 (a) Showing various grades of equinus in the articulated skeleton of normal foot and ankle: EQ1 at ankle, EQ2 at heel, EQ3 at intertarsal and tarsometatarsal joints, EQ4 at toe joints, and EQ5 also at ankle due to oversized talus vis-à-vis ankle mortis. EQ1 is lowest grade as G1 and EQ5 is highest as G5. This may be present in increasing severity as only EQ1 or as severest form as EQ5. (b) Bowstring/keloid surgical scar. (c) Unique congenital forefoot plantar skin contracture. (d) Keloid, bowstring scars of two surgeries on posterior and medial side. (e) Extensive adherent surgical scar, medial side. (f) Bowstring keloid surgical scar. (g) Extensive adherent medial and posterior surgical scars. (h) Multiple keloid and bowstring surgical scars with cock-up big toe and acute cavus. (i) Very extensive adherent multiple posterior and medial surgical scars.

foot gait with a large weight-bearing area on the dorsolateral aspect (Figure 4.5e). The second unusual case was of a 7-year-old female child with extremes of equinus, varus, and midfoot cavus as shown in Figure 4.5f. X-rays also showed extreme equinus with vertically positioned tali on both sides (Figure 4.5g,h). There was an abnormal thick slip of the tendon going in to the sole and getting inserted to the base of proximal phalanx of great toe (Figure 4.5i). Treatment of these 2 cases will be discussed in Chapter 5.

Tendoachilles percutaneous tenotomy scar: A densely-adherent 3″-long scarred area after triple percutaneous heel cord tenotomies with a gross deformity in a 2.5-year-old. The details of this unique case with three tendoachilles scars and its surgical treatment by innovative technique are shown in case descriptions in Chapter 5. There

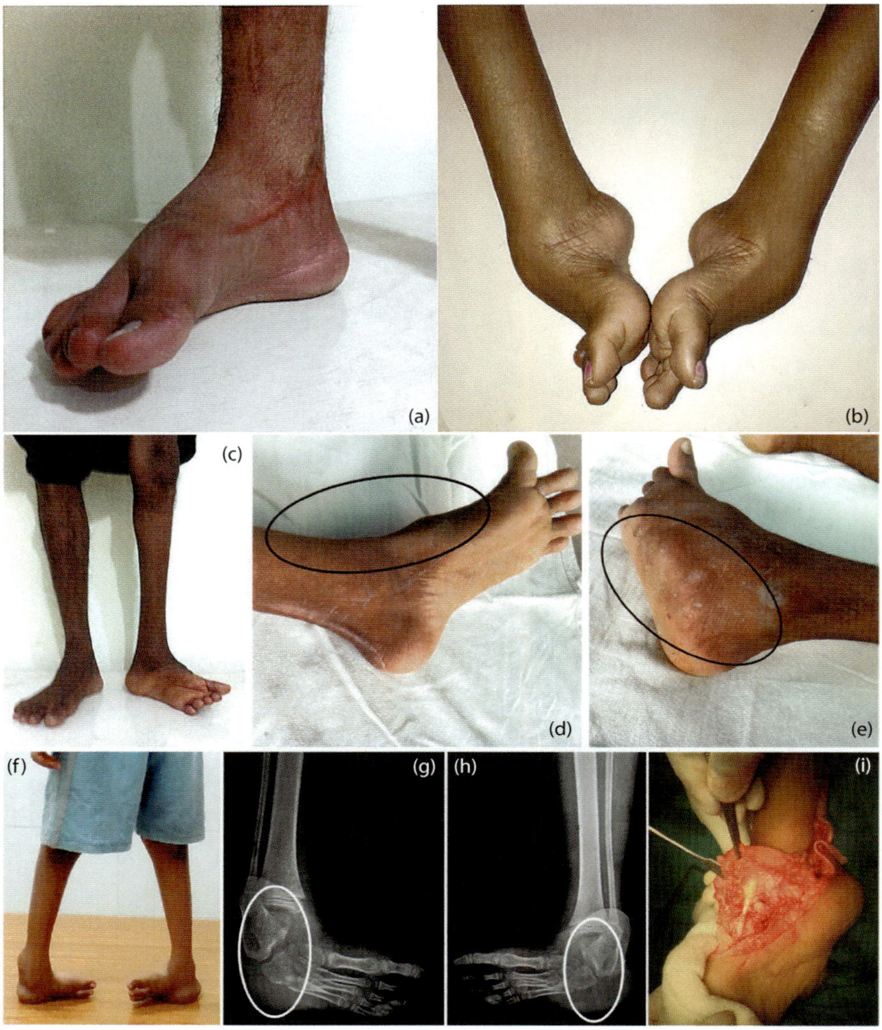

Figure 4.5 (a) Residual hallux varus. (b) Midfoot cavus with hyperextended MP joints and flexed IP joints (EQ4). (c–e) Overactive tibialis anterior with bizarre deformity, reversed foot gait, scars (bowstring) of earlier surgery, and highlighted depigmented weight-bearing area on dorsolateral aspect of foot. (f) Hyperacute equinus (EQ4) with huge callosities. (g) and (h) X-rays both feet with both tali vertical with head down below the ankle mortis and huge callosities at weight-bearing areas on talar head, cuboid, and anterior end of calcaneum in both feet. (i) Intraoperative abnormal tibialis anterior insertion going into the sole.

have been many cases of relapses due to this complication, which have been treated.

4.4.3.8 DORSOLATERAL HUMP

In clubfoot, depending upon the severity of the deformity, a dorsolateral hump is present in children, adolescents, and adults, which increases with duration of weight bearing. With increasing inversion, its site shifts more and more from the lateral to the dorsal side (Figure 4.5f). It is nature's attempt to decrease the stress of weight bearing by forming a bursa and thickening of skin, because dorsal skin is not the natural area of weight bearing. When the callosity is smaller with more cavus, a bursa is more likely to form and its size is also bigger, while with wider callosity, a bursa may not be present but only thickening of skin. Initially there is cornification of the outer skin and then a bursa under this provides a cushion effect for the weight-bearing area. With more weight bearing, this bursa may become inflamed, infected, and may even give way to pus discharge and even become chronic, especially in paralytic clubfoot due to spina bifida with sensory involvement.

4.4.3.9 SYMPTOMATIC GENU RECURVATUM

Residual equinus is a frequent residual deformity in treated clubfoot, conservatively or by surgery, and this, invariably, will result in compensatory hyperextension at the knee. Besides this, often in untreated clubfoot, it is a common observation for such patients to walk with asymptomatic hyperextended knees, but the foot is plantigrade, with occult equinus without any symptoms. This becomes a reason for not seeking treatment and continues until late age. Sometimes, they become symptomatic with various symptoms: a visible awkward gait making the patient or parents self-conscious, an inability to run, locking with pain and constant apprehension regarding falling. Intervention is certainly required in such cases. I have seen two such cases and treated them. One was a 12-year-old boy with unilateral residual equinus operated 10 years ago with an awkward gait and inability to run, and the other was an 18-year-old male with bilateral clubfeet, operated twice in early childhood with residual equinus (EQ3) with high dome and severe genu recurvatum with painful locking and instability with a history falling and constant apprehension. Their feet were treated, but not the knees, and the knees corrected of their own in due course. They will be shown in Chapter 5.

4.4.3.10 NUMEROUS UNUSUAL PATHOANATOMICAL PROBLEMS WITH MORBIDITY

With increasing awareness and unusual cases coming in, a large number of many more unusual pathoanatomical features have been discovered in recent years while treating these patients. Due to increased awareness, about 20 complications, hitherto ignored, have actually been seen by the author with reasons to operate for better quality of life in these cases: painful walking (due to inflamed bursa, bunion, infection, scar, ulcer); painful and unstable genu recurvatum and other knee deformities; stress fracture of the fifth metatarsal; heterogeneous scars (extensive, adherent, keloid, bowstring scars of earlier surgeries); marital problems (before and after); additional congenital defects (coalitions); polydactyly; arthrogryposis multiplex congenita; residual hallux varus; early osteoarthritis in the foot, knee, and spine; post-trauma problems; and others. All these complications have been seen by the author and have been documented in the recent international publication Mittal[32] and shown in Chapter 5. Many times, fear of surgery also plays an important role in untreated deformities until late age. Nothing concrete is available in the literature, except a few passing references, which advise arthrodesis of foot joints, for many of the above complications, resulting in a shortened stiff foot. In the present well documented techniques, triple arthrodesis is avoidable in the majority, with occasional exceptions. With additional skin expanders, bones and soft tissues can be comfortably accommodated in the opened-out position with maximum foot length with preserved flexibility.

These issues relate to physico-psycho-socioeconomic problems. Patients face physical handicap for running and jumping, awkward gait, inferiority complex, social problems such as social stigma and pre- and post-marital issues, less earning than typical individuals. Taken individually, the unique morbid anatomical features with their presenting complaints are described next, as each one is different. As these complicating issues of clubfoot have always remained neglected, they must be understood with actual case descriptions:

1. *Proximal joints*: Sometimes, there are associated congenital genu varum or genu valgum. Even in clubfeet persisting until late age, there is early onset of symptomatic osteoarthritis of not only the feet and knee joints but even the spine. Such cases have been seen by the author, and they increase loss of DALYs and consequently the GBD. This only shows that clubfeet should always be treated, even in late age, to avoid complications, as these newer techniques, with satisfying results, are meant for such cases and satisfying. As an example, the author has recently seen, in April 2018, a case of a 52-year-old female with extreme unilateral clubfoot deformity of right foot with genu valgum. She was going on with this highly rigid grade 3 extreme deformity of the right foot, as it was painless. Moreover, no satisfactory treatment was offered to her. Now,

Skin contracture was found to be the most important factor of pathoanatomy, based on evidence, which had always remained neglected worldwide. All the deeper soft tissues, as well as osseous structural abnormalities too, were contributing to the whole deformity: contractures of fasciae, various muscles, ligaments, bones, and joints were also present. The major components of the deformity revolved around the ankle, subtalar, and midtarsal joints, which have been described in detail along with their biomechanics. They were then analyzed in all the details with their clinical applications. Finally, considering the three-dimensional nature of the deformity and the prime importance of skin contracture, the first-generation new surgical technique was evolved which was three-dimensional correction of the skin contracture by a dorsolateral fasciocutaneous thick flap of loose skin, rotated posteromedially, where the skin is tight, called DOrsoLAteral Rotation skin flap for any and every resistant clubfoot in children. The acronym DOLAR was later used for this long name. Along with the release of skin contracture, the deeper correction of the posterior, medial, and lateral sides was called subtotal subtalar release or SSR, which was more than the partial subtalar release of Turco and less than the complete subtalar release of Simons.

This research has been executed in three, need-based phases and proved on ample evidence. The first-generation technique continued to be used for more than 20–25 years with gratifying results. Gradually, more severely contracted clubfeet in older children and adolescents started coming for treatment, which led to more research in further lengthening of skin. This led to evolution of the second-generation surgical technique with the addition of Z plasty on the medial side to provide more skin length. So, the DOLAR incision became DOLARZ, with highly gratifying results in older age groups. This also continued to be used for about one and a half decade. Because of the high impact of the Internet and other electronic and print media, the real breakthrough in research started and more patients with severe deformities at all ages from early childhood to late adults started coming for advice and treatment. This led to rethinking and discovery of newer vistas in pathoanatomy, and the era of evolution of the third-generation surgical technique started.

After this, there was a tremendous change in the concept of pathoanatomy. There were innumerable new concepts, which have been discussed in detail. **Each clubfoot is different** has been proved with numerous evidences. A generic name of "extreme clubfoot deformities" was given to scores of confusing names in the literature for resistant deformities. They were divided into three grades: trimorphic deformities grade 1–3 with different age groups with varying rigidity. For an all round universal three-dimensional expansion of skin, an abundance of evidence from the plastic surgery literature has been collected. Based on this evidence, V-Y plasty was incorporated in this DOLARZ incision to make it a unique three-in-one technique, used for the first time in clubfoot.

After the evolution of the third-generation surgical technique, there has been a nonstop deluge of new pathoanatomical features in relation to clubfoot. More and more cases with new problems are pouring in, all of which have been discussed above and will be further described in the next chapter. Even the latest one, discovered only in April or May of 2018, has been described. The most important of them all, that **each clubfoot is different**, has been discussed in detail with all the abundant evidence. Equinus, the most important element of the deformity, has been evaluated in a new light in a wider angle to achieve better correction of all plantar flexions from the ankle to distal interphalangeal joints. Heterogeneity of scars has been emphasized. In this category, many cases of Ponseti's casting with percutaneous heel cord tenotomy with resultant scar, as a cause of relapse, have been seen and treated successfully. Other morbid anatomy features such as deformities of toes, abnormalities of muscles, dorsolateral hump, and symptomatic knee deformities have been discovered and were discussed. As more and more extreme deformities presented, many more new features were discovered and treated: unusual tarsal dislocations, stress fractures, post-trauma effects on clubfoot, coalitions, plantar horn, high dome deformity, polydactyly, and osteoarthritis in proximal joints such as in knees have been discovered and treated. The value of scoring systems in extreme deformities has been considered, and this cannot be applied in these cases because of countless variables and each case being different. A latest case seen and treated in May 2018 has been a case of calcaneovarus due to heel cord tenotomy after Ponseti casting and a stretched-out heel cord, with an extensive scar lower down. With this solid background of pathoanatomy, we will now proceed to Chapter 5.

REFERENCES

1. Decker GAG, Du Plessis DJ; *Lee McGregor's synopsis of Surgical Anatomy* with a Foreword by Myberg JA (Indian Edition); Varghese Publishing House. Hind Rajasthan Building, Dadar, Bombay 400 014, 1995.
2. Bertetson A; Treatment of congenital clubfoot; *J Bone Joint Surg*; 1957;39-B:599.
3. Singer M, Fripp AT; Tibialis anterior transplant in congenital clubfoot; *J Bone Joint Surg*; 1958;40-B:252–255.
4. Turco VJ; Resistant congenital club feet. One stage posteromedial release with internal fixation. A follow up report of a fifteen-year experience; *J Bone Joint Surg*; 1979;61-A:805–814.
5. Huang YT, Lei W, Zhao L, Wang J; The treatment of congenital clubfoot by operation to correct deformity and achieve dynamic muscle balance; *J Bone Joint Surg*; 1999;81-B:858–862.
6. Tarraf and Carroll 1992 quoted by; Huang YT, Lei W, Zhao L, Wang J; The treatment of congenital club foot by operation to correct deformity and achieve dynamic muscle balance; *J Bone Joint Surg*; 1999;81-B(5):859–862.
7. Shands AR Jr.; *The Early Orthopaedic Surgeons of America*. St. Lousie: C.V. Mosby; 1970.
8. Stewart SF; Clubfoot; its incidence, causes and treatment. An anatomical physiological study; *J Bone Joint Surg*; 1951;33-A:577–590.
9. Flinchum D; Pathological anatomy in talipes equinovarus; *J Bone Joint Surg*; 1953;35-A(1):111–114.
10. Fried A; Recurrent congenital clubfoot. The role of M. tibialis posterior in etiology and treatment; *J Bone Joint Surg*; 1959;41-A:243–252.
11. Bissell TB; The morbid anatomy of congenital talipes equinovarus. *Arch. Paediatr*; 1888;5:406–418.
12. Irani RN, Sherman MS; The pathological anatomy of clubfoot; *J Bone Joint Surg*; 1963;45-A:45–52.
13. Waisbrod H; Congenital club foot. An anatomical study; *J Bone Joint Surg*; 1973;55-B(4):796–801.
14. Settle GW; The anatomy of congenital talipes equinovarus: Sixteen dissected specimens; *J Bone Joint Surg Am*; 1963;45(7):1341–1354.
15. Bechtol CO, Mossman HW; Clubfoot an embryological study of associated muscle abnormalities; *J Bone Joint Surg*; 1950;32-A:827–838.
16. Wiley AM; Clubfoot. An anatomical and experimental study of muscle growth; *J Bone Joint Surg*; 1959;41-B:821–835.
17. Turco VJ; Surgical correction of resistant club feet; *J Bone Joint Surg*; 1971;53-A:477–497.
18. McKay DW; New concept of and approach to morbid anatomy of clubfoot—Section I: Principles and morbid anatomy; *J Paediatr Orth*; 1982;(2):347–356.
19. McKay DW; New concept of and approach to morbid anatomy of clubfoot—Section II: Correction of the clubfoot; *J Paediatr Orth*; 1983;3:10–21.
20. Simons GW; Complete subtalar release in clubfoot part I; *J Bone Joint Surg*; 1985;67-A(7):1044–1055.
21. Simons GW; Complete subtalar release in clubfoot, part II; *J Bone Joint Surg*; 1985;67-A(7):1056–1065.
22. Goldner JL; Congenital talipes equinovarus-Changing concepts during the past twenty five years; *Orthop Trans*; 1979;3:306–307.
23. Hippocrates; *Great Books of the Western World*. Vol. 10, P. 110. Chicago: Encyclopedia Britannica; 1952.
24. McKay DW; New concept of and approach to clubfoot treatment—Section III: Evaluation and results; *J Paediatr Orth*; 1983;3:141–148.
25. Ghali NN, Smith RB, Clayden AD, Silk FF; The results of pantalar reduction in congenital talipes equinovarus; *J Bone Joint Surg*; 1983;65-B(1):1–7.
26. Scarpa A, Leonard FP; A memoir on the congenital club feet of children, and of the

mode of correcting that deformity; *Clin Orthop Relat Res*; Nov. 1994 Section I: Symposium: The Classic.
27. Windisch G, Anderbuber F, Haldi-Brandle V, Exener GU; Anatomical study for an updated comprehension of clubfoot. Part I: Bones and joints; *J Child Orthop*; 2007 Mar;1(1):69–77.
28. Windisch G, Anderbuber F, Haldi-Brandle V, Exener GU. Anatomical study for an updated comprehension of clubfoot. Part II: Ligaments, tendons and muscles; *J Child Orthop*; 2007;1(1):79–85.
29. Pinto JA, Hernandes AC, Buchaim TP, Blumetti FC, Chertman C, Yamane PC, Fernandes ADRC; Radiographic abnormalities of the talus in patients with clubfoot after surgical release using the McKay technique; *Rev Bras Ortop* [online]. 2011;46(3): [cited 2018-02-08], 293–298.
30. Mittal RL, Makhni SS, Sidhu GS; Morbid anatomy of congenital clubfoot; *Ind J Orthop*; December 1981;15(2):129–135.
31. Mittal RL; The surgical management of resistant clubfoot by rotation skin flap and extensive soft tissue release; *Int Orthop*; 1987;11(3):189–192.
32. Mittal RL; Trimorphic extreme clubfoot deformities and their management by triple surgical skin expanders: DOLAR, DOLARZ and DOLARZ-E (evidence based mega-corrections without arthrodesis); *Internat Orthop (SICOT)*; 2018. Online first. 20.2.2018 http://link.springer.com/article/10.1007/s00264-017-3741-6. and print version June issue (2018) 42:1297–1306 https://doi.org/10.1007/s00264-017-3741-6
33. Ponten B; The fasciocutaneous flap: Its use in soft tissue defects of lower limb; *Brit J Plast Surg*; 1981;34:215–220.
34. Bhattacharya V, Watts RK, Reddy GR; Live demonstration of microcirculation in the deep fascia and its implication; *European J Plas Surg*; 2005;(115):458–463.
35. Bhattacharya V, Barooah PS, Nag TC et al.; Detail microscopic analysis of deep fascia of lower limb and its surgical implication; *Ind J Plas Surg*; 2010;43:135–140.
36. Bhattacharya V; Experimental and clinical evidence based rationality of incorporation of deep fascia in tissue transfer for reconstructive surgery; *Ann Natl Acad Med Sci (India)*; 2016;52(4):222–231.
37. Cormack GG, Lamberty BGH; The fasciocutaneous system of vessels. The arterial anatomy of skin flap. Churchill Livingstone, 1986. https://www.amazon.com/Arterial-Anatomy-Skin-Flaps/dp/0443032149.
38. Beatson TR, Pearson JR; A method of assessing correction in clubfeet; *J Bone Joint Surg*; 1966;48B(1):40–50.
39. Antonio Scarpa (1752–1832) quoted by Grzybowski A, Sak J; *J Neurol*; 2013 (2);260:695–696.
40. Muller T; An anatomical study and discussion of congenital clubfoot in three neonates, Seven Foetuses and One Calf. *Medical Proceedings*; 1968;14:333. Quoted by Waisbrod 1973 at ref no 13.
41. Lloyd-Roberts GC; Congenital club foot. *J Bone Joint Surg*; 1964;46-B:369. Quoted by Waisbrod 1973 at ref. no 13.
42. Kite JH; Non-operative treatment of congenital club foot. *Clin Orthop*; 1972;84:29–38.
43. Shapiro F, Glimcher MJ; Gross and histological abnormalities of congenital club foot; *J Bone Joint Surg*; 1979-A; 61:522–530.
44. Mittal RL; Obstinate clubfoot with triple plus dislocation; *J Foot Ankle Surg (Asia-Pacific)*; 2014:1(2):72–77.

5

Extreme clubfoot deformities and their management

5.1 BACKGROUND

This is a highly important chapter, because extreme deformities are very prevalent, at all ages, right from birth to later age. They are much more common, especially in LMICs, where about 80% of the world population lives. They do need treatment to improve the patient's physico-psycho-socio-economic health.

In spite of voluminous literature on clubfoot, it still remains an unsolved problem. This had been stressed time and again in the literature, but never given its due importance and hence remained neglected. The problem is not with mild and moderate deformities of children, because they invariably get corrected with the various contemporary conservative and surgical methods. The real problem has been with the more severe deformities at all ages, from birth onward, wherein untreated, residual, and relapsed deformities keep showing up with increasing age after previous conservative and/or surgical treatments. More and more such reports are appearing in the literature, some even reporting as high as 95% relapse rate (Tarraf and Carroll[6]). This aspect of clubfoot has always remained a field of uncertainties and dilemmas, more so in extreme deformities in older age groups, syndromic deformities and many other rare problem cases. For such cases talectomy has been recommended frequently in the literature (Solund[10], Byington[11]), for improving the quality of life, but complete correction cannot be achieved. The author has been researching this very gray area for almost half a century and has achieved a breakthrough as shown in a landmark publication. An online first comprehensive article has recently been published, in the highly reputed *SICOT* journal *International Orthopaedics* in February 2018, and its print version in the June 2018 issue (Mittal[4]). The pathoanatomy of clubfoot has been conceived in a new perspective and based on this. Surgical techniques have been evolved for any conceivable clubfoot deformity, at any age with the best patient satisfaction. The most important strength of this research has been that it is based on ample evidence of pathoanatomy from anatomical dissections and consolidated on long-term clinical experience of surgical corrections in a large series. For these reasons, this book should prove to be a global resource for the future, with the latest material on clubfoot, as was also the observation of some of the reviewers at the proposal stage of this book stage for this book.

In order to help the readers fully understand these techniques along with their rationale, it is highly imperative to describe every possible detail in this chapter, because the recent publication had very brief descriptions of everything due to limitations of space. There may be many repetitions, which have been considered essential, keeping in view the importance, convenience and better understanding for the readers, regarding the newer and changing concepts about clubfoot.

Scores of confusing terms have been appearing in the literature for innumerable types of problematic clubfoot patients with various stages of rigid and severe deformities, each with a different name, as discussed in Chapter 4. However, they all converge to a common aim of good correction. Therefore, highly simplified and unifying names have been proposed for such deformities, as well as their surgical treatments. They have been **named Trimorphic Extreme Clubfoot Deformities with three hierarchic grades (1–3) and their management by triple surgical skin expanders.** All the details on pathoanatomy have already been discussed in Chapter 4, but they do need a review.

That each clubfoot is different is a hard fact, proved by evidence and documented in the *SICOT* publication too. This difference is evident even at birth, and it not only continues during childhood, adolescence and adulthood, but this variation goes on increasing due to variable factors in each patient. Although it was appreciated by Hippocrates as early as 400 BC when he said, "It appears that no two clubfeet are similar," this was a casual statement, which was disregarded and went into oblivion. It has now been proved by the author with concrete and plentiful evidence. Although discussed in Chapter 4, it is quite pertinent to briefly recapitulate its evidence based salient points:

1. Each of the four **components of deformity, namely equinus, adduction, inversion, and cavus**, varies in amount and rigidity in every newborn child.
2. This variation further increases with growth due to static effects and dynamic influences of weight bearing until late age, contributing their share of modifying effects on the severity and rigidity of deformity.
3. Effects of casting treatments, Ponseti and others, varying from case to case, with or without percutaneous tenotomy.
4. Effects of various surgeries (single or multiple) with heterogeneous scars leading to residual or recurrent deformities.
5. Other causes of clubfoot, for example, paralytic (flaccid and spastic) and traumatic, with specific disease-related variation of dynamic and static influences.
6. Large number of early and delayed complications, related to the deformed foot itself or problems arising in proximal joints. All these have been seen by the author and will be described in detail in this chapter. Therefore, considering all the myriad variables in clubfoot, this could, in fact, be **considered as "Clubfoot Disease"** with every conceivable equinovarus deformity falling under this. There is only one conclusion from all this discussion: each case needs individual assessment as a separate entity and then its correction should be planned. There cannot be a "one size fits all" policy in clubfoot. **This is a well-considered view and will help in better management of all clubfoot deformities.**

Presentation of clubfoot in such myriad variables was the reason to study the morbid anatomy of clubfoot by anatomical dissections in stillborn fetuses and gain a basic knowledge of the morbid anatomy of the disease. This has been consistently reinforced with evidence-based, clinical experience, gained from patients of different age groups with all their variations. It was concluded that, unless we correct the pathoanatomy as completely as possible, from skin to deep fascia, bones, and joints, we will not be successful in correcting the deformity. Enlargement of the skin chamber assumes the highest priority to achieve all the patient acceptability goals, which include a longer foot, mobile joints, cosmetically good shape, and improved function over the long term. None of the earlier surgical treatments could achieve all these goals, which mostly advocated arthrodesis or talectomy, but ignored the skin contracture. **If the container is small, the contents will always remain cramped.**

This research has evolved in three stages, being need based, with a distinct timeline with some overlap. First-generation research continued for about 25 years, second-generation for about 10 years, and third-generation has been going on for about 7–8 years and is still continuing. In fact, **the third-generation research has opened the floodgates for this research with unending possibilities.** Research is an ongoing process, especially in a disease like clubfoot, where variation is so wide. Even during the course of writing this book over the last one year, newer vistas have been constantly opening up in pathoanatomy as well as in the surgical steps needed for correction, and I have included **a couple of such cases, even without much follow-up, just to showcase these new things, never heard or seen earlier.** However, with the evidence at hand, there has always been an optimistic outlook of the results from previous experience, provided one is meticulous in technique and a dedicated outlook to improve.

5.2 EVOLUTION OF TRIPLE SURGICAL TECHNIQUES

First-generation research was carried out in two parts: the first part was the complete study of pathoanatomy as described in Chapter 4, which was well documented (Mittal[1]). The second part was evolution of a surgical technique based on the pathoanatomy. These patients were children, who were undercorrected/relapsed by earlier available conservative or surgical techniques or remained untreated. They were resistant to all other available methods of treatment. **The cutting edge concept** of this technique was first to correct the posteromedial skin contracture by rotating the loose skin from the dorsolateral side medially and backward, followed by the deeper correction. Correction of the skin contracture is the most important and very first thing to do, as emphasized earlier. As clubfoot is a three-dimensional deformity from skin to deeper tissues, its correction should also be three dimensional. The container has to be wider to accommodate the contents in an orderly arrangement. This was published in *International Orthopaedics*.[2] To give it a crisp and catchy name, the technique was later named using the acronym DOLAR (from **DO**rso-**LA**teral **R**otation), giving importance to the skin contracture in clubfoot correction. The deeper releases of posterior, medial, subtalar, and lateral were also given a technical name, Subtotal Subtalar Release, or SSR, in contrast with the Partial Subtalar Release and Complete Subtalar Releases, PSTR and CSTR, of Turco[12] and Simons[13], respectively. The advantage of SSR over the other two is: That in partial subtaslar release, talus is not sufficiently moblie, because lateral release i.e. interosseous talocalcanean ligament is not touched at all and hence talus is not sufficiently free to rotate over calcaneum due to this intact tough ligament; whereas CSTR is too aggressive, must be done under X-ray control, and even then often leads to overcorrections, as reported by Simons himself. As the need arose for improvement for more rigid deformities, this was followed by second-generation research with better measures to expand the skin and deeper structures. Demand arose for even grade 3 rigid deformities and the third-generation research got under way, which further opened the vast horizon with more and more scope for improving things.

5.2.1 First-generation (DOLAR) surgical technique

This was the first innovation in this chain of surgical techniques, which was started in grade 1 extreme deformities as described in detail here.

All operations are done under pneumatic tourniquet. As these are extensive surgeries, they have to be meticulous, preserving the smallest neurovascular structures. The incision consists of two parts: a semicircular part on the dorsum and medial side of the foot and the longitudinal part on the leg. For a beginner at this technique, a roughly semicircular mark is made on the foot with the dividers of a geometry box. One prong of the dividers is placed over the center of the ankle joint in front and the other prong is opened out to reach behind the fifth metatarsal base. A semicircle is marked over the dorsum, toward the medial side, to reach near the insertion of the tendoachilles behind the medial malleolus. As one gets experienced in marking the semicircular part of the incision, it can be done with a free hand and dividers will no longer be needed. This is then prolonged proximally in a longitudinal direction, on the medial side of the leg, in front of the tendoachilles, for about four inches. A limited and thick fasciocutaneous flap is raised for only 1.5–2 centimeters. All the posterior, medial, plantar, subtalar, and lateral releases, along with talo-navicular reduction and tarsometatarsal mobilization are done through this incision. Even other procedures such as a dorsolateral wedge resection are done through it, whenever required. **It is important to describe each step of the surgical procedure in order to be able to correct these extreme deformities:**

1. The first step is Z plasty of the tendoachilles, dividing the medial half from the calcaneum so as to undo the adverse, inverting effect of this abnormal medial insertion of the heel cord.
2. The hypertrophied abductor hallucis is released forward with fine dissection to annul its adverse effect of adduction contracture on the midfoot.
3. After that, the tibialis posterior tendon is exposed from behind the medial malleolus in its groove and all its nine insertions to various bones are traced in the sole of the foot

and divided, remaining close to the bones. In a small child, it will be difficult to identify the nine insertions, but it is important to reach the depth to release these. At the other end of the scale, in adults, it is much easier to identify the attachments and deal with them. This step is important in correction of varus (inversion and adduction) and midfoot cavus (Figure 5.2b).

4. Flexor hallucis longus and flexor digitorum tendons are divided at Henry's knot.
5. After that and after retracting all tendons and neurovascular structures forward behind the medial malleolus, the next step is dealing with the "trio," i.e., the conjoint posterior capsule of the ankle and subtaloid joint, its continuation medially with the posterior part of the deltoid ligament and laterally with the posterior talofibular ligament (posterior part of the lateral collateral ligament of the ankle), forming a thick continuous capsular sheet significantly responsible for equinus, especially heel equinus (EQ2). This is divided completely from medial to lateral side to open up the ankle and subtaloid joint under vision and to see both joints moving; otherwise EQ2 will not be corrected fully.
6. Steindler's release of the plantar aponeurosis and flexor digitorum brevis from under the calcaneum is performed.
7. The spring ligament (plantar calcaneo-navicular ligament) is now exposed by retracting all other tissues away from the bones. It will be seen below the navicular and sustentaculum tali as a thick sheet, the bony landmarks lying close to each other. Normally it forms a wide triangular area between these two attachments for the head of the talus to rest on it. A significant fact of pathoanatomy that is not often appreciated is that there are usually three articular areas at the plantar aspect of the talo-calcaneo-navicular joint for the talus, one each at the navicular and sustentaculum tali and the third at the spring ligament lying between them, its attachments. In clubfoot, there are only two articular areas; the one for the spring ligament is missing and the sustentaculum tali is lying close to the navicular. This is divided completely from lateral to medial side to open up the space between the navicular and sustentaculum.
8. The interosseous talo-calcaneal ligament is now divided by inserting a tenotomy knife blindly in the sinus tarsi from the lateral side at its normal surface marking as a shallow depression, after pulling the skin slightly forward to prevent adhesion there, because on releasing the pulled skin, normal skin will come over the deeper cut. This will free the talus sufficiently (subtotal), more than partial but less than complete, so that it can be manipulated easily to reduce talo-navicular dislocation, mostly present in clubfoot.
9. Tarsometatarsal mobilization is done by dividing the appropriate ligaments after Kendrick et al.,[14] in cases where rigid metatarsus varus is present.
10. For severe varus and in children over four years of age, the modified Dillwyn Evan procedure, i.e., excision of a dorsolateral wedge from the cuboid is done and not from the calcaneocuboid joint, in order to retain movements at the calcaneocuboid joint.
11. Talo-navicular dislocation is now reduced by pulling the talar head medially and plantarward with a curved artery forceps around its neck on the lateral side and abducting and elevating the forefoot to bring the navicular in front of the talar head in its normal position, and it is fixed with a K-wire passed from in front into the talus.
12. The cuboid open wedge is closed with two K-wires at different angles.
13. At this stage, when the surgery is complete, the tourniquet is deflated, circulation is ensured, and complete hemostasis is secured to minimize postoperative edema. Sometimes, in less severe cases, the foot can be fully corrected without any force and with good circulation.
14. For closure of the wound, the amount of possible rotation of the flap can be roughly assessed by passively manipulating the flap medially and posteriorly before starting stitching. **In this surgery, stitching is not started from one end to the other as in other surgeries.** Maximum rotation of the skin flap is crucial here, and hence, closure of the wound is started around the middle on the medial side of the foot at an appropriate place.
15. **Placement of the first stitch is important so as to bring about maximum rotation of the flap.**

16. The dog ear left on the distal side at the lateral end of the dorsolateral flap is adjusted gradually by taking a wider bite on the dog-ear side and a lesser bite on the proximal side.

The rotation-flap incision details are shown in diagrammatic representation in Figure 5.1. (Figure 5.1a–d: After the diagram, the same is also being shown in the photographs on an actual clubfoot for better understanding [Figure 5.1e–g].)

Postoperative management: After wound closure, no force is required to keep the foot in the corrected position in less-resistant deformities with good circulation in the foot up to the toes, including the flap area. A well-padded, below-knee plaster cast is applied. Stitches are removed at three weeks along with the K-wire (sometimes later in more severe deformities) and a plaster cast reapplied. The period of immobilization varies from two to three months, depending upon age and severity of the deformity. A more severe deformity in an older child needs longer immobilization, with more cast changes. In more rigid and severe deformities in older children, force is required to keep the foot in the corrected position, with risk of circulatory embarrassment by postoperative edema. In such cases, a well-padded cast is given in the undercorrected position and reapplied in a more-corrected position every 2–3 weeks until full correction is achieved. After removing the plaster cast, the child usually walks about in ordinary shoes, except in some cases in which talipes shoes with a straight inner border and a shoe raise on the outer border are used to avoid recurrence of deformity. Regular follow up, with increasing intervals, is important for a couple of years.

Hidden equinus: This is an important consideration in clubfoot, because it is not only the plantigrade foot, but full restoration of dorsiflexion of about 20° after correction of the deformity, which

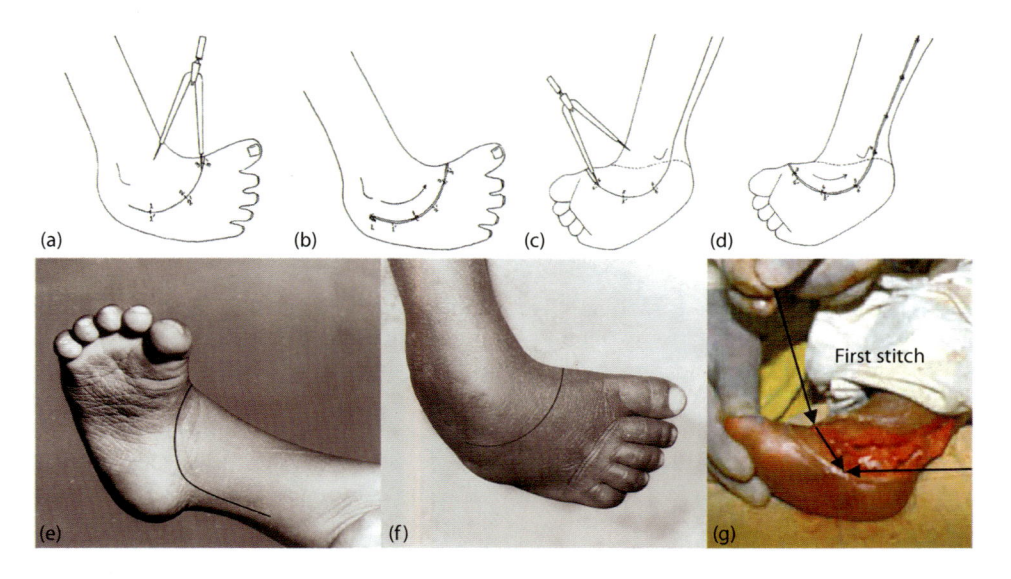

Figure 5.1 **(a–g)** Diagram and actual clubfoot **(a–d)** showing the skin flap marked out with the help of dividers and the amount of rotation at the end of operation: **(a)** Dorsal surface with incision mark. **(b)** Medial and planter side of foot with incision mark. **(c)** Dorsal surface with the rotated flap and arrow showing the direction of rotation. The distal portion of skin covering the dorsolateral aspect becomes loose after closure as depicted by letter **L** as shown in figure in **(b)**. **(d)** Medial and plantar aspect of foot after rotation of flap and wound closure with arrow depicting the direction of rotation and the numbers showing the amount of rotation achieved. **(e)** Incision mark on the posteromedial aspect of a rigid clubfoot in a one-year-old child. **(f)** Incision mark on the dorsolateral aspect. **(g)** Intraoperative in a case, showing application of first stitch and the amount of rotation of the skin flap which can be brought about. (Figure 5.1(a–d): Reprinted/adapted by kind permission and courtesy from Springer Nature and Copyright Clearance Center's RightsLink. From author's own published article; Mittal RL. *Int Orthop (SICOT)*;1987;11(3):189–192. For the book *Clubfoot: A Comprehensive Approach* (past present and future) for the publisher Taylor & Francis Group by Dr. R. L. Mittal. 2018–2019.)

is to be achieved for an excellent result. Lesser dorsiflexion, even if the foot is neutral on standing, means hidden equinus is present. There is a simple test to detect hidden equinus: in standing position with feet fully plantigrade; if the patient sits on the ground with fully flexed knees (an important position for ADL in India), both the feet will be fully plantigrade if there is no hidden equinus. This position is possible only if there is 20° of dorsiflexion at the ankle. If hidden equinus is present, the heel of that side in a unilateral case and of both sides in bilateral clubfoot will become raised from the ground. This distance from the ground to the heel can be measured in inches, and it is reproducible with accuracy. This test is very authentic, being subjective as well as objective. Patient will often complain about it specifically as heel/heels not touching the ground, as this is an important position in India for ADL. The other test, by passively dorsiflexing the foot in the lying down position, with knee flexed, is only a rough objective sign with individual variation. The hidden equinus and its correction after surgery at follow-up will be seen in the photographs of many individual cases later in this chapter. Specifically, this may be seen in Case No. 15.

Criteria for grading the results: The criteria used for grading the results in the first-generation research were as follows. **Excellent**—Healthy scar, deformity fully corrected with fully plantigrade foot without any hidden equinus. **Good**—Healthy scar, foot fully plantigrade without hidden equinus, but minor degree of metatarsus varus present. **Poor**—Partial correction of deformity with contracture of scar or overcorrection with valgus foot. These criteria were published in *International Orthopaedics* in 1987 in a series of 100 feet. Surgery was performed after the walking age and not before it: in 80 feet of patients between one and four years of age, twelve feet of patients between four and eight years of age, five feet of patients between eight and ten years of age, and only three feet of patients between nine months and one year of age. Besides a good clinical assessment, radiological assessment was done by measuring calcaneometatarsal angle in the anteroposterior view and talo-calcanean alignment in anteroposterior and lateral skiagrams.[5] Radiological assessment was found to be useful in deciding the amount of dissection required in each case. However, it did not correlate with clinical correction of the deformity, as there may be radiological undercorrection with excellent clinical correction and vice versa. The follow-up period in this published series varied from one to nine years, with an average of 43 months, and in 50% follow-up was for more than five years. Results of this series were 52% excellent, 42% good, and 6% poor. The assessment criteria were modified with the changed concept of clubfoot and were formulated on the patient satisfaction level. He or she is the beneficiary and is the best judge of the benefits.

This publication of *International Orthopaedics* in 1987, served as an incentive to continue further. First of all, a crisp and catchy acronym name, DOLAR skin flap, was given to the procedure. For almost 20–25 years, this era continued.

5.2.2 Second-generation research and the DOLARZ surgical technique

With continued involvement in clubfoot surgeries and spreading public awareness through hearsay, print media, or direct evidence from a treated patient to an untreated patient, more and more uncorrected or undercorrected, rigid deformities with many other complications in older age groups, and even in some younger children, started coming for treatment. Being more rigid and more severe, they could not be corrected by only the DOLAR technique. This prompted a newer thought process. However, the attention was again on how to expand the skin further to achieve better deeper correction. Because of the rationale and success of the rotation skin flap, a Z plasty was added on the medial side of the incision with its thick fasciocutaneous flap, to make it **a 2-in-1 procedure** (Figure 5.2a). Deeper corrections were also more extensive in such cases. In older patients, the nine insertions of tibialis posterior could be traced better in the sole and divided (Figure 5.2b). With more experience and more successful results, two Z plasties were being added more frequently for more medial lengthening (Figure 5.2a). Occasionally, in older patients with a larger foot, even a third Z plasty could be added. Thus the second-generation technique, DOLAR + Z plasties, or DOLARZ, technique evolved. This was a thick fasciocutaneous flap, meticulously carried out, with the least undermining in order to preserve the lifeline of the flap.

Many unusual radiological features were discovered, which too were corrected by innovative procedures. As a typical example, there was a unique case

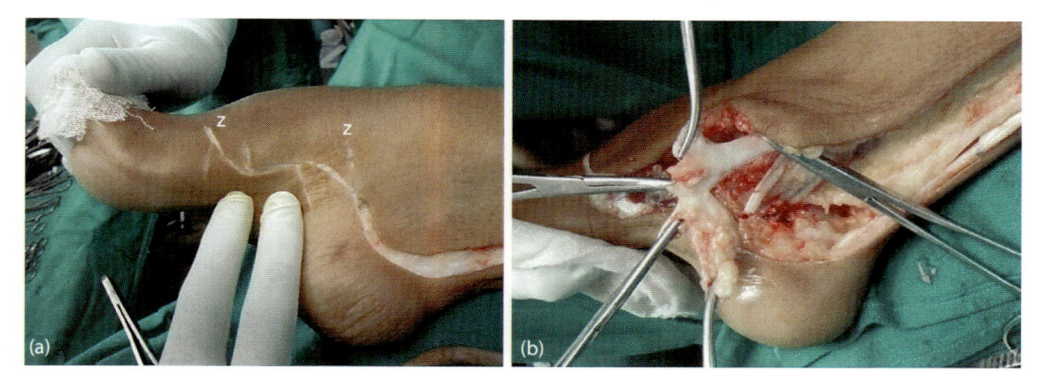

Figure 5.2 (a) An extremely rigid clubfoot in an adult with extreme cavus and varus with rotation and two Z plasty incisions are seen. (b) Nine insertions of tibialis posterior released from its attachments in the sole of the foot can also be seen.

of triple plus dislocation, which was corrected by sliding osteotomy of the cuboild. This case has been discussed in detail, and photographs of this case can be seen later in this chapter in case descriptions of Case 14 and Figure 5.16A. Plantar and medial ligaments also required more thorough attention for correction. The talo-navicular dislocation was not always present, but other tarsal malalignments were present, which were corrected in the best possible way.

5.2.3 Third-generation research and the DOLARZ-E surgical technique

There were a large number of newer pathoanatomical features, discovered by the author, which were described in detail in Chapter 4. With the success of the second phase of research and highly gratifying results with the 2-in-1 (DOLARZ) skin expansion technique, the third phase of three-dimensional skin expansion started. There were a large number of newer pathoanatomical features, discovered by the author, which were described in detail in Chapter 4. With further spread of public awareness, even more extreme cases of grade 3, with undercorrected or uncorrected deformities in adolescents/adults, and some even very young children, started presenting for treatment. This led to the evolution of the third-generation surgical techniques, the DOLARZ-E, i.e., DOLAR + Z + V-Y plasty, all three plastic surgery procedures in the same incision to provide the real universal expansion of skin in three dimensions. From concrete evidence in many reports in plastic surgery journals worldwide, it was considered appropriate to add V-Y plasty also to this incision in clubfoot. For the first time, the author used all three plastic surgery procedures: rotation flap, Z plasty, and V-Y plasty, as 3-in-1, in the same incision in highly meticulous surgeries in clubfeet. Instead of adding V-Y as a suffix, the letter E has been used to denote Extended in a broader sense, because this includes not only V-Y plasty of the skin but also other minor skin procedures for facilitating skin cover, rather than using major V-Y plasty, for example, a small partial-thickness skin graft (Thiersch graft) or a proximal relaxing incision for facilitating small-wound closure at the surgical site or even for facilitating a closure of a V-Y plasty flap, or multiple small lazy Z plasties instead of one big one and even a fillet flap where filleting is indicated, which will be described later in this chapter. The gap at the site of the relaxing incision can be closed by a little undermining as the skin is healthy and elastic there. In one case in an adult with a rigid grade 3 extreme deformity with extensive scars, a double V-Y plasty, one with a distal base and the other with a proximal base, were used (Case 26). This was done in a meticulous technique preserving the neurovascular and lymphatic networks with their perforators. Besides these skin procedures, numerous deeper surgical steps, many different innovative ones, have been used to obtain a desired deeper correction. There are many other issues required to be dealt with when the associated complications also have to be treated. This could be done by a large number of surgical procedures under the heading of DOLARZ-E which are not related directly to the foot deformity, but result as complications from the foot deformity. They too must be treated. There has been an influx of such cases of uncorrected or undercorrected clubfeet at all ages, presenting various complicating issues for treatment. Numerous new ideas have emerged in the pathoanatomy of clubfoot during this third phase research.

Each new case had something different to diagnose and treat. From this evidence-based insight, the whole concept of pathoanatomy of clubfoot and its surgical management has been reorganized in a new perspective, which was published recently (online first in February 2018) as a comprehensive article in *International Orthopaedics* and now in its print version in June 2018. Pathoanatomy of these new features has been described, in detail, in Chapter 4. The number of surgical steps/procedures is so large that it would be difficult, as well as out of context, to describe each of these procedures in one paragraph, as they are so diverse. Hence, after the description of basic V-Y plasty, it will be interesting to describe each of these procedures in the actual description of each patient, making them easily understandable. Such cases are very frequently seen in all ages in all LMICs of Asia and Africa, and many other LMICs, but have remained neglected or inadequately treated for want of good treatment.

Shaping of VY-plasty Flap: The third-generation, or DOLARZ-E, surgical technique is a 3-in-1 surgical incision for grade 3 extreme deformities (see pathoanatomy), present from birth as untreated or with scars of one or more earlier surgeries at all ages, in children as well as adults. In most of the cases, it is three-in-one skin expanding incision, but sometimes, innovations have to be used to close the wound; e.g. adding fillet flap to make it 4-in-1 or a double V-Y plasty etc. As a rule, V-Y plasty is added to the incision after all corrections, when a gap in the wound is under tension and cannot be closed after rotation + Z-plasty (one or more) incision in rigid grade 3 deformities and where scars have been excised.

Wound closure is started by rotating the flap on the medial side of the foot and on the leg from the proximal to the distal side. An elliptical gap of variable size, below and behind the medial malleolus, remains unclosed. In such cases, depending upon the size of the gap, distal-based, inverted V-shaped incision is marked with a fine stab knife over the skin. Remaining superficial to the deep fascia, blunt dissection is meticulously performed, the skin of the flap made freely mobile, preserving every possible mini-vascular supply of the flap. This triangular flap is now pliable enough for closing. At this stage, the tourniquet should be released and complete hemostasis should be achieved. Close the V-Y flap first on the distal side and then on the other side. The V will thus be converted to Y, based distally. There should be no tension on this triangular flap, which is in complete continuity with the fasciae and with the rich vascular network. Occasionally, whenever in doubt, in very severe contractures, especially with scars, a relaxing incision at a distance on the proximal side may be required to loosen the proximal skin further and reassure circulation. This will also help in preventing postoperative edema by providing an outlet for edematous fluid.

Deeper dissection in grade 3 extreme deformities is more extensive with regard to tendons, ligaments, and bony corrections, which varies from case to case. A well-padded plaster cast is given, usually below the knee. The patient must be kept under observation, with the foot elevated, for 2–3 days, and slitting of plaster may be needed after 24 hours in order to accommodate postoperative edema. To avoid circulatory problems, the foot is kept undercorrected after surgery before applying the plaster cast.

The plaster is changed every 2–3 weeks to achieve full correction. Stitches are removed after three weeks and may occur in two or three stages. The total period of immobilization is 12–14 weeks. After that, sometimes, in older cases with very rigid deformities, patients may require protective shoes with foot–ankle orthosis for 2–3 months during initial weight bearing. This decision is made on a case-by-case basis, and there cannot be a fixed regimen.

Criteria for assessment and grading of results: For assessing the results, various popular assessment criteria, such as Demiglio's, Pirani's, and others, cannot be applied because each case is different and with countless variables. The differences are in age, severity, rigidity, components of deformity, previous treatment (casting and/or one or more surgeries), additional defects, complications, radiological variations, and so forth. The patient, who is the beneficiary, is the best judge for assessing the results. Therefore, their satisfaction level has been considered as the best way to assess the results. Various improvement parameters taken into consideration are foot length, cosmetic appearance of the foot, absence of pain, flexibility of the foot, and function of the foot. Three grades of assessing criteria have been formulated. In more than 40 years, 1,080 surgeries were performed in extreme deformities with adequate long-term follow-up in 800 feet from 6 months to 30 years and in 600 feet for more than 5 years, with an average of 12.5 years. Results obtained were 96% excellent/good with the patients satisfied on all the parameters. In good results, there was slight forefoot adduction and everything else was at full satisfaction of the patient. Fair/poor results were 4%, with overcorrection or residual adduction/inversion or overcorrection with or without infection. There was only marginal necrosis of skin in 3% of cases, healing in due course and not affecting the results. Such an extensive 3-in-1 incision, although it appears aggressive, is completely evidence-based from plastic surgery journals around the world, without compromising the circulation of flaps, as discussed in the pathoanatomy. This approach has been used for the first time in clubfoot to correct the rarest of the rare extreme clubfoot deformities.

As **each clubfoot is different**, also true for extreme deformities, the surgical steps are also variable for every case. Extreme deformities are quite prevalent, and they are as common in small children as in adolescents and adults. It will be interesting to describe case histories of extreme deformities from different age groups, ranging from one to 45 years of age, with very wide variation in morphology and widely different surgical steps in each. Many of these cases have been documented in the June 2018 print issue of *International Orthopaedics* (SICOT), with a highly abbreviated description of each in a consolidated table form. It is difficult to comprehend the detailed morphology and surgical treatment in such brief descriptions. Therefore, for better understanding by those interested in clubfoot, it appears essential to describe each of these unique cases separately with complete morphology and surgical corrections. Besides, these already documented cases, with an equal number of unique cases, some of which may be the first of their kind, are also described in detail.

CASE 1: CLUBFOOT WITH ADDITIONAL PLANTAR FASCIO-MYOCUTANEOUS CONTRACTURE OF FOREFOOT

AS, a 1-year-old male child with grade 3 extreme unilateral right clubfoot deformity with the usual equinovarus elements of deformity. The child had flail middle three toes, which were flexed toward the sole, more than 90°, with a unique fascio-myocutaneous plantar contracture of the forefoot, like a closed fist. The middle toes were smaller with rudimentary osseous nuclei and absent second and third metatarsals on skiagrams. This was corrected in three stages: the first stage utilized the usual DOLAR surgical technique and subtotal subtalar release. The second stage was to correct the plantar contracture of the forefoot by an innovative distal multipoint soft tissue distractor after a meticulously performed V-Y plasty of the plantar skin and the plantar fascia and gradually pulling the plantar skin and soft tissues of the foot distally, over a period of three weeks. The third stage was by a minor V-Y plasty of the plantar aspect of the second toe. The result was highly satisfying at four years follow-up (personal communication). The patient is walking about with a good correction as per verbal communication (Figure 5.3a–e).

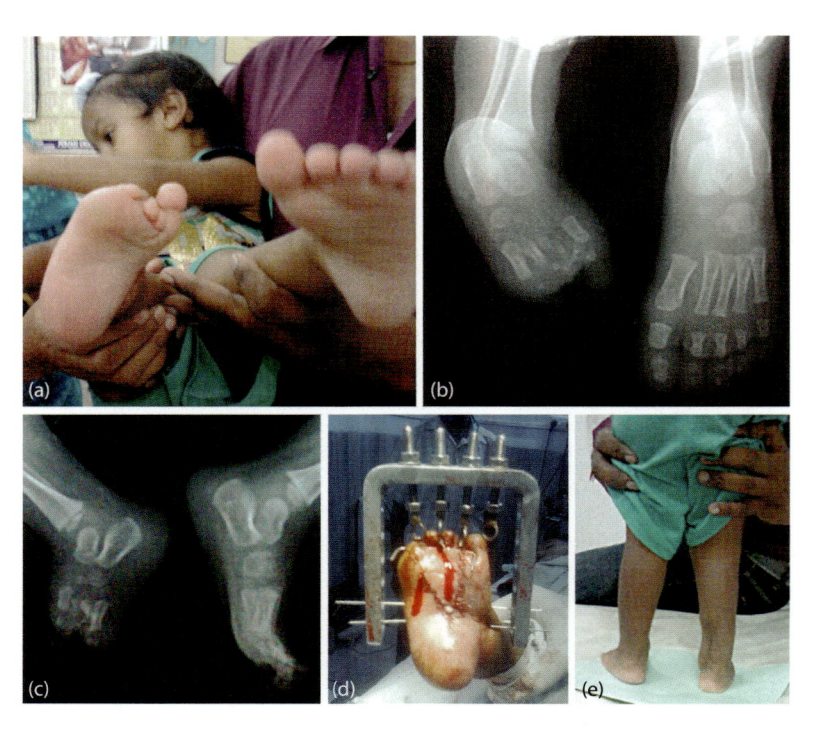

Figure 5.3 **(a)** Showing a unique congenital contracture with fascio-myocutaneous contracture with middle toes flexed toward the ball of the foot. **(b,c)** X-rays, AP and lateral views, showing absent middle two metatarsals and contracture. **(d)** Seen with the **Distal Soft Tissue Distraction External Fixator** with plantar V-Y plasty. **(e)** Follow-up photograph of patient. (Reprinted/adapted by kind permission and courtesy from Springer Nature and Copyright Clearance Center's RightsLink. From author's own published article; Mittal RL. *Int Orthop (SICOT)*, June 2018;42(6):1297–1306. For the book *Clubfoot: A Comprehensive Approach* (present, past and future), for the publisher Taylor & Francis Group by Dr. R. L. Mittal. 2018–2019.)

CASE 2: EXTREME GRADE 3 WITH UNUSUAL PATHOANATOMY IN A SMALL CHILD

P, a 2.5-year- old male child with untreated, bilateral grade 3 extreme deformities, with big callosities, compensatory hyperextended knees and genu valgum, and wasted legs. Skiagrams, AP and lateral views showed gross unusual abnormalities. Although navicular and cuneiform ossific nuclei had not appeared, yet from the position of the talus, dorsal as well as lateral talo-navicular

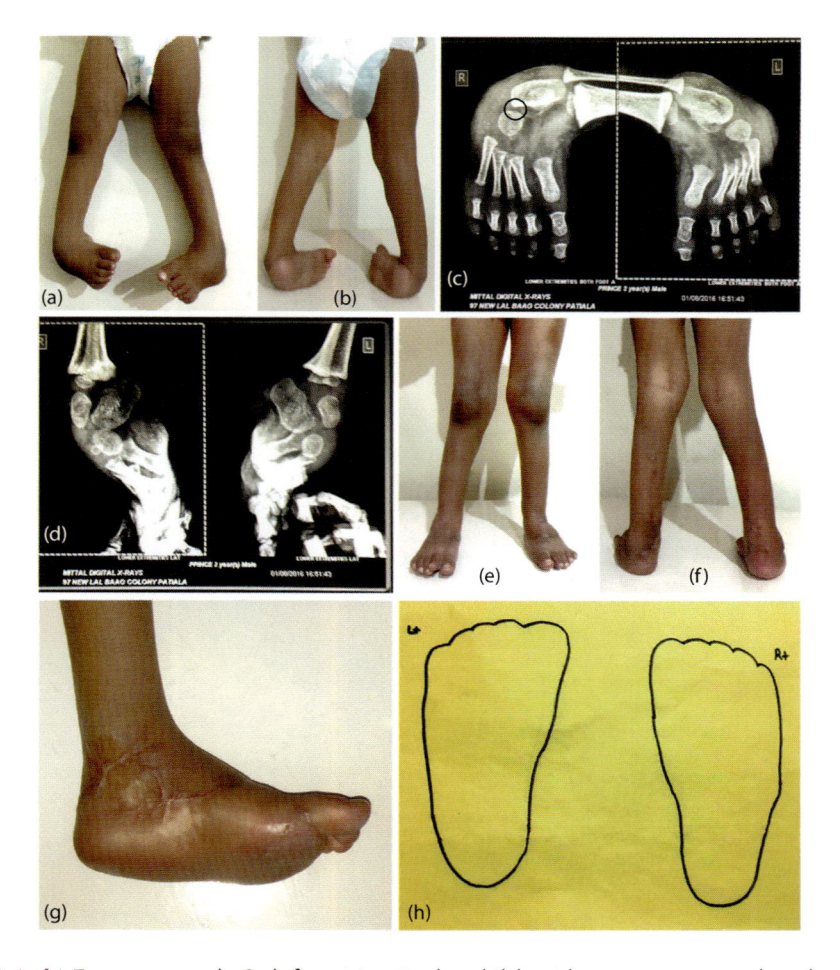

Figure 5.4 **(a,b)** Extreme grade 3 deformities, in the child, with acute cavus and cock-up big toes, big callosities more on left, weight bearing is entirely on dorsal surface on lateral side. **(c,d)** Skiagrams, AP and lateral views, showing calcaneocuboid and talo-navicular dislocations, hyperacute cavus deformities both sides (EQ4). **(e,f,g)** Showing excellent corrections for both feet and scar of DOLAR + Z + V-Y plasty incision with healthy scar mark on left foot. **(h)** Showing footprints of both well-corrected feet at one year follow-up. (Reprinted/adapted by kind permission and courtesy from Springer Nature and Copyright Clearance Center's RightsLink. From author's own published article; Mittal RL. *Int Orthop (SICOT)*, June 2018;42(6):1297–1306. For the book *Clubfoot: A Comprehensive Approach* (present, past and future), for the publisher Taylor & Francis Group by Dr. R. L. Mittal. 2018–2019.)

dislocation was appreciated. Calcaneocuboid and cuneonavicular dislocations were also present and appreciated in spite of the absence of ossific nuclei. There was hyper-acute cavus (EQ4) at the midfoot, more medial cavus at the first metatarsal, and hyperextended metatarsophalangeal joints, especially the first. At operation, all pathological features of soft tissues abnormalities, as described in the pathoanatomy, were on the posterior, medial, and lateral side. Surgical corrections were carried out through the DOLAR + Z + V-Y plasty on the left side and DOLAR + Z incision on the right side. The releases performed were abductor hallucis, tibialis posterior insertions, flexor hallucis and digitorum longus tenotomy, Z plasty heel cord, conjoint posterior capsule, spring ligament and all plantar and medial ligaments and the interosseous talo-calcanean ligament, including dorsolateral wedge resection from cuboid. The deformity was corrected and multiple K-wire fixations were done for maintaining the correction. The wound was closed after hemostasis, followed by well-padded casts, repeated at requisite intervals. The result was excellent in both feet at one year follow-up. However, only partial radiological correction could be achieved. Therefore, one should be prepared for unusual radiological features, and effort must be made to achieve as best correction as possible by extensive meticulous dissections. Patient had excellent clinical correction on both sides, but with radiological undercorrection. Various preoperative and postoperative photographs are given to see these unusual features (Figure 5.4a–h).

CASE 3: BILATERAL CLUBFOOT WITH MULTIPLE CONGENITAL CONSTRICTION BANDS

SD, a 1-year-old male child with bilateral rigid clubfeet, right more than left, with constriction bands on both sides and partial amputation of all toes on both feet with syndactyly also. The band on the right side was in zone 2 and it was grade 2; the band on the left side was grade 1 in the lower part of the leg above the ankle with a slight hourglass appearance, in addition to in utero grade 4 bands at distal parts of all toes leading to their congenital amputations. First, on the right leg, the band was excised around the whole circumference, and multiple longitudinal incisions were given in the deeper part of the band area to relax any remnant constrictions. After that, multiple Z plasties were done in four parts, starting from the anterior one-fourth circumference and going around the whole circumference, so that the same area of skin was opposed to the corresponding other side and there was no rotation of the skin. Left foot was operated first by soft tissue correction with the DOLAR technique. After three weeks, it was done on the right side. At six months follow-up, correction on the left side was excellent, but on the right side, there was partial relapse due to the deep constriction band of leg grossly affecting the deeper soft tissues and a second surgery was needed, for which the patient did not report (Figure 5.5a–e).

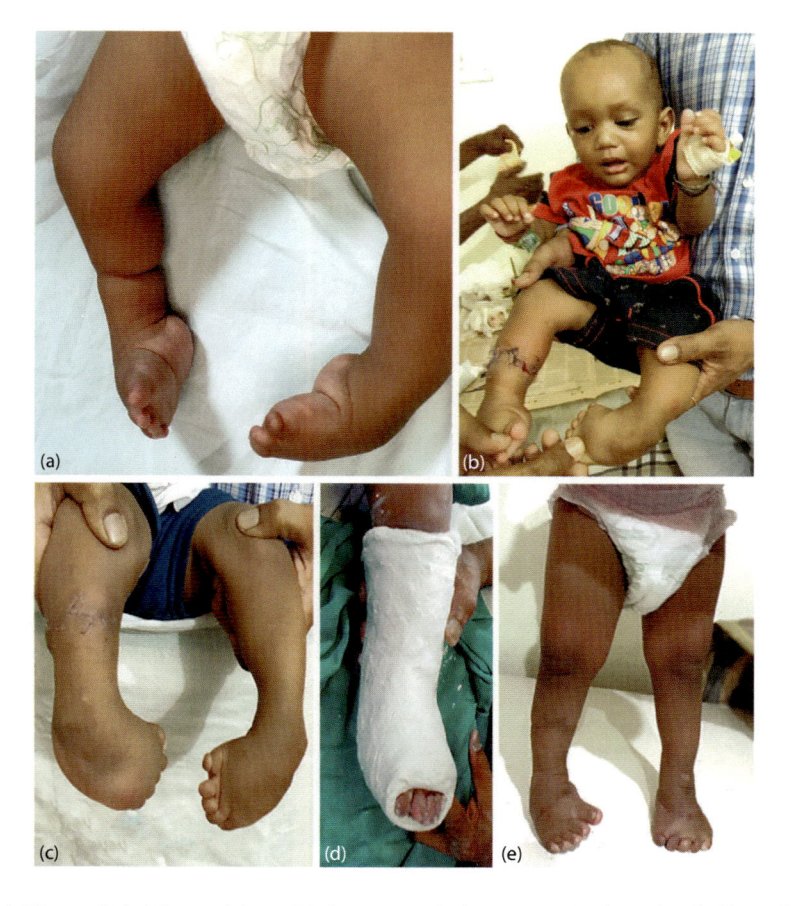

Figure 5.5 (a) Bilateral clubfoot with multiple congenital constriction bands of all grades, showing congenital amputations of toes (grade 4) both sides, very deep grade 2 constricting band on right leg and a shallow grade 1 band on left leg above ankle. (b) Multiple Z plasties of right leg at three weeks. (c) Correction of constriction of right leg with fine Z plasties scar. (d) Postoperative photograph of left foot. (e) At six months follow-up, left foot corrected, but right showing relapse.

CASE 4: UNIQUE CLUBFOOT WITH MULTIPLE CONSTRICTING BANDS OF ALL SEVERITIES

GKS, a 1-year-old male child with bilateral clubfoot. On the right side, he had multiple zone 2, 3, and 4 bands, as well as a deep zig-zag grade 3 severity constriction band near the ankle with lymphedema. On the right side, there were also grade 4 at the toes with their congenital amputations and absent foot bones, a disorganized ankle, and short tibia and fibula. On the left side, he had a zone 2 band at the leg and zone 4 bands at the toes with partial amputations, with additional bands at the remaining parts of some toes, along with a rigid clubfoot. The right side was operated on first, and all bands of the foot and ankle area were excised by multiple Z plasties with very good correction. After that, the left foot was operated on by rotation flap and extensive soft-tissue dissection with acceptable correction. He was given foot/ankle orthosis with an extended prosthetic on right side and a talipes shoe on the left side. The child is walking now with the extension prosthesis on the right side at 1 year and 8 months of follow-up. The child can also be seen standing on the left leg and short right lower limb with the unusual foot deformity. It is hoped that with growth, leg lengthening and some more correction of the right foot deformity may be possible for a better rehabilitation of the child (Figure 5.6a–h).

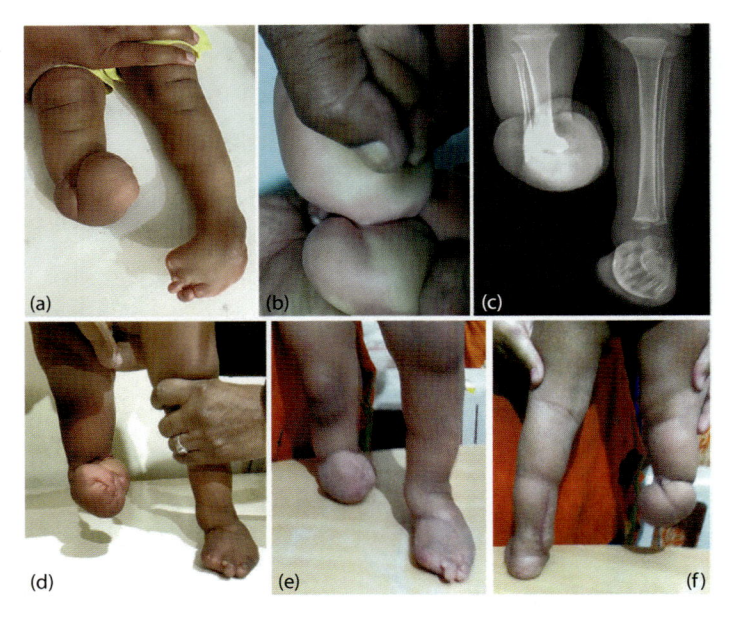

Figure 5.6 (a) Constricting bands of all grades and zones, both sides. Right foot unusual deformity with shortened leg bones with gross lymphedema of foot and leg with some hard ossicles in foot and ankle area felt in the depth with severe grade 3 and 4 bands. (b) A close-up of left foot area with grade 3 and 4 very deep constriction bands. (c) Skiagrams of both sides, showing the deformities, right leg bones short, and blurred ossific nuclei of ankle and metatarsals are seen. (d) Multiple Z plasties done on right side and left foot operated through DOLAR skin expanding incision with reasonably good correction with patient standing on both feet. (e) Patient can put some weight on right foot also with support. (f) From the back, patient standing on corrected left foot with support and shortening of right leg seen at six months follow-up. The child has not started walking yet.

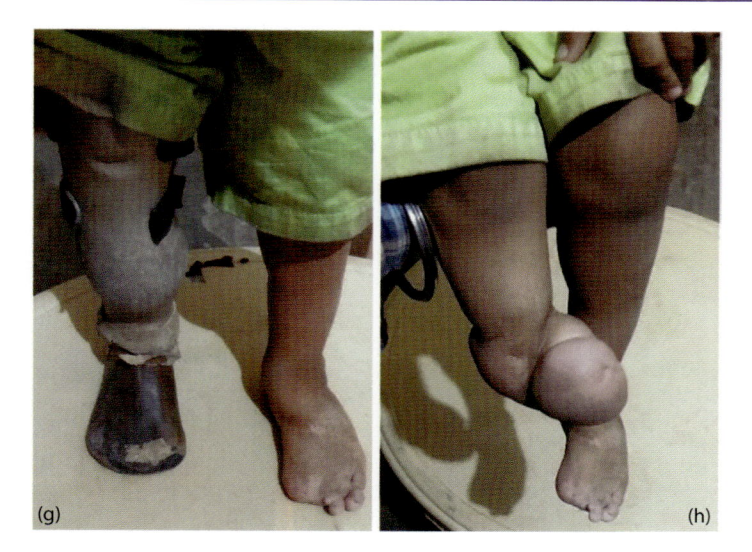

Figure 5.6 (Continued) **(g)** At 1 year and 8 months follow-up, the child is now walking with an extension prosthesis. **(h)** Seen without prosthesis standing on left operated foot.

CASE 5: HIGHLY RIGID DEFORMITY AFTER PONSETI WITH THREE HEEL CORD TENOTOMIES

Roh, a 2.5-year-old male child, started Ponseti casting treatment at 1.5 years for about a year with three heel cord tenotomies at short intervals (can be seen better with a magnifying glass), and the deformity increased even more than before. On examination, there was grade 3 extreme deformity

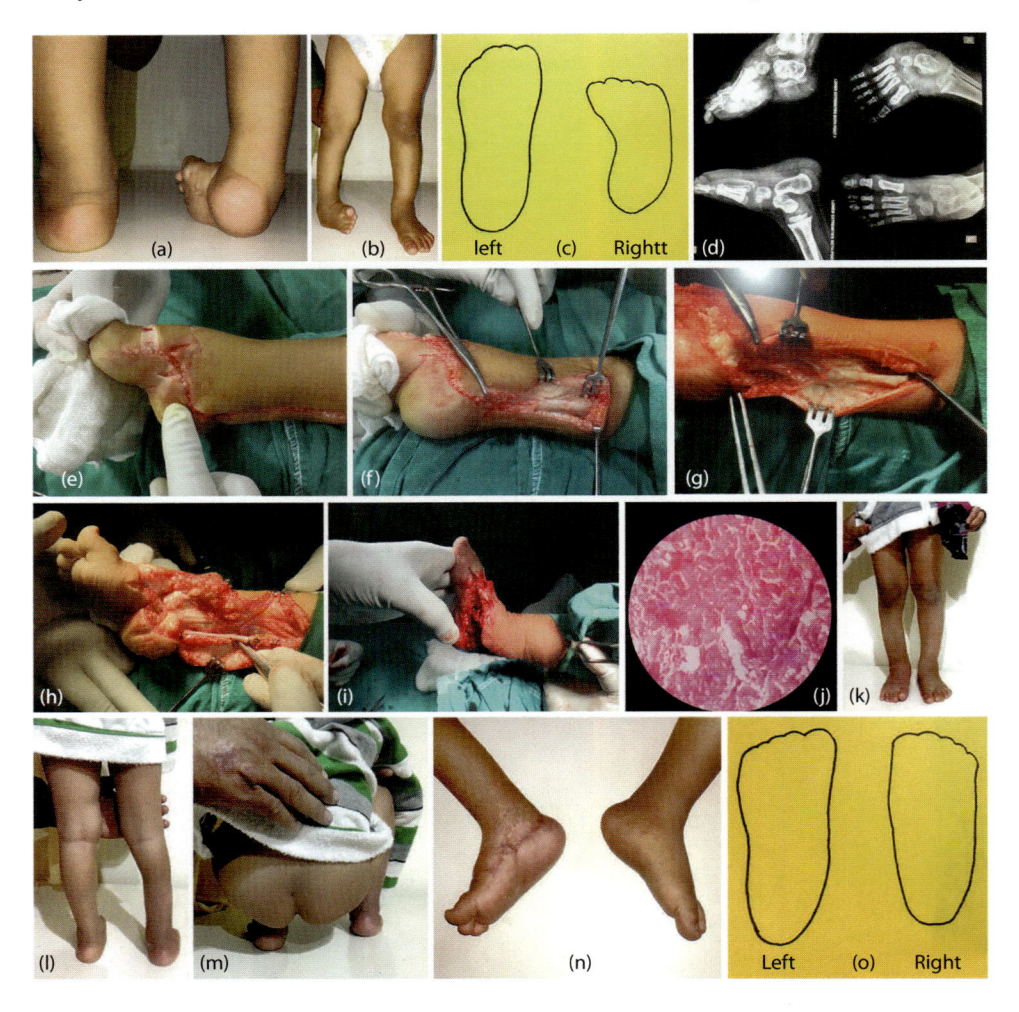

Figure 5.7 **(a)** Showing, from the back, scars of three heel cord tenotomies with rigid grade 3 deformity, better seen with a magnifying lens. **(b)** Deformity seen from front with dorsolateral callosity. **(c)** Footprints of plantar surfaces (not weight bearing). **(d)** Skiagrams, AP and lateral views, showing talo-navicular dislocation, calcaneocuboid and cuneonavicular malalignments with severe cavus and varus. **(e)** DOLAR + double Z plasty. **(f,g)** Showing dull, grayish, thick adherent extensive scar from skin too deep in about 4″ of heel cord area, from shining heel cord above to calcaneum below. **(h)** Excision of scar and free flexor hallucis longus tendon graft taken after its tenotomy at Henry's knot. **(i)** Corrected deformity with two K-wires *in situ*; **(j)** Histopathology of the excised scar showing dense irregular collagen tissue. **(k–m)** Showing deformity corrected including hidden equinus. **(n,o)** Corrected deformity with healthy scars of surgery and footprints of weight-bearing typical sole area now at six-months follow-up.

(very rigid and severe) with three heel cord tenotomy scars and a thickened and scarred heel cord area. Skiagrams, anteroposterior and lateral views, showed marked cavovarus (EQ3), talo-navicular dislocation, forward subluxated talus at the ankle and subtaloid joint, calcaneocuboid subluxation (**triple plus dislocation**) and possibly subluxation at the cuneonavicular joints. The operation was performed through a DOLAR + Z plasty incision. The abductor hallucis was slided forward, the tibialis posterior insertions were divided at their bony insertions; flexor hallucis and digitorum longus were divided, at the Henry's knot; Steindler's release was performed; spring ligament, plantar ligaments, and medial capsules of the first metatarsophalangeal joint were divided, tarso-metatarsal mobilization was done as per Kendrick et al.,[14] and the interosseous talo-calcanean ligament was released. **The most important finding in this case was in the heel cord area**: it showed an extensive adherent scar in an approximately 4" area, recognizable by its dull white look as compared with the shiny white look that is usually seen. The scar was excised as required, and the tendoachilles gap was reconstructed by a free graft obtained from the tenotomized flexor hallucis longus tendon. Bony alignments were corrected to the best possible extent and fixed with multiple K-wires through the first tarsometatarsal and through the talo-navicular and calcaneocuboid joints. The wound was closed in the corrected position after hemostasis. The foot was immobilized in a well-padded, below-knee cast with total immobilization for three months. The histopathology of the heel cord showed irregular fibrous tissue, unlike typical tendon tissue. Follow up at six months showed excellent correction (Figure 5.7a–o).

CASE 6: RESIDUAL DEFORMITY AFTER PONSETI ADHERENT HEEL CORD TENOTOMY

Rash, a 3-year-old male child, came with rigid, severe (extreme grade 3) clubfoot, had Ponseti casting treatment and heel cord tenotomy during the first year of life, with partial correction of the equinus. On examination, there was grade 3 extreme deformity (very rigid and severe) with a heel cord tenotomy scar and EQ3. Skiagrams, anteroposterior and lateral views, showed marked cavovarus (EQ3) with extreme medial cavus and talo-navicular dislocation. Surgical correction was performed through a DOLARZ incision. Hypertrophied abductor hallucis, tibialis posterior insertions, flexor hallucis, digitorum longus, and Steindler's releases were performed. The heel cord area showed adherent dull white scar continuing with shining tendon above. Tendoachilles adherent was released from adhesions by a sharp dissection, and Z-lengthening was performed,

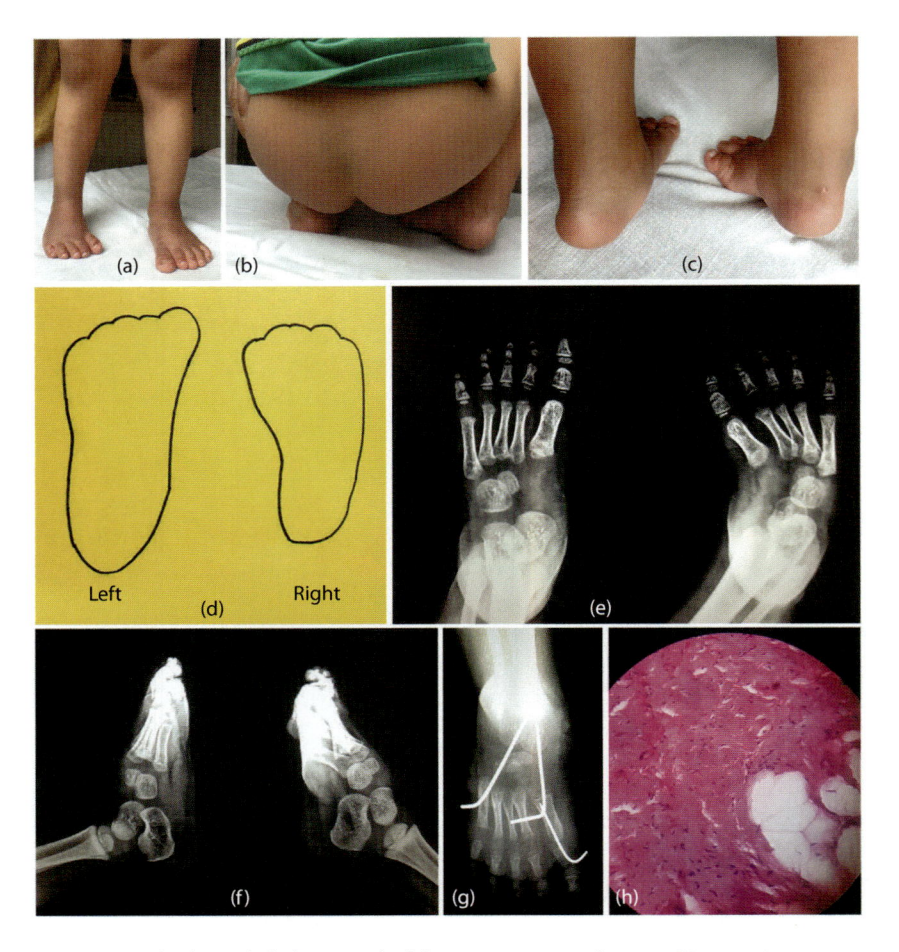

Figure 5.8 **(a–c)** Residual rigid deformity, hidden equinus, and scar of Ponseti percutaneous tenotomy. **(d)** Footprints showing the residual deformity. **(e,f)** X-rays showing talo-navicular and calcaneocuboid subluxation with marked cavus and cock-up big toe on abnormal side. **(g)** Showing postoperative X-rays with three K-wires fixing the corrected foot, including cock-up big toe. **(h)** Histopathology of scar taken from heel cord scarred area after Ponseti's tenotomy, showing irregular collagen.

as there was continuity. Conjoint posterior capsulotomy, spring ligament, plantar ligaments, and interosseous talo-calcaneal ligaments were released like in other cases. A dorsolateral wedge from the cuboid was excised. The deformity was corrected and fixed with multiple K-wires in the talo-navicular, first metatarsophalangeal joint, and calcaneocuboid joints, and the wound was closed with adequate skin lengthening. A well-padded, below-knee plaster cast was given for three months and K-wires were removed at four weeks, with plaster immobilization for three months. Results were excellent at one year of follow-up and full satisfaction with telephone personal communication (Figure 5.8a–h).

CASE 7: PONSETI HIGHER HEEL CORD TENOTOMY

IK, a 2.5-year-old male child with residual and recurring left clubfoot, was treated by Ponseti casting for about six months and heel cord percutaneous tenotomy one year previously. On examination, the foot appeared plantigrade with hyperextended knee with poor appearance of the rigid residual varus and hidden equinus. There was a scar from the heel cord tenotomy about 2.5" above the insertion of heel cord and there was adherent thickening in the middle. The footprint of weight-bearing area was smaller, wider, and in varus. Surgery was done through a DOLAR surgical incision. The adhesions were freed and the scar excised. Conjoint posterior capsulotomy was done to correct heel equinus. On the medial side, abductor hallucis release, tibialis posterior release, Steindler's release, and tenotomy of the flexor hallucis and digitorum longus were carried out at the Henry's knot. The spring ligament, other plantar ligaments, and the interosseous talo-calcanean ligament were done. Lengthening of the heel cord was done by extending half of the thickness of the tendon from below as well as from above and side-to-side stitching in the middle. Talo-navicular dislocation was reduced and fixed with K-wire like others. Correction was excellent with typical-looking footprint at one year follow-up (Figure 5.9a–i).

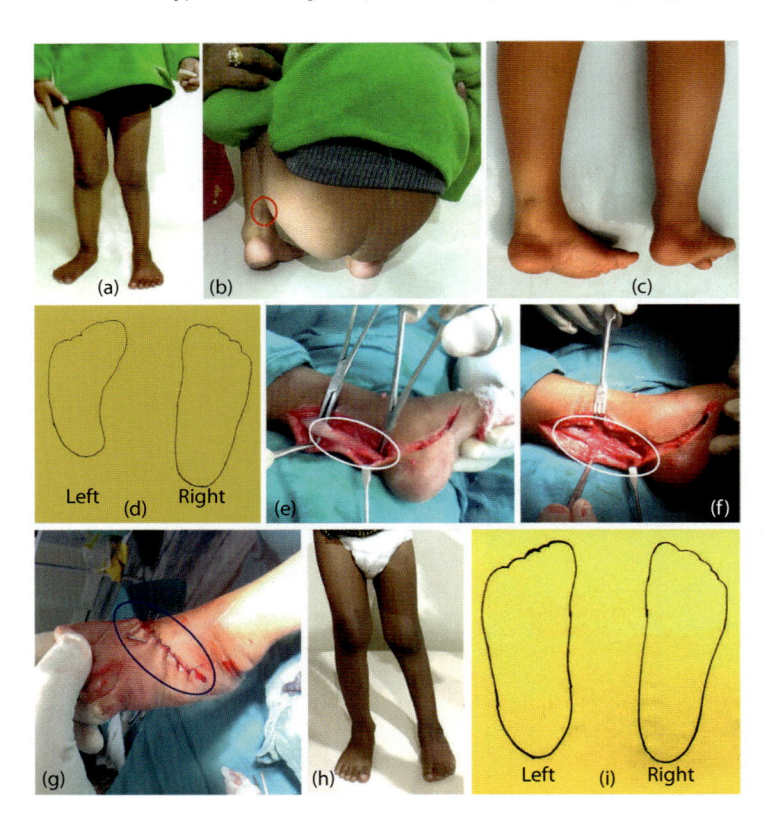

Figure 5.9 (a) Deformity seen from front. (b) Patient sitting on feet showing hidden equinus and highlighted heel cord tenotomy scar. (c) Ponseti scar and deformity seen from behind. (d) Footprints of weight-bearing soles showing smaller, deformed, and splayed-out left foot. (e,f) Intraoperative Ponseti's heel cord tenotomy scar as dull, whitish-gray and adherent heel cord area with shining tendoachilles above. (g) Corrected deformity after closure of rotation flap wound with a K-wire seen with reduced talo-navicular dislocation. (h) After operation at six-months follow-up, patient standing with corrected deformity. (i) Typical-looking footprints of weight-bearing areas of both feet.

CASE 8: RESIDUAL AND RELAPSED DEFORMITY AFTER PONSETI WITH OLDER CHILD

HspK, a 5-year-old female child, with grade 2 extreme deformity had Ponseti casting treatment and heel cord percutaneous tenotomy in the first few months of age with residual equinovarus deformity, and the deformity was increasing with age along with hidden equinus. The foot looked plantigrade on standing with hyperextended knees. She had talo-navicular dislocation also. This was corrected by a DOLAR + Z plasty incision. The heel cord in the sectioned area was scarred and adherent. Adhesions were released by meticulous sharp dissection. Z-lengthening of tendoachilles, and conjoint posterior capsulotomy was done to open up subtaloid, and ankle joints to correct hidden equinus with all other steps of subtotal subtalar release. Dorsolateral wedge resection from the cuboid was done along with K-wire fixation of the talo-navicular joint and cuboid. The wound was closed after hemostasis, and a well-padded, below-knee plaster cast was given. Total period of immobilization was for three months. Excellent correction, including hidden equinus, was evident at one year of follow-up (Figure 5.10a–g).

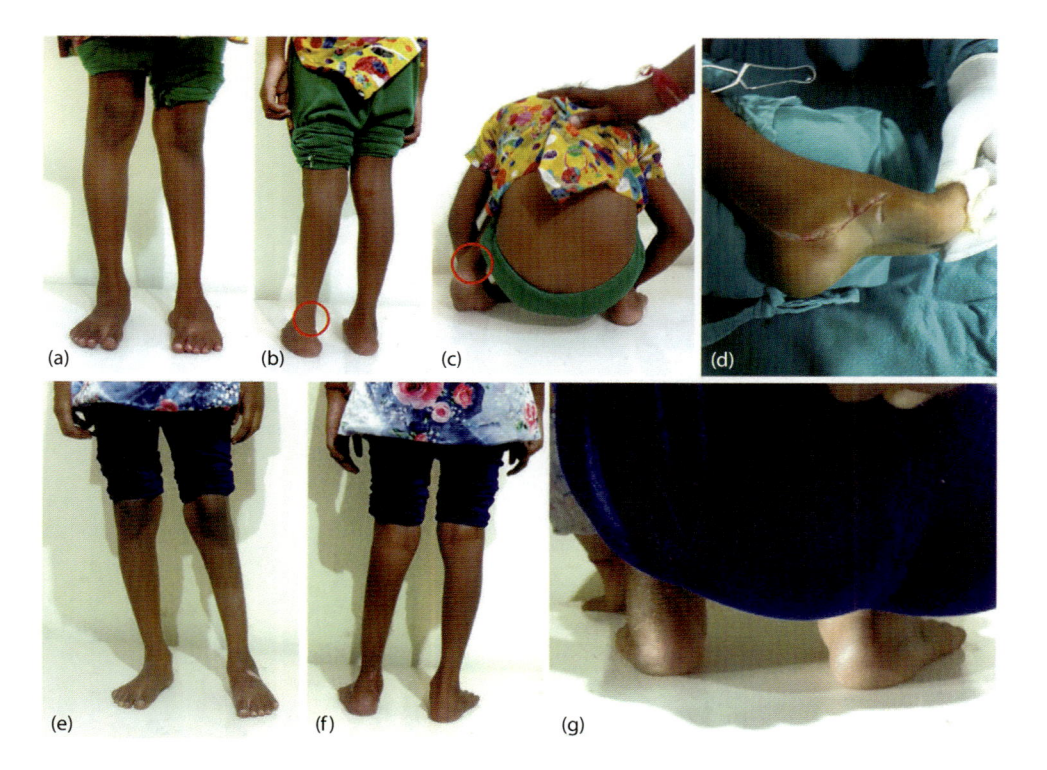

Figure 5.10 **(a)** Residual deformity seen from front. **(b)** Varus deformity seen from behind with heel cord tenotomy scar (seen better with magnifying lens) and Ponseti casting treatment. **(c)** Hidden equinus seen with patient on feet with knees flexed (position for ADL in India) and heel cord tenotomy scar highlighted. **(d,e)** Deformity corrected by DOLARZ technique seen from front and back. **(f)** Hidden equinus also corrected with the patient sitting on both feet.

CASE 9: OLDER CHILD WITH FAILED SURGERY SCARS

LS, a 7-year-old male child, with extreme grade 3 deformities with scars of earlier posteromedial release (PMR) on both sides at the age of six months, with the right foot more severe and walking with equinovarus gait. Talo-navicular dislocation was present on both sides. Surgery of right foot was started through a DOLAR + Z incision initially, and at closure of the wound, V-Y plasty was also done due to a gap there (DOLARZ-E). Scars were excised, and Z plasty of the heel cord, posterior capsulotomy of the ankle and subtaloid joints to correct heel equinus, Steindler's release, hypertrophied abductor hallucis release, meticulous release of all nine insertions of the tibialis posterior tendon in the sole which grasp and pull the bones toward the medial malleolus like nine tentacles (highlighted blue in Figure 5.11(A) h), plantar ligament release, interosseous talo-calcanean ligament release through sinus tarsi on the lateral side, dorsolateral wedge resection from the cuboid

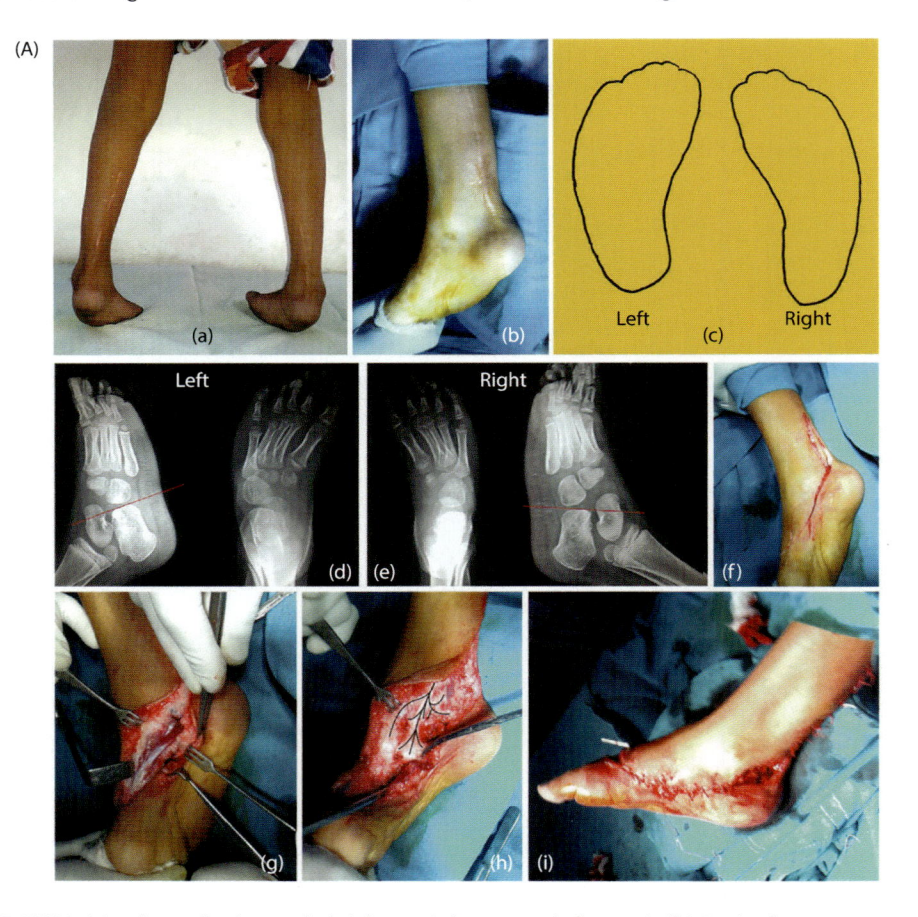

Figure 5.11(A) (a) Bilateral relapsed clubfoot, right more deformed. (b) Right foot prior to surgery with adherent posterior and medial scars. (c) Footprints of weight-bearing areas, right is more deformed. (d,e) Skiagrams of both feet, AP and lateral views, right side showing more intertarsal disruptions and even anteriorly subluxated talus from ankle and subtaloid joints. (f) DOLAR + Z incision initially with excised posterior scar. (g) Hypertrophied short abductor hallucis muscle. (h) Tenacious all nine tibialis posterior insertions exposed in the sole (highlighted) and released. (i) Talonavicular dislocation reduced and fixed with K-wire and an elliptical unstitched wound gap below and behind the ankle medial side, which was closed by V-Y plasty.

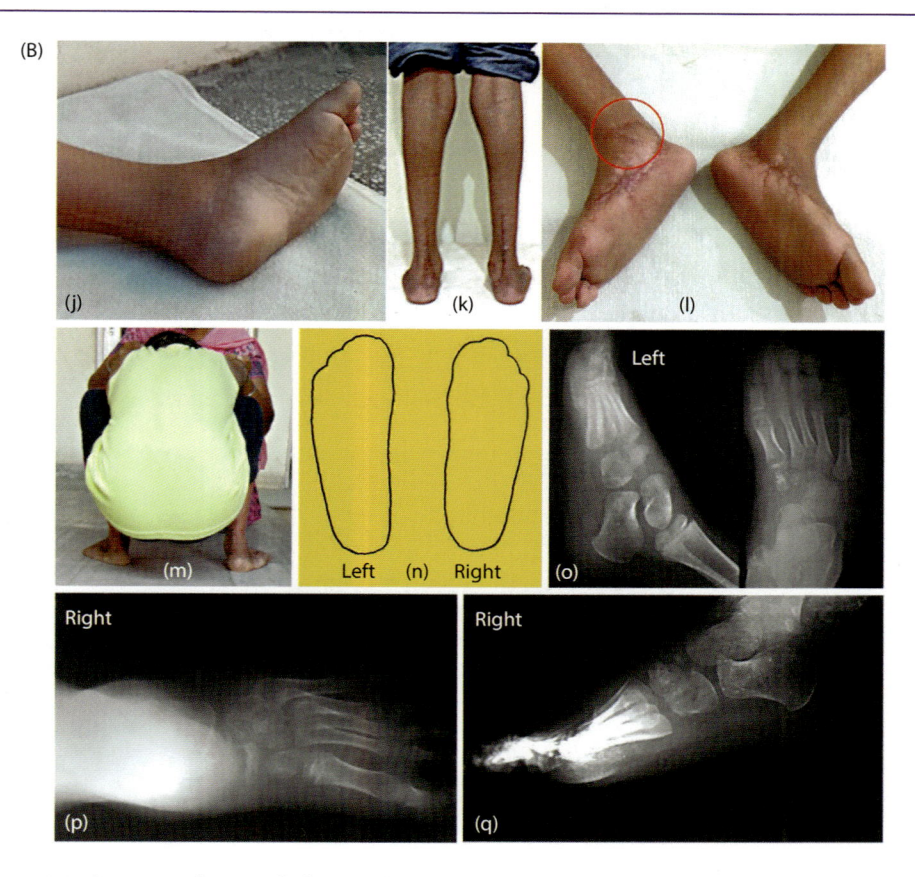

Figure 5.11(B) (Continued) **(j)** Left foot with old scars not so deformed as right. **(k)** Both feet corrected seen from back. **(l)** Both feet corrected close-up with healed scars, V-Y scar on right foot highlighted. **(m)** Sitting on feet with hidden equinus also corrected. **(n)** Footprints both feet, typical looking. **(o)** Skiagrams, left foot showing corrected deformity. **(p,q)** Skiagrams, right foot showing corrected deformities. (Reprinted/adapted by kind permission and courtesy from Springer Nature and Copyright Clearance Center's RightsLink. From author's own published article; Mittal RL. *Int Orthop (SICOT)* 1987;11(3):189–192; For the book *Clubfoot: A Comprehensive Approach* for the publisher Taylor & Francis Group by Dr. R. L. Mittal. 2018–2019.)

were all done. Talo-navicular dislocation was reduced and the dorsolateral wedge was closed and they were fixed with K-wires to maintain correction. A well-padded cast was given after hemostasis. The left foot was operated through DOLAR + Z plasty only, but all other similar surgical steps were carried out. At 3.5 years mean follow-up for both feet, the result was excellent for both feet with hidden equinus also corrected. The appearance of follow-up footprints of weight-bearing area was normal as compared with the preoperative prints [Figure 5.11(A)a–i and (B)j–q].

CASE 10: EXTREME DEFORMITY WITH EXTENSIVE SCARS

MhpK, a 3-year-old female child with grade 3 relapsed and rigid clubfoot, right side, after two failed surgeries, at the age of four months and then nine months, with multiple adherent scars on the medial and posterior sides, with hidden equinus and extreme cavus. X-rays showed extreme cavus and varus. The deformity was corrected by excision of adherent scars and DOLARZ-E (3-in-1) skin expander incision. Extensive deeper meticulous dissections included Z plasty of heel cord and capsulotomy of conjoint posterior capsule and abductor hallucis, tibialis posterior insertions, Steindler's, flexor hallucis and flexor digitorum longus releases. The spring ligament, all plantar and medial ligaments, the interosseous talo-calcanean ligament were released and a dorsolateral wedge from the cuboid was also excised. Osseous corrections were fixed with K-wires. At two-years follow-up, there is excellent correction with good shape of the foot with high patient satisfaction (Figure 5.12a–n).

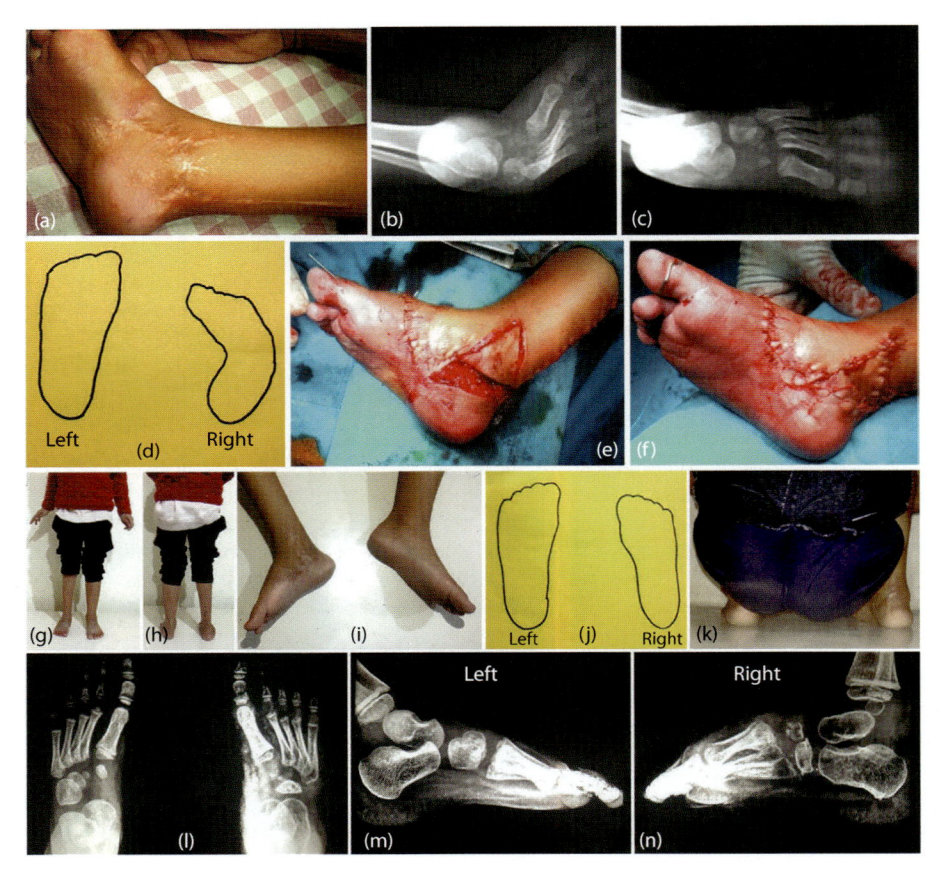

Figure 5.12 **(a)** Deformed right foot with extensive adherent multiple scars. **(b,c)** X-rays showing talo-navicular dislocation with extreme varus. **(d)** Footprint showing the deformity of weight-bearing area of left foot on standing. **(e)** 3-in-1 skin expanders by DOLAR + Z + VY plasty incision and excised scars. **(f)** Closure of extensive wound after excised scars. **(g,h)** Good shape of corrected foot with heeled scars compared with typical from front and back. **(i)** Close-up of both feet from medial side showing very well healed 3-in-1 scar. **(j)** Footprints of weight-bearing areas of both feet. **(k)** Patient sitting on heels seen from back with hidden equinus also corrected. **(l–n)** X-rays showing correction of deformity, but radiological undercorrection and a flat-topped talus on affected side.

5.2 Evolution of triple surgical techniques 123

CASE 11: EXTREME UNCORRECTED DEFORMITY IN A SMALL CHILD

MjtK, a 1.5-year-old, with grade 3 bilateral extreme deformities. The right foot was operated on using DOLAR + Z + V-Y plasty technique with extensive deeper dissection by Z plasty of tendoachilles. Posterior capsulotomy of conjoint posterior capsule, Steindler's release, abductor hallucis release, tibialis posterior insertions, and flexor hallucis and flexor digitorum longus release at Henry's knot, spring ligament and all plantar ligaments and interosseous talo-calcanean release were performed. Initially, only rotation and Z plasty incision was given, and later on, after all intraoperative corrections, when closure of the wound was not possible due to the gap below and behind the ankle, V-Y plasty was also added. **V-Y plasty is always added while closing the wound, if needed**. There was excellent correction at 1.25 years follow-up. The later photographs also show excellent results. The other foot is yet to be operated (Figure 5.13a–o).

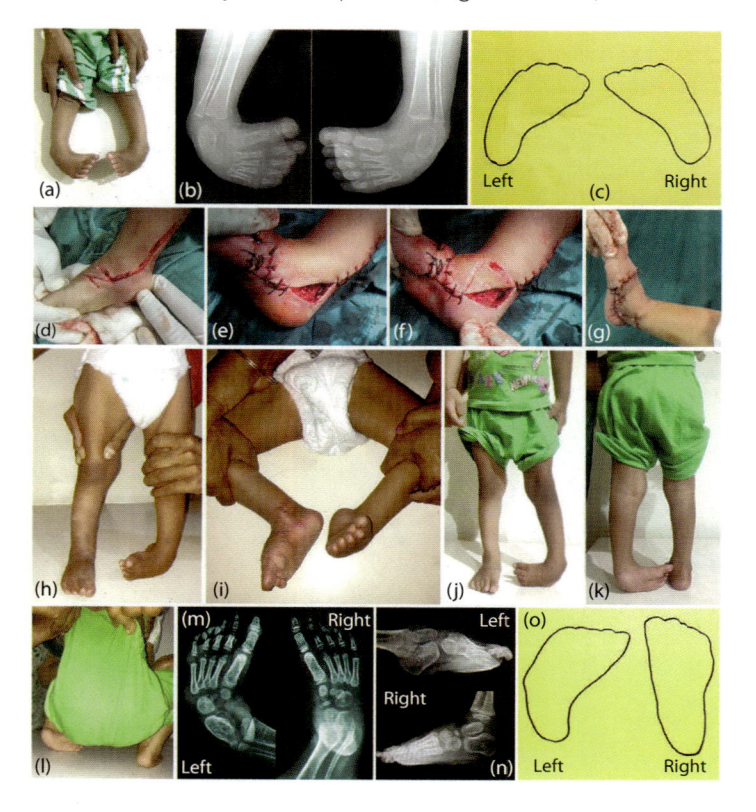

Figure 5.13 (a) Grade 3 deformities both feet. (b) X-rays showing calcaneocuboid dislocation with positional possibility of talo-navicular dislocation also, because ossific nucleus is still not present. (c) Footprints of both feet in adducted positions. (d) DOLAR + Z plasty incision of right foot intraoperative. (e) Closing the wound with leaving a gap. (f) V-Y plasty added to the incision (DOLARZ-E) below and behind the medial malleolus to facilitate wound closure. (g) At the operation table, wound closed easily without tension at the skin margins. (h,i) Deformity corrected in standing position and as seen from medial side with close-up of nicely healed triple skin expanding incision at five-months follow-up. (j–l) At 15-months follow-up, right foot looking typical as seen in standing position from front and behind; heel equinus too corrected as seen in sitting position from behind. (m,n) X-rays, AP and lateral views, right foot showing excellent clinical as well as radiological correction. (o) Footprints of weight-bearing areas showing excellent correction at 15-months follow-up. Left foot is yet to be operated, as and when the family chooses.

CASE 12: CLUBFOOT WITH VERY EXTREME EQUINUS (EQ4)

AS, a 7-year-old female with grade 3 rigid bilateral deformities of both feet with huge callosities, high-end extreme equinus (EQ4) with tali vertical in the ankle mortis on X-rays (shown in Chapter 4 also). Most of the weight is borne on the head of the talus, the anteroinferior end of the calcaneum, and the posteroinferior end of the cuboid, resting on the thick dorsolateral callosity and anterior part of the lateral border of the foot touching the ground. Besides talo-navicular dislocation, there was disruption of calcaneocuboid and cuneonavicular relationships. Surgery was performed, on both sides, by the DOLAR + Z + V-Y plasty approach under tourniquet. There was abnormal insertion of the tibialis anterior tendon going into the sole to the metatarsal bases, which was released. Abductor hallucis, all tibialis posterior insertions, flexor hallucis longus, and flexor digitorum longus were released. Conjoint posterior capsule was completely divided, including the posterior part of the deltoid ligament and the posterior part of the lateral collateral ligament of the ankle joint (posterior talo-fibular ligament). Both ankle and subtaloid joints were opened and confirmed by seeing both moving, which indicated the correction of the heel equinus fully. Steindler's

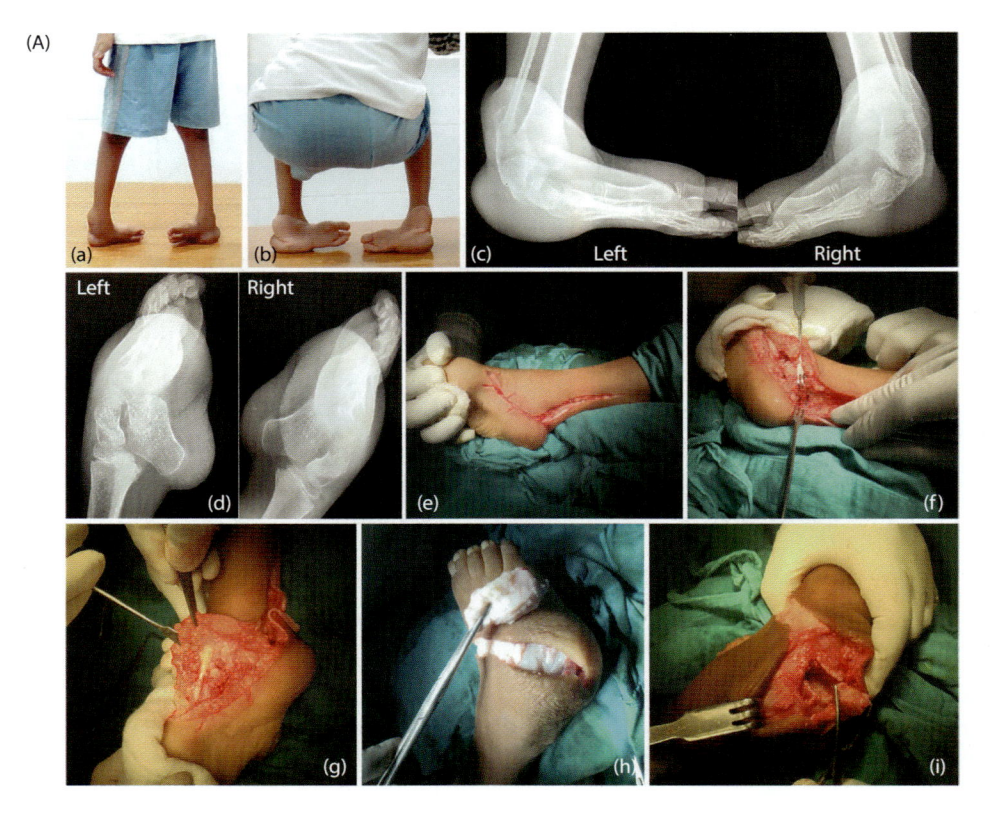

Figure 5.14(A) (a) Grotesque, most extreme, and awesome bilateral deformities. (b) Seen from back, patient trying to sit on feet, to depict the severity better, including hidden equinus, both the heels are vertical to the ground. (c,d) Skiagrams showing both tali vertical in 90° equinus with head down and all other osteoarticular abnormalities. (e) Showing DOLAR + Z incision. (f) Showing opened-out ankle and subtaloid joints after dividing the conjoint posterior capsule. (g) Showing abnormal tibialis anterior tendon going into the sole. (h,i) Excised bursa and dorsolateral wedge from cuboid.

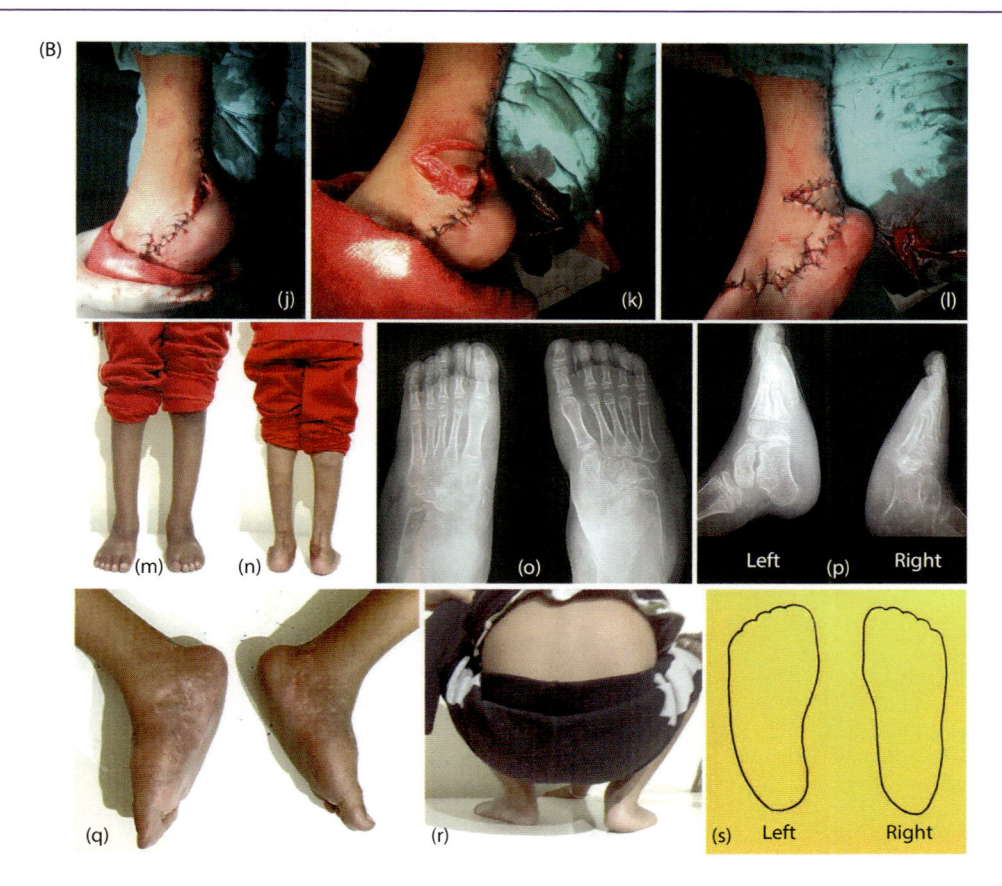

Figure 5.14(B) (Continued) **(j–l)** Showing tight wound gap behind the ankle and V-Y plasty skin flap facilitating wound closure. **(m,n)** Corrected both feet at follow up from front and back at one-year follow-up. **(o,p)** Skiagrams, AP and lateral views, showing radiological undercorrections. **(q)** Close-up both feet showing good corrections with healthy scars at one-year follow-up. **(r)** Sitting on feet showing corrected hidden equinus. **(s)** Good-looking footprints of weight-bearing area.) (Reprinted/adapted by kind permission courtesy from Springer Nature and Copyright Clearance Center's RightsLink. From author's own published article; Mittal RL. *Int Orthop (SICOT)*; June 2018;42(6):1297–1306; For the book *Clubfoot: A Comprehensive Approach* for the publisher Taylor & Francis Group by Dr. R. L. Mittal. 2018–2019.)

plantar release was adequately performed. The spring ligament and other plantar ligaments were also released. The interosseous talo-calcanean ligament was divided through sinus tarsi, blindly from the lateral side. The dorsolateral bursa and a wide dorsolateral wedge from the cuboid were excised. The deformity could be corrected with closing of the wedge and talo-navicular reduction. Hemostasis was secured before closing the wound, and K-wires were used for fixation. The wound was closed and a well-padded plaster cast given. As the dissection was very extensive, the cast was applied in undercorrection to avoid circulatory problems. This was gradually corrected with new plaster casts every two weeks. Both feet were operated similarly and the total period of immobilization was three months in each. Excellent clinical correction with high patient satisfaction at one-year follow-up was achieved. However, there was radiological undercorrection [Figure 5.14 (A)a–i and (B)j–s].

126 Extreme clubfoot deformities and their management

CASE 13: KLIPPEL–FEIL SYNDROME WITH MULTIPLE DEFORMITIES AND CLUBFOOT

SPS, a 9-year-old male, with a case of Klippel–Feil syndrome with multiple deformities and grade 3 extreme clubfoot, right side, with big callosity, weight bearing on the lateral border foot from little toe to cuboid area, indicating more equinus deformity. Other congenital defects were webbing of the neck with cervical fusion, hypoplastic pectorals and winging of the scapulae, undescended testes (inguinal), flexion deformity of the left knee, and lateral subluxation of the right patella. X-rays showed cuneonavicular and calcaneocuboid dislocations and acute cavovarus (EQ4), but talo-navicular dislocation was apparently present with no ossific nucleus of the navicular. Surgery

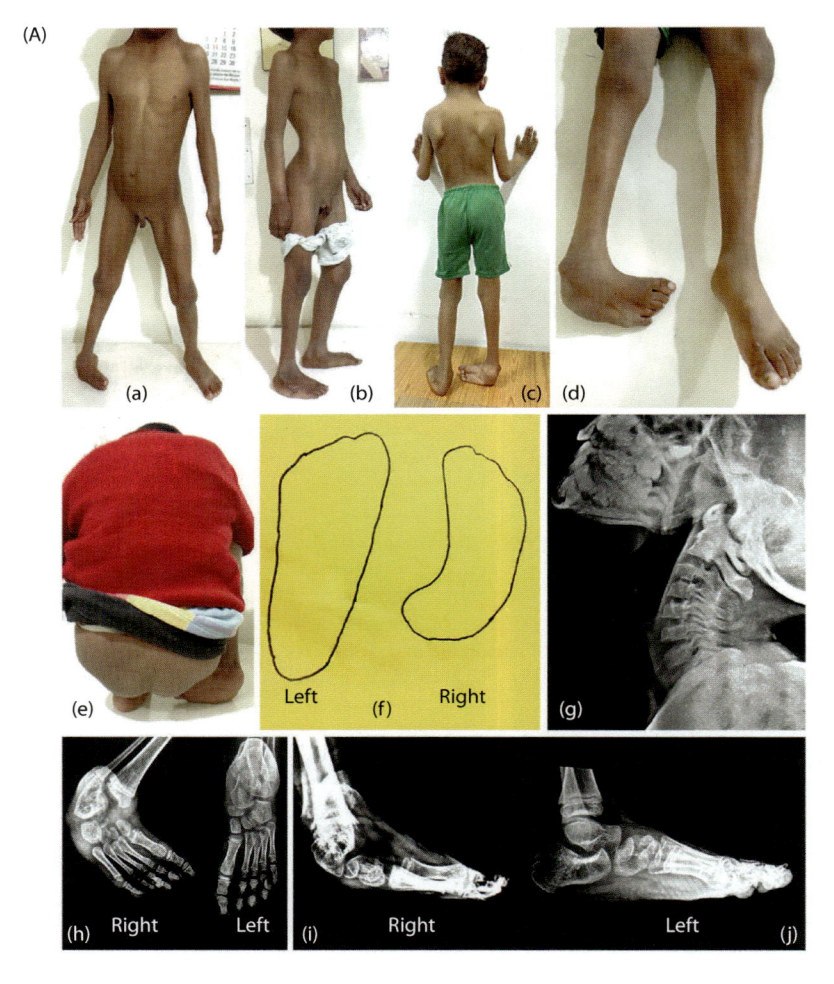

Figure 5.15(A) (a–d) Showing right side clubfoot with large callosity, webbed neck, winged scapulae, hypoplastic pectorals, undescended testis, flexion deformity in left knee, right patella subluxated laterally, right foot is flat. (e) Patient sitting, showing hidden equinus deformity from back. (f) Preoperative footprints of weight-bearing area. (g) Lateral X-rays showing atlantoaxial fusion, as well as lower cervical region. (h–j) X-rays, AP and lateral views, both feet showing right foot with calcaneocuboid dislocation and presumed positional cuneonavicular and talo-navicular dislocations (ossific nucleus of navicular still not there), acute cavovarus (EQ4).

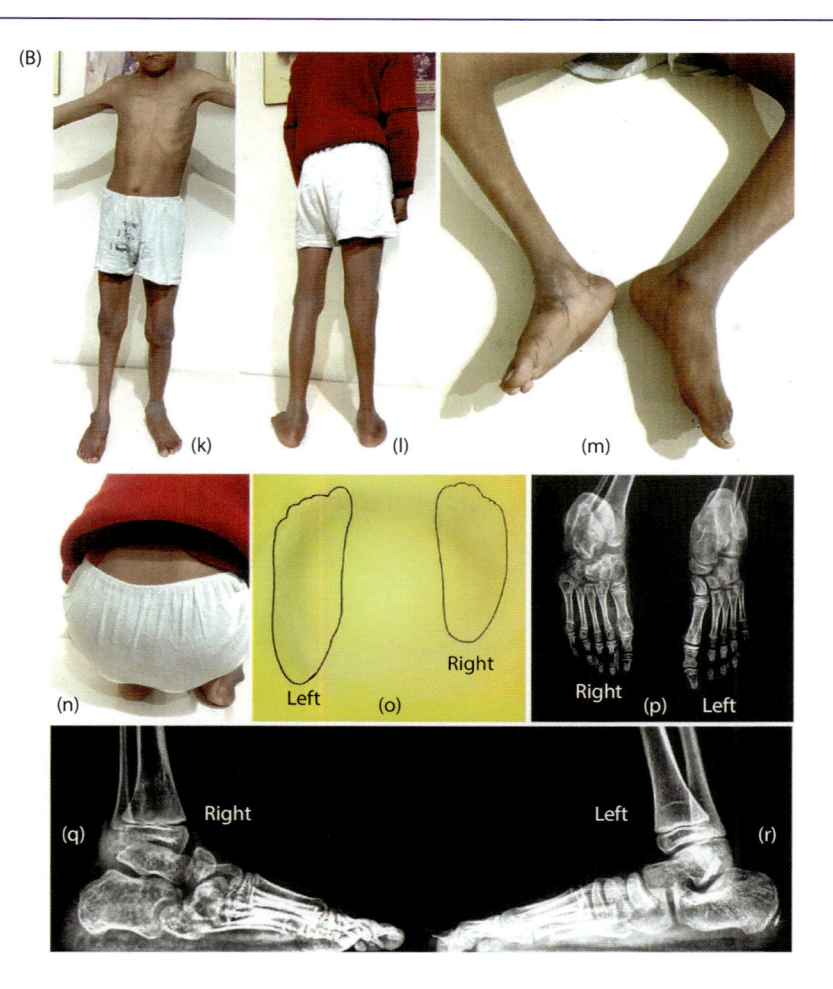

Figure 5.15 (B) (Continued) (k,l) Excellent result seen from front and back at two-years follow-up, pectoral hypoplasia more on right side also seen. (m) close-up of feet with scars of DOLAR + Z + V-Y plasty. (n) Patient sitting on feel, required for ADL in India (compare with image e above). (o) Footprints of weight-bearing area. (p–r) Post-op follow up, AP and lateral X-rays showing calcaneocuboid dislocation corrected, but others only partly corrected with navicular bone now visible. (Reprinted/adapted by kind permission courtesy from Springer Nature and Copyright Clearance Center's RightsLink. From author's own published article; Mittal RL. *Int Orthop (SICOT)*; June 2018;42(6):1297–1306; For the book *Clubfoot: A Comprehensive Approach* for the publisher Taylor & Francis Group by Dr. R. L. Mittal. 2018–2019.)

was performed by the DOLAR + Z + V-Y plasty approach with all the extensive deeper dissection surgical steps: abductor hallucis release, Z plasty of tendoachilles, conjoint posterior capsulotomy, Steindler's release, release of nine tibialis posterior insertions, flexor hallucis and digitorum longus release at Henry's knot, spring ligament and all plantar and medial release, interosseous talo-calcanean ligament release, dorsolateral wedge resection from the cuboid, with adequate tarso-metatarsal mobilization. K-wire fixations were done after correcting the osseous defects, reducing talo-navicular dislocation and closing the cuboid wedge gap. A well-padded plaster cast was given after hemostasis. At three years follow up, the correction was clinically excellent, the foot of course shorter but with high patient satisfaction, and the testes also descended by themselves. However, there was obvious radiological undercorrection [Figure 5.15 (A)a–j and at follow up (B)k–r].

CASE 14: A UNIQUE CASE WITH TRIPLE PLUS DISLOCATIONS

Dhr, a 9.5-year-old male child, a unique case, presented with a very rigid right side unilateral clubfoot (grade 3 extreme deformity) with adherent bowstring scars from two previous surgeries done at six months and seven years of age. The deformity had further increased, especially after the second surgery. On inspection, there was wasting of the leg, with a widened ankle mortis as compared with the left, and the child was walking with an awkward gait. Parents and the child were dejected

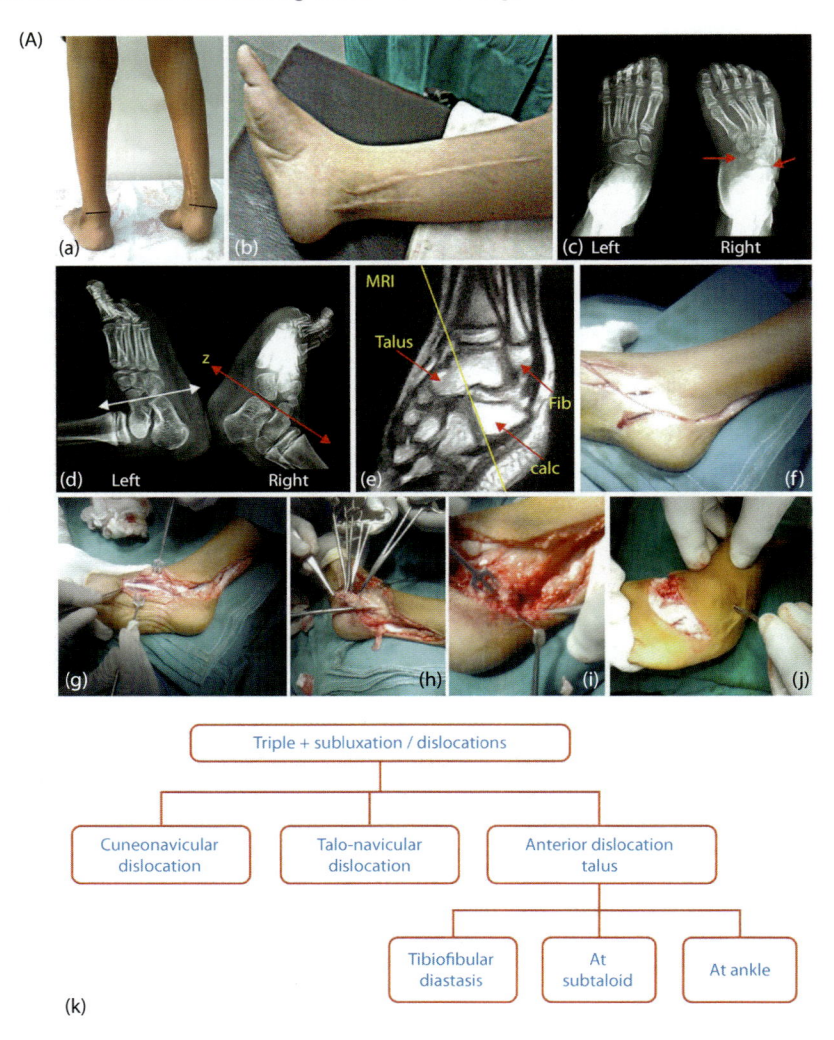

Figure 5.16(A) (a,b) Showing broader ankle mortis and posterior shift of lateral malleolus, rigid deformity with keloid and bowstring scars of two earlier surgeries. (c–e) X-rays and MRI showing flat-topped talus and triple plus dislocations as described in the text and in the flow chart at k. (f) Showing rotation and double Z plasty incision. (g) Hypertrophied abductor hallucis. (h) Nine tibialis posterior insertions shown after having been divided. (i) Conjoint posterior capsule divided, opening up ankle and subtaloid joint correcting heel equinus. (j) Blind interosseous talo-calcanean ligament division at the sinus tarsi, moving the overlying skin backwards to avoid adhesions (Subtotal Subtalar Release). (k) Flow chart showing the details of three components anterior dislocation of talus to make it triple plus dislocations.

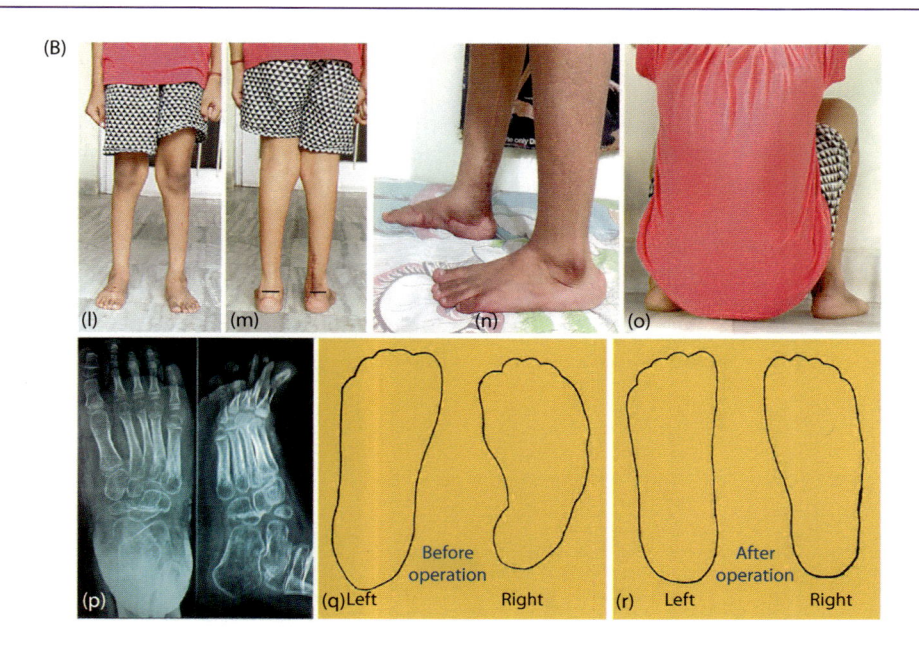

Figure 5.16(B) (Continued) **(l,m)** Showing patient standing, seen from front and back with deformity corrected. **(n)** Close-up of foot from medial side showing scar. **(o)** Patient sitting on feet with flexed knees, a position of ADL in India, corrected hidden equinus too. **(p)** Full radiological correction with sliding osteotomy of cuboid united; **(q,r)** Footprints of weight-bearing areas, before and after operation, with full correction at three years follow-up. (Figures 5.16A and B with flow chart above have been reprinted/adapted by kind permission & courtesy from Jaypee Brothers Medical Publishers Pvt LTD from author's own published article R.L. Mittal: Obstinate club foot with triple plus dislocations - a case report (Unique patho-anatomy & its correction by DOLARZ Surgical Technique); *J Foot Ankle Surg* (Asia Pacific), 2014:1(2):72–77. For the book *Clubfoot: A Comprehensive Approach* for the publisher Taylor & Francis Group by Dr. R. L. Mittal. 2018–2019.)

and felt helpless when they presented to the author. Skiagrams (AP and lateral views) and MRI demonstrated many unique findings: a flat-topped talus and apparent triple sublux/dislocations (cuneonavicular, talo-navicular, and anterior dislocation of the talus). However, the anterior dislocation of the talus was a complex dislocation affecting all three joints connected with it, that is, anterior subluxations at both the ankle and subtaloid joints as well as inferior tibio-fibular diastasis. The lower end of the fibula is lying far posterior to the tibia in the lateral X-ray as compared with unaffected ankle joint. MRI further confirmed the plain skiagram findings. That is why this unique type of dislocation has been given the name of **triple plus dislocation**. This pathoanatomical feature has never been reported before and has been published by the author (Mittal[3]) along with the unique treatment of this case. Surgery was performed through a DOLAR + double Z plasty incision with excision of earlier scars and extensive deeper dissection steps: abductor hallucis release, tibialis posterior release of its nine insertions, dividing both flexor hallucis and digitorum longus, Steindler's release, spring ligament, other plantar ligaments, conjoint posterior capsule, and interosseous talo-calcanean ligament releases. A dorsolateral wedge was excised from the cuboid with its complete osteotomy to correct the intertarsal malalignments. Reduced talo-navicular dislocation and other malalignments were fixed with K-wires after laterally sliding the distal segment of the cuboid (innovative sliding osteotomy of the cuboid). Excellent result with full patient satisfaction and good cosmetic and functional result, including radiological correction, was achieved at three years follow-up [Figure 5.16(A)a–k and (B)l–r].

CASE 15: PRE-ADULT RESIDUAL/RELAPSE, GRADE 3, WITH GENU RECURVATUM

RjS, a 16-year-old male, with bilateral rigid relapsed, grade 3 extreme deformity with scars of earlier surgeries performed during the first year of age on both feet, left more severe than right. Deformity has been increasing with age including genu recurvatum. There was marked medial cavus (EQ3), more on the left side, talo-navicular and cuneonavicular subluxations in X-rays, the left more so. Left foot was operated on three years previously, through DOLAR + double Z plasty

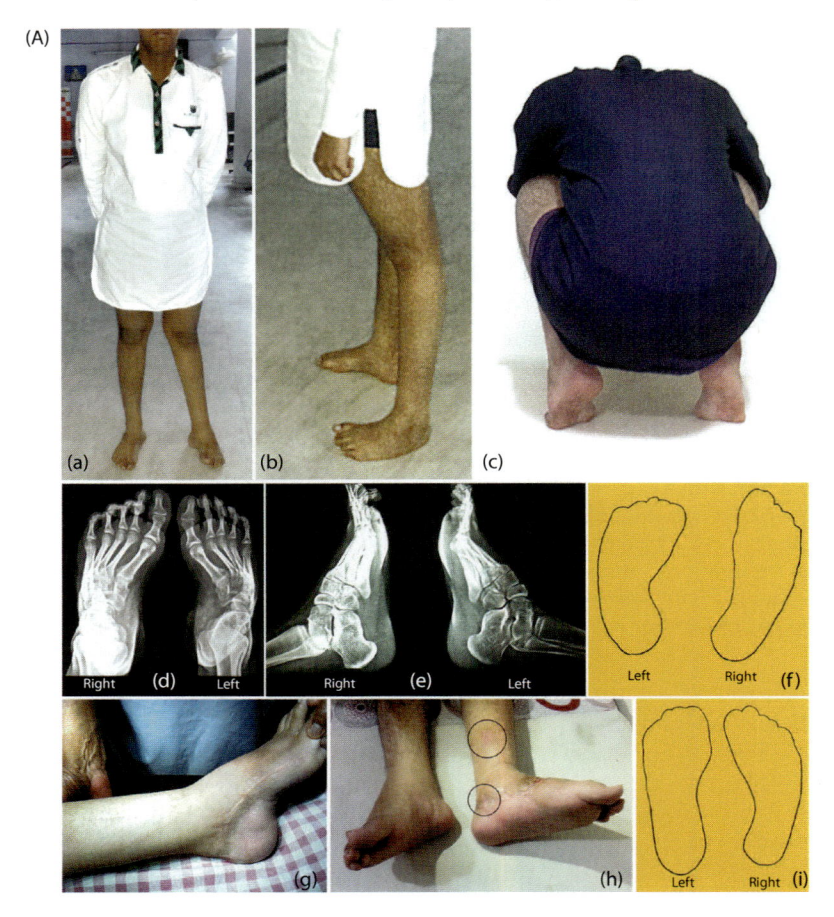

Figure 5.17(A) (a–i) (left foot) **(a and b)** Bilateral deformity seen from front and side, left more with genu recurvatum and valgum. **(c)** Showing hidden equinus (as genu recurvatum). **(d,e)** Skiagrams, AP and lateral views, showing talo-navicular dislocation and cavovarus, left much more than right. **(f)** Footprints, left more deformed than right. **(g)** Close-up of left foot with old scar. **(h)** Deformity corrected, also showing donor as well as recipient sites for small Thiersch skin graft; **(i)** Footprints at three-years follow-up showing correction of left foot. (Reprinted/adapted (left foot surgery figures) by kind permission courtesy from Springer Nature and Copyright Clearance Center's RightsLink. From author's own published article; Mittal RL. Trimorphic extreme clubfoot deformities and their management by triple surgical skin expanders—DOLAR, DOLARZ and DOLAR-E (evidence based mega-correction without arthrodesis). Mittal RL. *Int Orthop (SICOT)*, June 2018;42(6):1297–1306. For the book *Clubfoot: A Comprehensive Approach* for the publisher Taylor & Francis Group by Dr. R. L. Mittal. 2018–2019.)

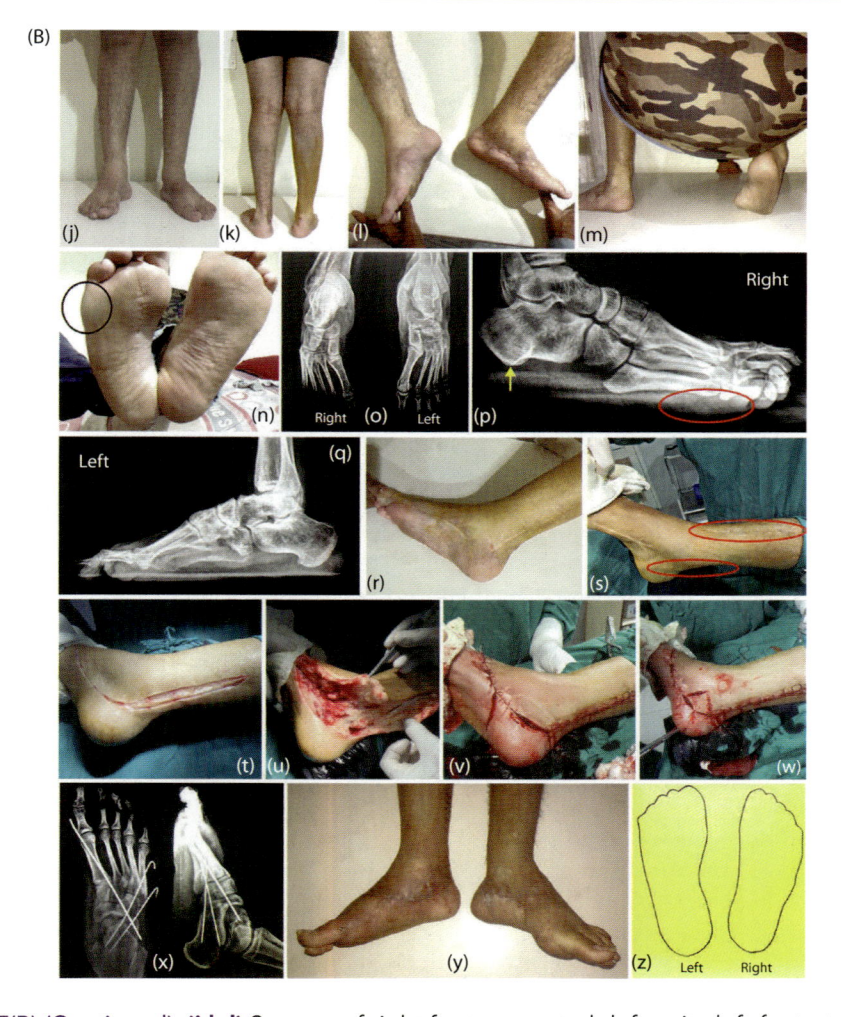

Figure 5.17(B) (Continued) (j,k,l) Surgery of right foot; corrected deformity left foot at three-years follow-up, seen from front, behind and close up of zig-zag healed scar. Right foot does have some deformity seen in standing position. (m) Hidden equinus also corrected on left side; on right side it is still persisting as uncorrected (this position is required for ADL in India. (n) After 3 years, painful callosity on the right foot seen as highlighted under the lateral side ball of right foot, forcing the patient for surgery on right side too. Medial cavus is also seen. (o–q) AP and lateral skiagrams both feet, left foot showing corrected cavus with foot lengthened without arthrodesis, excised dorsolateral wedge form cuboid and cuneiform also seen. On right foot in lateral X-ray heel equinus and painful callosity sites are highlighted. (r,s) Showing scars on medial, posterior, and anterior side. (t) Showing excised posterior scar. (u) Showing all medial, plantar joints opened up with corrected deformity. (v,w) Showing corrected deformity with an unclosed tight skin wound gap, facilitated by V-Y plasty flap being closed with good circulation. Tourniquet has been removed before closure of wound. (x) Postoperation X-rays showing correction with K-wires in place. (y,z) Three months after surgery, wound well-healed including V-Y plasty, deformity corrected with patient lying down, footprints of weight-bearing area, far better than before surgery at i.

incision, the scar was excised and subtotal subtalar release with all deeper dissections: Z plasty of tendoachilles, conjoint posterior capsulotomy. Abductor hallucis release, Steindler's release, tibialis posterior insertions release, flexor hallucis, and flexor digitorum longus releases were carried out. Spring ligament, all plantar and medial intertarsal and tarsometatarsal mobilization and interosseous talo-calcanean ligament releases were carried out. On closure, a small partial thickness skin graft taken from the lower part of same leg was applied below the medial malleolus instead of V-Y plasty, as the area was very small. Excellent correction of the foot deformity was achieved including hidden equinus. With equinus fully corrected, genu recurvatum corrected by itself in due course. At three years follow-up, the patient is highly satisfied with correction of the left foot. He has now been forced to get surgery for the right foot too. This surgical result was published in the *International Orthopaedics* publication of June 2018.

After three years, this patient developed **a painful callosity** on the right foot underneath and lateral to the head of the fifth metatarsal, which troubled him during walking. He also reported stiffness, difficulty with footwear, and dissatisfaction with the shape. He came to seek treatment for the right foot also now. He had been operated on the right foot recently in April 2018 initially only through DOLAR incision, but while closing the wound V-Y plasty was also required below and behind the medial malleolus. In deeper dissections, the scar was excised and abductor hallucis release, Z plasty of heel cord, and posterior capsulotomy of conjoint posterior capsule were done. The tibialis posterior tendon was not found and was probably divided at previous surgery, but flexor hallucis longus and flexor digitorum were divided at the Henry's knot, Steindler's release, spring ligament, and all plantar and medial ligaments and interosseous talo-calcanean ligaments were divided, besides excision of a dorsolateral wedge from the cuboid. Multiple K-wires were used for fixing and maintaining all corrections, including talo-navicular joint. Wound closure was done after hemostasis and a well-padded plaster cast was applied. Slitting of cast after 24 hours was also done, to forestall circulatory problems. Excellent correction has been achieved at the table. Follow up at three months after surgery shows excellent correction of this foot, comparing both feet lying down, as well as in footprints in the photographs w and x. This case proves that complications keep on coming up as the deformity persists in later age. All these are shown in the photographs in [Figure 5.17(A)a–i and (B)j–z]. This case, with inadequate follow up, has been shown to actually display this rare complication and its satisfactory management even at late age without any arthrodesis procedure, with highly satisfied patient.

CASE 16: 17-YEAR-OLD BILATERAL EXTREME CLUBFOOT WITH BIG CALLOSITIES

The author went to Indonesia in 1996 as a visiting professor, on a World Orthopaedic Concern assignment, at the University of Ujung Pandang (Sulawesi Province) to set up the postgraduate facility in their department. A 17-year-old poor Indonesian boy with bilateral severe rigid deformities with big callosities was operated on there by the author by only a first-generation rotation flap incision technique without any triple arthrodesis. At that time, the second- and third-generation techniques had not been innovated, and the deformity must have been grade 1 extreme deformity. Even at the operating table, the deformity was very well corrected. The follow-up protocol was explained to the Indonesian doctors, as the author's stay there was only two weeks. However, the author has no follow-up of this case, but it should be good from his experience. (See photograph in Figure 5.18.)

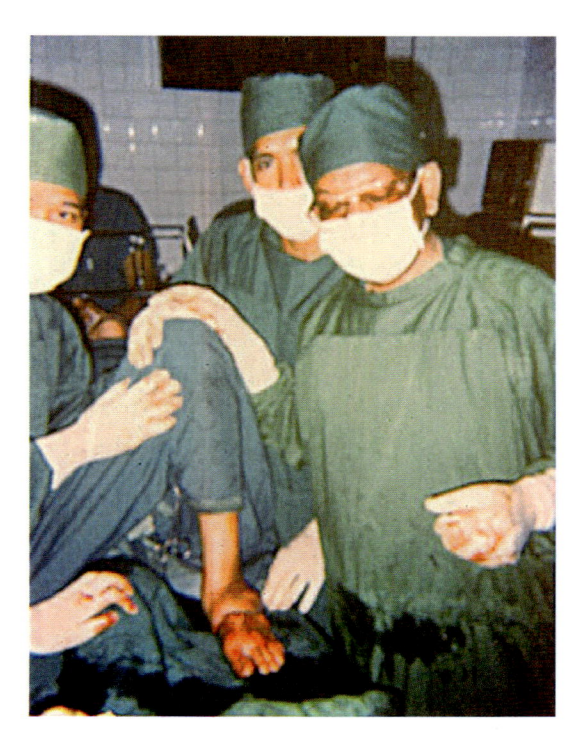

Figure 5.18 Indonesian patient grade 3 extreme deformity with huge dorsolateral callosity, corrected by the DOLAR technique, without any arthrodesis, seen at the operation table before applying plaster cast.

CASE 17: OCTOPUS CLUBFOOT IN ADULT: A UNIQUE DEFORMITY AND THE FIRST CASE WITH A NEW NAME AND UNIQUE SURGERY

RK, an 18-year-old female with unusual, first of its kind multiple deformities was published in the June 2018 issue of *International Orthopaedics* and is being described in full detail here. On clinical examination, there was 2.5" shortening of the left lower limb and equinovarus deformity the left foot with eight toes (octopus clubfoot). The extra toes were two preaxial and one

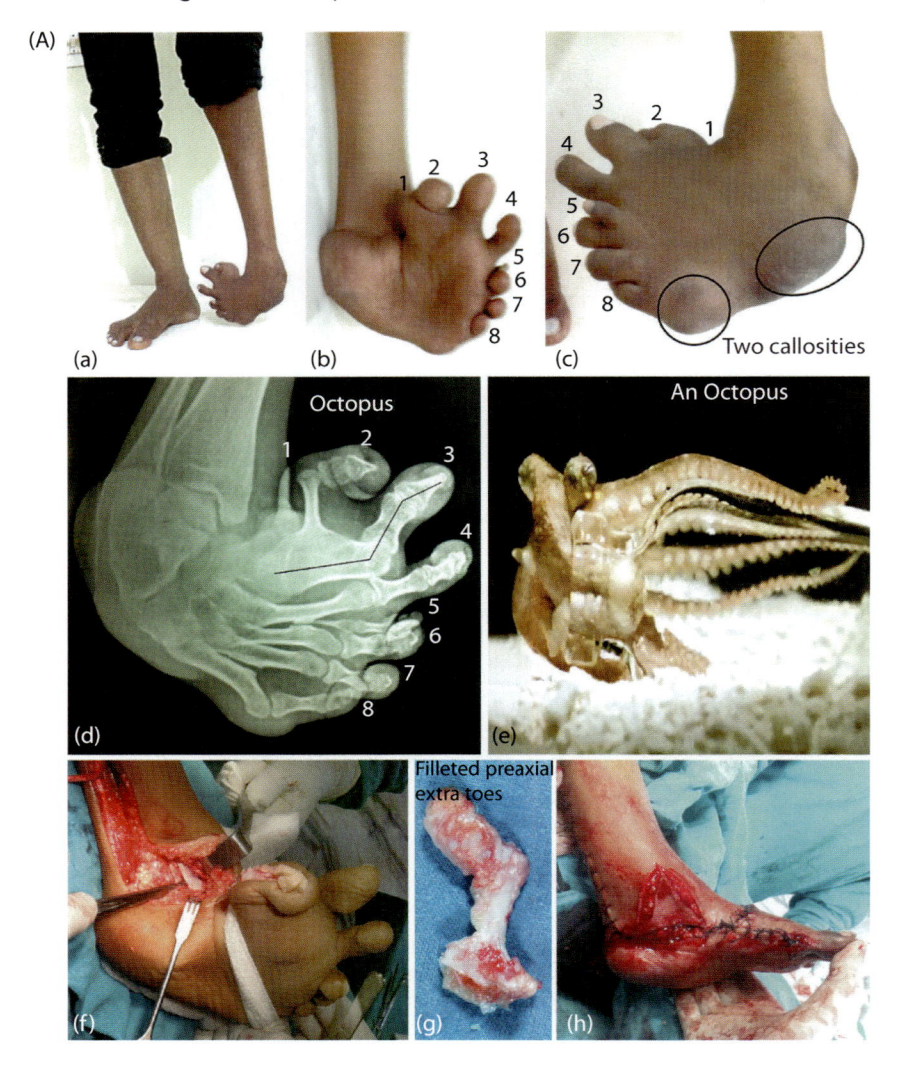

Figure 5.19(A) **(a–c)** Clubfoot with eight toes, coupled rotation deformity of foot at 90° on double axes with dorsum facing directly forward, sole backward and two highlighted weight bearing callosities. **(d)** X-ray showing eight toes and varus of great toe with angular deformities of metatarsals and coalitions are seen. **(e)** An octopus with semblance of its body parts to foot bones in X-ray can be seen in one's imagination. **(f)** Highly contracted and short tibialis posterior fanning out into the sole. **(g)** Excised/filleted-out bones (pre-axial extra toes from the fused first metatarsal) from the fillet flap. **(h)** 4-in-1, i.e., DOLAR + Z + VY + fillet flap were used to provide adequate skin cover for total all-around correction.

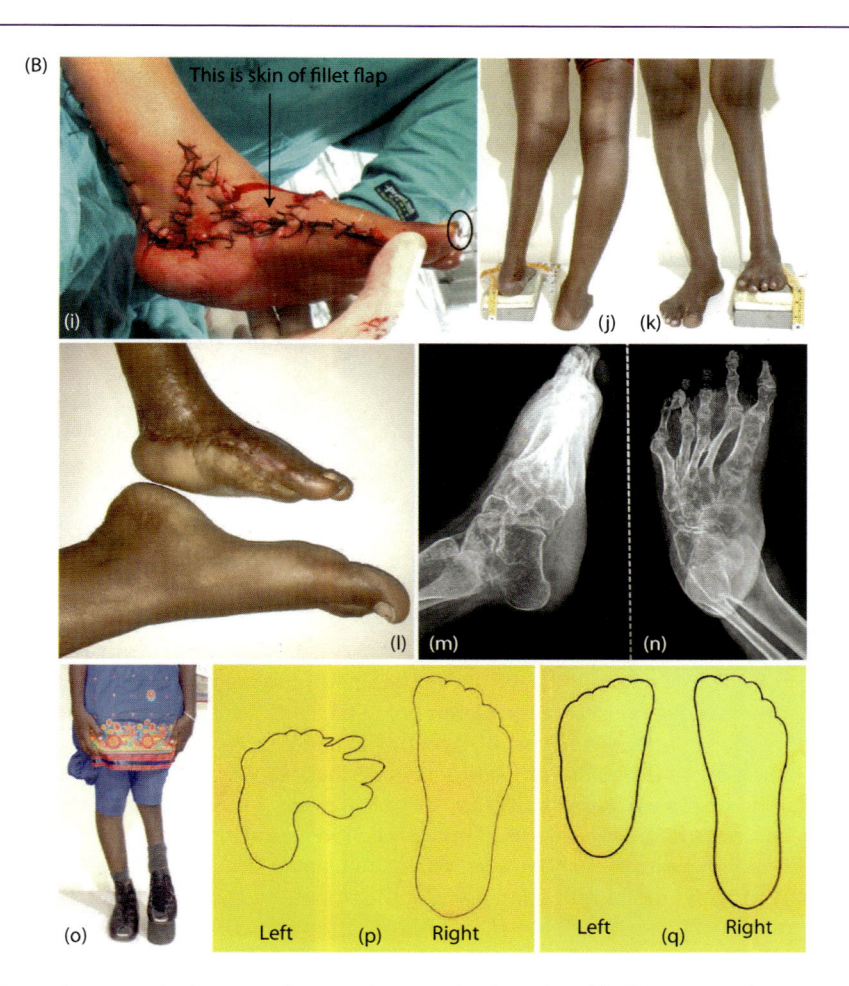

Figure 5.19(B) (Continued) (i) 4-in-1 flaps with wounds closed and hallux varus also corrected with a highlighted K-wire in the great toe. (j–l) Showing corrected deformity in various views, with 2½ inches shortening with patient standing and wind-swipe deformity. (m,n) Skiagrams, AP and lateral views, showing corrected deformity and intertarsal coalition with angulated fifth metatarsal as the second callosity site. No arthrodesis procedure has been done. (o) At one-year follow-up, patient walking with 2″ shoe raise. She is highly satisfied, not willing to undergo limb lengthening for the present. (p,q) Footprints of weight-bearing areas of deformed foot and corrected foot compared with the normal side. Deformity has been very well corrected except for a smaller foot size. (Reprinted/adapted by kind permission courtesy from Springer Nature and Copyright clearance centre of RightsLink. From author's own published article; Mittal RL. Trimorphic extreme clubfoot deformities and their management by triple surgical skin expanders—DOLAR, DOLARZ, and DOLAR-E (evidence based mega-correction without arthrodesis). Mittal RL. *Int Orthop (SICOT)*, June 2018;42(6):1297–1306. For the book *Clubfoot: A Comprehensive Approach* for the publisher Taylor & Francis Group by Dr. R. L. Mittal. 2018–2019.)

rudimentary toe on the inner side of the third toe, extending between the third and fourth metatarsals. The patient was standing on the lateral border of the foot with double callosities, one at the calcaneocuboid area and other at the head of the fifth metatarsal. There was complex rotational deformity, around both the anteroposterior and vertical axes through 90° each, with the sole facing backward and the dorsum facing forward. There is marked wasting of the left lower limb as a whole, with wind-swipe deformity of the knees to the right. There was marked hallux varus deformity of the right great toe also. Skiagram showed two accessory toes arising from the first metatarsal with marked hallux varus, intertarsal fusions varus at the second, third, and fourth metatarsals, and the fifth metatarsal bent laterally at the mid-shaft with varus at its metatarsophalangeal joint with a callosity there. There is inversion of the heel with callosity at the calcaneocuboid joint. A footprint of the sole had a highly unusual appearance, like an octopus. A highly meticulous surgery of about 3.5 hours, with good planning, was required to correct this deformity through a DOLAR + Z + VY plasty incision with the **addition of the well-known concept of the fillet flap of plastic surgery** (removing the bones but preserving all the soft tissues with the skin cover for use on an uncovered area) as reported by Kuntscher et al.[7] and Eliezer et al.[8]: excision of the preaxial extra toes by filleting and using the proximally based fasciocutaneous flap (fillet flap) to cover the raw area after full correction and supplementing the rotation, Z, and V-Y plasty, thus using for the first time, the innovative **4-in-1 evidence-based concept**, for providing extra skin cover for use over extensive raw area left after correcting this unusual deformity. Z plasty of the heel cord was done, the conjoint posterior capsule was divided completely to correct hidden equinus, the spring ligament, plantar ligaments medial capsule of the great toe, interosseous talo-calcanean ligament, and flexor hallucis brevis, knot of Henry, the grossly contracted fan shaped insertions of the tibialis posterior were divided, Steindler's plantar stripping was done, and a dorsolateral wedge from the cuboid was excised. The deformity was corrected including hallux varus and fixing by multiple K-wires for hallux varus, talo-navicular dislocation and calcaneocuboid area. Excellent correction was achieved at one year of follow-up, with the patient walking with a 2″ shoe raise, due to two and a half shortening with hypoplasis of whole limb. Although limb lengthening can also be done, the patient was not willing and was extremely happy to walk about with the shoe raise. The foot, of course, is still smaller in length, despite the maximum length achieved without any arthrodesis procedure. Because of intertarsal fusion, flexibility of the foot bones is also restricted, which can be further improved by removing the coalitions. Preoperative, intraoperative and follow up photographs show all the details [Figure 5.19(A)a–h and (B)i–q]. This is the first such case in the world literature, treated with the innovative 4-in1 skin expansion technique and without any arthrodesis procedure.

CASE 18: ADULT GENU RECURVATUM WITH PAINFUL LOCKING AND INSTABILITY

PS, an 18-year-old male with residual deformities of both feet with severe cavus and equinus with marked symptomatic genu recurvatum, right more than left, with painful locking and instability and fear of falling down. Feet were plantigrade. Patient was brought for the knee symptoms and they were unaware that the knee problem was the result of something wrong with the feet, because they felt the feet were already operated on nicely in early childhood and were straight. On examination,

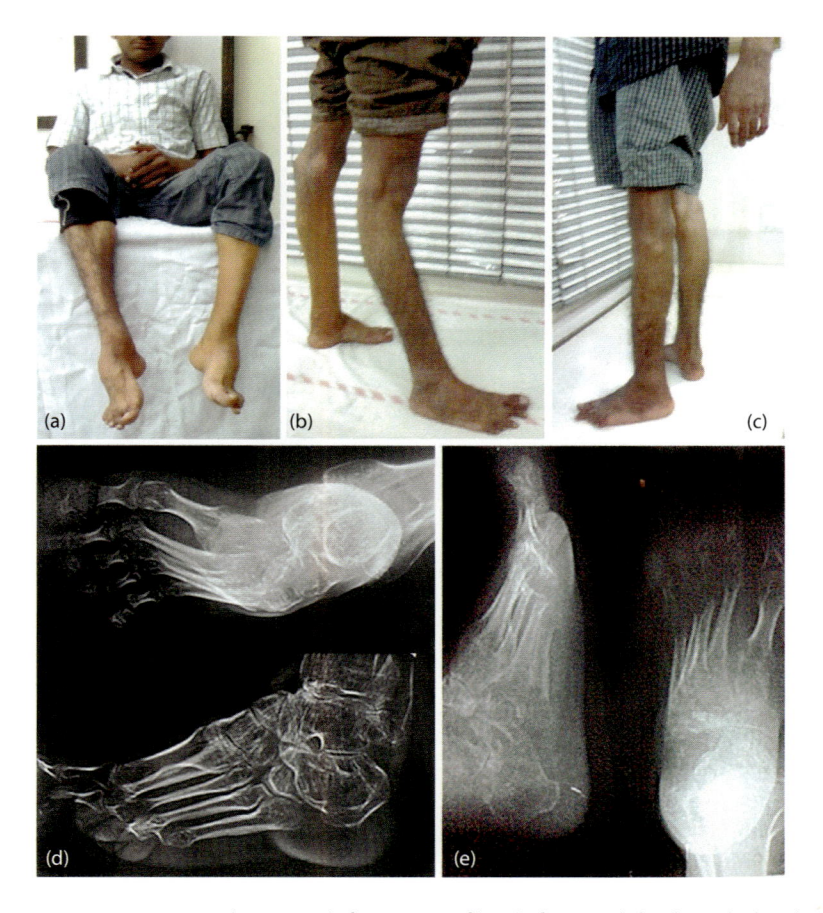

Figure 5.20 (a) Patient sitting, showing deformities of both feet with high arch, heel equinus, hyperextension at metatarsophalangeal joints, and flexion at interphalangeal joints. (b) On standing, equinus both sides with bilateral genu recurvatum and posterior subluxation both sides, right side more. (c) After surgery by DOLAR technique, at follow-up, foot as well as knee deformity corrected. (d) Preoperative X-rays showing the deformity. (e) Follow-up X-rays showing corrected deformities without arthrodesis. (Reprinted/adapted by kind permission courtesy from Springer Nature and Copyright Clearance Center's RightsLink. From author's own published article; Mittal RL. Trimorphic extreme clubfoot deformities and their management by triple surgical skin expanders—DOLAR, DOLARZ, and DOLAR-E (evidence based mega-correction without arthrodesis). Mittal RL. *Int Orthop (SICOT)*; June 2018;42(6):1297–1306; For the book *Clubfoot: A Comprehensive Approach* for the publisher Taylor & Francis Group by Dr. Mittal RL. 2018–2019.)

there were rigid heel equinus, marked medial cavus, cock-up deformity of the big toe, flexion at the interphalangeal joints (EQ4), knees showed anteroposterior laxity, posterior subluxated tibia with McMurray's test positive; all the findings were more severe on the right side. With great difficulty, the parents were convinced that the feet needed treatment and not the knee. The right foot was operated on first with this technique with all the extensive deeper dissections: heel cord Z plasty, conjoint posterior capsulotomy, Steindler's release, tibialis posterior and Henry's knot release, and dorsolateral wedge resection from the cuboid with fixation with K-wires, but without any arthrodesis procedure. At five years of follow-up, there was excellent correction of the foot deformity and the knee corrected itself in due course of time, as seen in the photographs (Figure 5.20a–e).

5.2 Evolution of triple surgical techniques 139

CASE 19: ADULT WITH GRADE 3 RIGID FOOT

NS, a 19-year-old male with rigid grade 3 left clubfoot with a big callosity on the dorsolateral aspect in the calcaneocuboid area and marked cavus and cock-up of the big toe with wasting left leg. Skiagrams, AP and lateral views, showed acute cavus (EQ4) and cock-up of the big toe. As it was an extremely rigid, severe deformity, surgery was planned in two stages in order to offer the patient a longer, well-shaped foot without arthrodesis. The first stage was done by a DOLAR + Z plasty incision to start, but during closure, V-Y plasty had to be added. The following deeper corrections were done: heel cord Z plasty, conjoint posterior capsulotomy to open ankle and subtaloid joints for correcting hidden equinus, abductor hallucis release, Steindler's release, all tibialis posterior

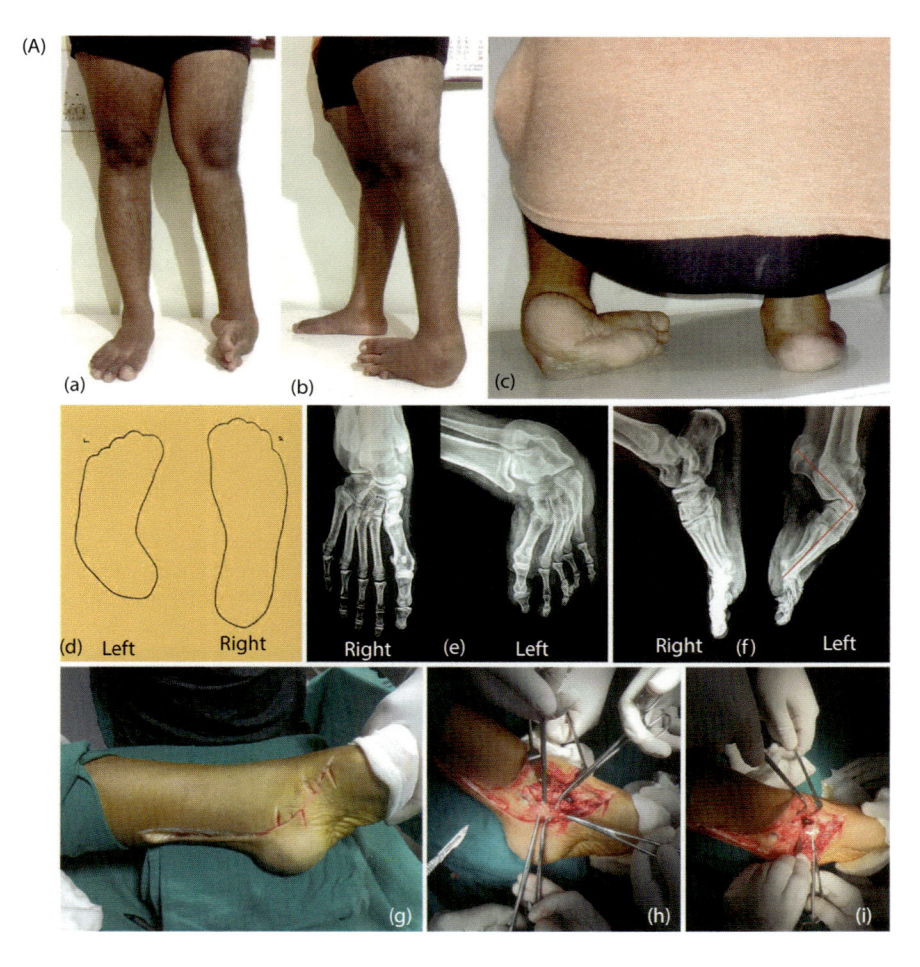

Figure 5.21(A) **(a)** Showing a very severe rigid grade 3 deformity. There is external rotation of the knee indicating bi-axial rotation of the foot. **(b)** Showing the deformity from the lateral side. **(c)** Sitting on feet showing the callosity and heel equinus deformity. **(d)** Footprints of plantar surfaces of both feet. **(e)** Skiagrams, AP views, compared with typical, showing not only talo-navicular dislocation, but also some intertarsal subluxations at other joints as well as tarso-metatarsal subluxations. **(f)** Lateral X-rays showing extreme cavus (EQ4) and cock-up big toe. **(g)** Incision mark with two Z-plasties. **(h)** Divided fan-shaped all nine tibialis posterior insertions held with multiple artery forceps. **(i)** Flexor hallucis longus and flexor digitorum longus at the knot of Henry to be divided.

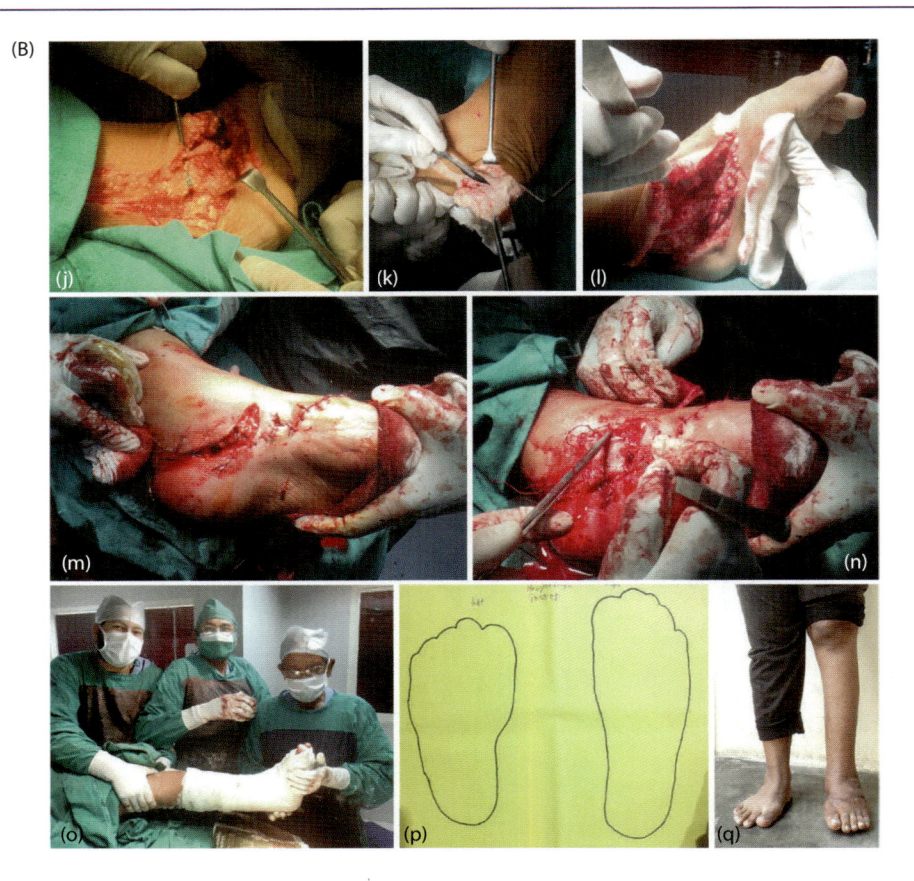

Figure 5.21(B) (Continued) (j) Showing opened up subtalar and ankle joint after posterior capsulotomy. **(k)** Showing excising dorsolateral bursa. **(l)** Showing all medial side joints opened out with varus corrected. **(m)** Showing unclosed tense gap ready for V-Y plasty flap. **(n)** V-Y plasty flap being closed. **(o)** Well-padded plaster cast in undercorrection to forestall circulatory problems. **(p)** Footprints of weight-bearing areas at three-months follow-up. **(q)** Patient standing at three-months follow-up with good partial correction.

insertions in the sole released, Henry's knot division, spring and other plantar and medial side ligaments, tarsometatarsal mobilization, interosseous talo-calcanean ligament release, dorsolateral wedge resection from the cuboid, and fixation with K-wires to correct the cock-up of the big toe, talo-navicular dislocation, and cuboid wedge closure. Hemostasis was secured and a well-padded plaster cast was given in the maximum safe correction.

The second stage of the surgery was done after about three months, through a small posterior incision releasing all tendoachilles adhesions and conjoint posterior capsule for correcting remaining equinus. A separate medial incision was given, and all dissections were done remaining close to bones, releasing all plantar and medial ligaments once again. A third incision, approximately one inch, was given over the calcaneocuboid area, and a complete osteotomy of the cuboid was done to move it freely, and the interosseous talo-calcanean ligament was once again divided. Multiple K-wires were used for fixing various bones and joints to achieve full correction

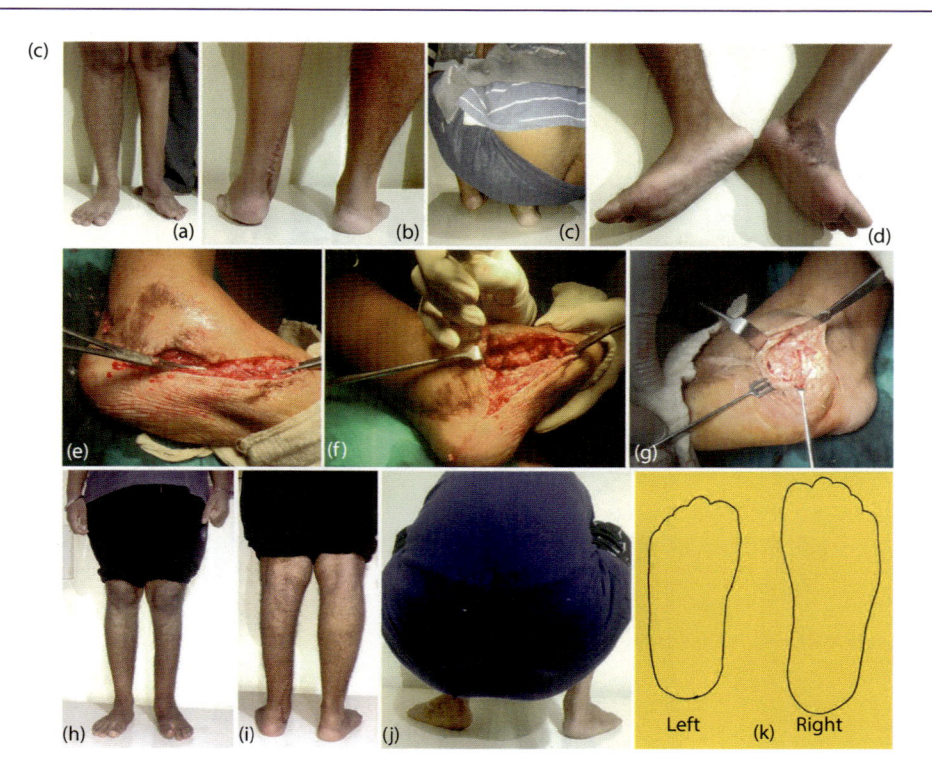

Figure 5.21(C) (Continued) (a–c) Preoperative photographs of both feet from front and back, **before second surgery**, patient standing and sitting on feet, showing good partial correction but some deformity still left. (d) Close-up of both feet from medial side with well-healed scars of DOLAR + Z + V-Y plasty incision and part of equinovarus deformity still left. (e, f) Second surgery through a small posterior incision releasing the adhesions of heel cord and medial incision releasing all soft tissues remaining close to bones and opening of all joints from medial side by dividing their ligaments. (g) Osteotomy of cuboid again. (h,i) Deformity well corrected, seen from front and back in standing position, at six months follow-up after second surgery, on comparing with preoperative pictures a, b, above. (j) Hidden equinus also corrected, comparing with preoperative picture at c, above. (k) Usual-appearing footprints of weight-bearing areas of both feet at last follow-up.

and maximum length of the foot. All wounds were closed after hemostasis, and the foot was immobilized for three months with changes at a 3–4 week interval, and after that, a protective foot–ankle brace was worn for another three months. Excellent correction with full patient satisfaction has been achieved at six months of follow-up after the second surgery; the patient is fully satisfied and walking freely now [Figure 5.21 (A)a–i, (B)j–q and (C)a–k].

CASE 20: ADULT WITH HIGH DOME, SMALLER FOOT WITH PSYCHOSOCIAL PROBLEM

RS, a 23-year-old adult equinovarus right foot with very severe medial cavus (EQ4) with hidden equinus also. He was resigned to the deformity. He could manage everything except the unsightly appearance of a smaller foot, especially now at adulthood, and the problem in finding a good marital match. This was a compelling psychosocial handicap to justify correction. On clinical examination, he had a rigid deformity, with hidden equinus with foot plantigrade in the standing position, high dome with marked medial cavus, cock-up of the big toe and thus EQ4 deformity. X-rays, lateral views, compared with the unaffected foot showed medial cavus with beaking at the head of the talus and calcaneum anterosuperior end, a stress-riser, and early sign of osteoarthritis. Surgery in this case was not rotation flap incision, but the usual posteromedial release with all the releases of Subtotal Subtalar Release (SSR), correcting the hidden equinus by heel cord

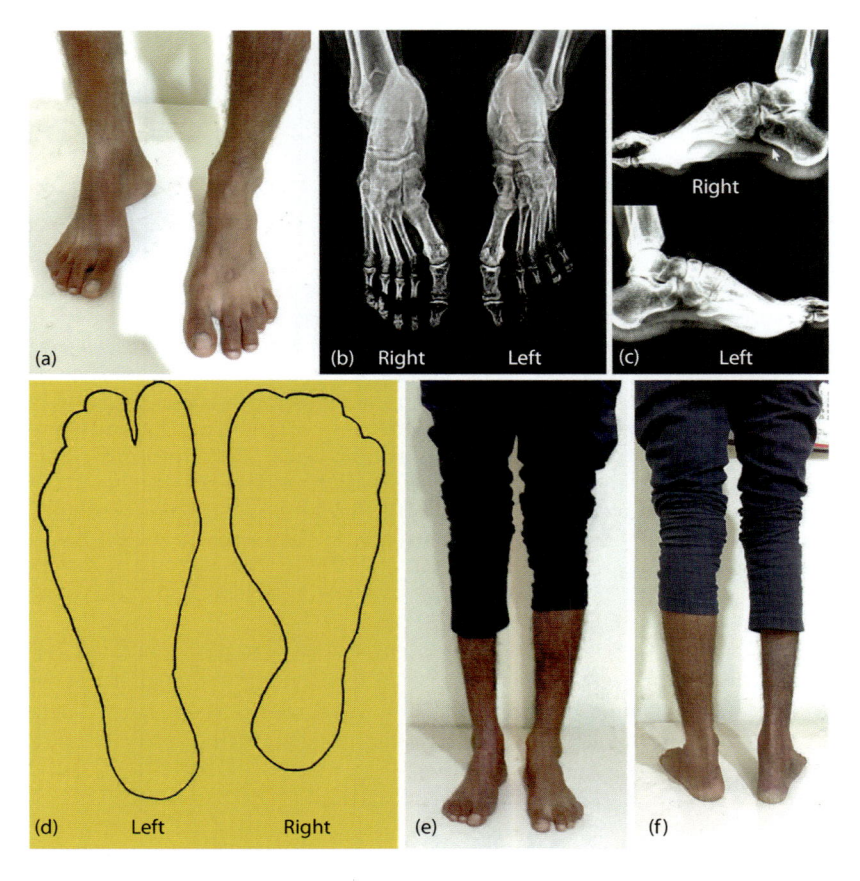

Figure 5.22 (a) Smaller splayed-out left foot with marked cavovarus (high dome) and heel equinus since birth and psychosocial problem in finding a match for marriage. (b,c) X-rays compared with typical; there is high dome as compared with typical. (d) Footprints of weight-bearing areas showing splayed-out foot with varus and high medial arch. (e,f) After surgery, by DOLAR incision approach at one year follow up, showing excellent correction without any arthrodesis.

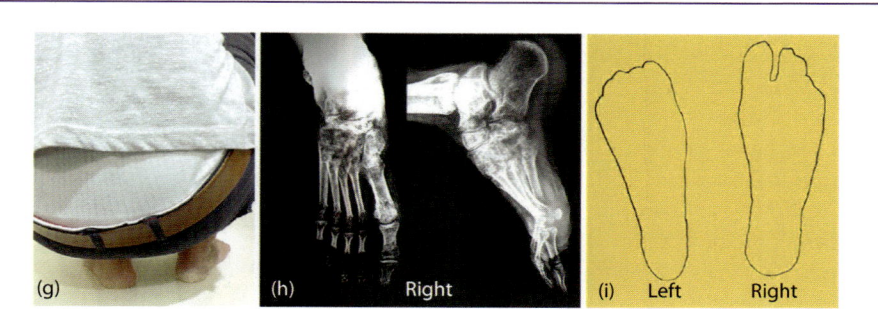

Figure 5.22 (Continued) **(g)** Hidden equinus also corrected with both feet plantigrade in sitting in this position. **(h)** X-rays of deformed foot after surgery at follow-up showing correction without arthrodesis. **(i)** Footprints showing good shape of deformed foot at follow-up. (Reprinted/adapted by kind permission courtesy from Springer Nature and Copyright Clearance Center's RightsLink. From author's own published article; Mittal RL. *Int Orthop (SICOT)*; June 2018;42(6):1297–1306; For the book *Clubfoot: A Comprehensive Approach* for the publisher Taylor & Francis Group by Dr. R L Mittal. 2018–2019.)

lengthening and conjoint posterior capsule release, tibialis posterior, flexor hallucis and longus release at Henry's knot, Steindler's release, spring and other plantar ligaments release, interosseous talo-calcanean ligament release, modified Robert Jones procedure for cock-up big toe, and dorsolateral wedge resection from the cuboid, thus mobilizing all the bones and joints. The deformity could be corrected without any arthrodesis procedure. Corrected foot bones were fixed with three K-wires: in the big toe going through the first metatarsal to correct the cock-up deformity, through talo-navicular joint correcting its subluxation, and through the cuboid laterally correcting varus. At one-year follow-up, the patient was extremely satisfied with a flexible, longer, good-looking, and better-functioning foot, as seen in the photographs (Figure 5.22a–i).

CASE 21: ADULT UNUSUAL 180° EVERTED FOOT AND A COLOSSAL DORSAL CALLOSITY

RI, a 23-year-old male, with extreme grade 3 deformity after childhood surgery and keloid/bowstring scars, grade 3 extreme equinovarus deformity, with grossly wasted leg, walked completely on dorsum in a reversed foot gait with huge dorsal and posterior painful callosity, extending from the dorsum posteriorly behind the ankle, which is the major weight-bearing area. Cock-up deformity of the big toe was also present. There was one-inch shortening of the limb. X-rays showed the major weight-bearing bones being the talus and calcaneocuboid area, which are in line with the ankle joint with the externally rotated leg. It is extremely important to analyze the pathoanatomical factors and correct each one of them to get good results. Correction was achieved by a DOLAR + Z + V-Y plasty incision, correcting heel equinus by heel cord lengthening and complete conjoint posterior capsulotomy to open up the subtaloid and ankle joint. The tibialis posterior insertions were released, flexor digitorum and flexor hallucis longus were divided, Steindler's was release, and spring and other plantar ligaments and interosseous talo-calcanean ligaments were divided. A dorsolateral wedge was excised from the cuboid. K-wire fixations with three wires were done. A well-padded plaster cast was given after wound closure. The period of immobilization was three months. The result was excellent with a highly satisfied patient at six months follow-up. He has a longer and flexible foot with far better function and looks as seen in the photographs (Figure 5.23a–l):

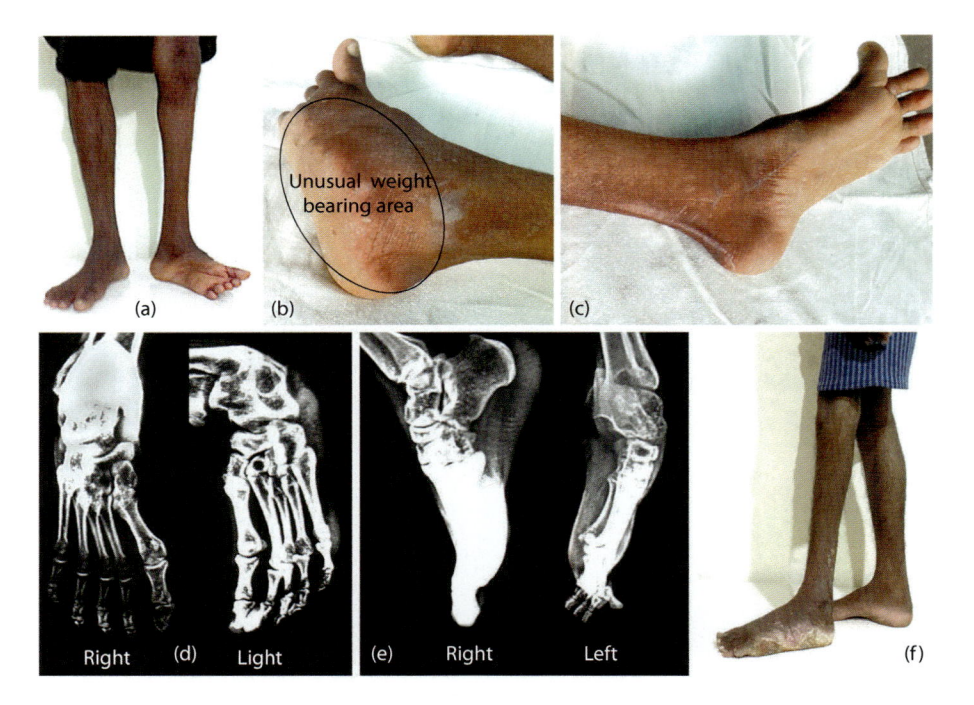

Figure 5.23 (a) Patient in standing position with reversed foot gait, weight borne completely on posterodorsal area. (b) Showing a huge callosity as a discolored dorsal area at the weight-bearing site. (c) Seen from medial side old bowstring keloid scar, tibialis anterior standing out with dynamic contracture, cavus, and cock-up big toe. (d) AP view X-rays compared with normal, there are talo-navicular calcaneocuboid subluxation and other tarsal disruptions. Lateral views showing extreme deformity with talar head dislocated and in vertical position in the weight-bearing area.

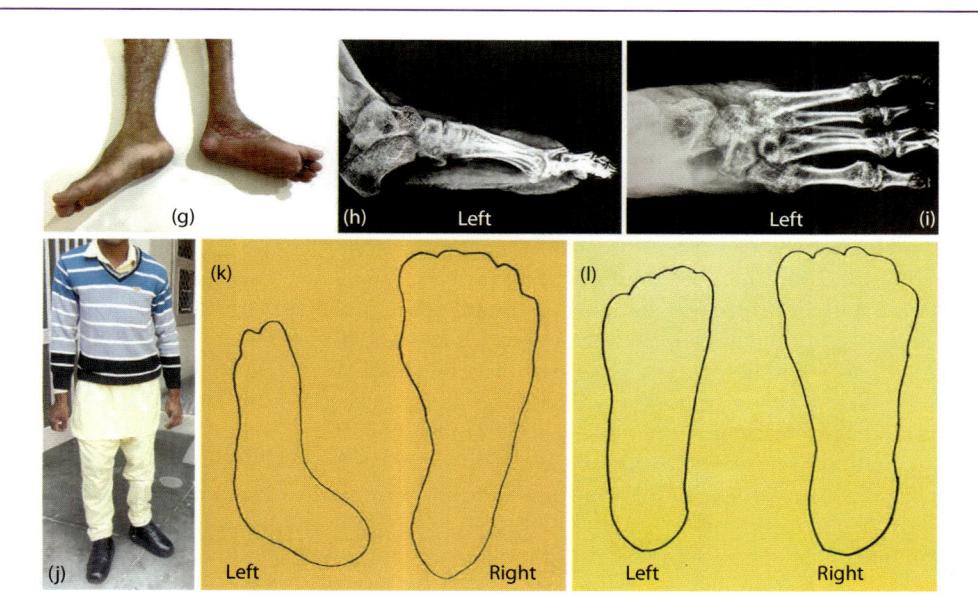

Figure 5.23 (Continued) **(g)** Deformity corrected without any fusion. **(h,i)** X-rays, AP and lateral views, showing deformity corrected without arthrodesis. There is radiological undercorrection. **(j)** Patient standing with normal shoes. **(k,l)** Footprints before and after operation at follow-up. (Reprinted/adapted by kind permission courtesy from Springer Nature and Copyright Clearance Center's RightsLink. From author's own published article; Mittal RL. *Int Orthop (SICOT)*; June 2018;42(6):1297–1306; For the book *Clubfoot-A Comprehensive Approach* for the publisher Taylor & Francis Group by Dr. R. L. Mittal. 2018–2019.)

CASE 22: ADULT CLUBFOOT WITH EXTENSIVE COALITIONS AND ADHERENT SCARS

RS, a 24-year-old male, had extreme grade 3 left-sided clubfoot with very rigid foot with adherent scar of surgery in early childhood and a jog of movement in some foot bones. On the left side, there were syndactyly, irregular coalitions of intertarsal and tarsometatarsal joints, interosseous tibiofibular fusion, exostosis seen in the left foot and an absent fourth metatarsal in X-rays and CT scan. His right foot also had congenital missing rays and syndactyly, but plantigrade. The patient was resigned to his fate, but with awareness spreading about the availability of these newer techniques, he consulted the author. He was offered a two-stage arthrodesis procedure to be able to preserve the maximum length, and he agreed. The first stage was DOLAR + triple Z incision with excision of the scar, as the anatomy was disturbed, the following deeper dissections were carried out remaining close to bones: complete release of tibialis posterior insertions, and cutting deep fascia, ligamentous, and other flexors meticulously, but trying to preserve even the smallest neurovascular structures. A dorsolateral wedge was also removed to get some mobility with partial correction. Fixing with K-wires stabilized this corrected foot. Closure of the wound was possible with lengthening of the skin pouch by a skin-expanding incision (DOLAR) after excising the scar. After three weeks, the second stage of intertarsal fusion with very little excision of bony tissue was done through a second rotation and Z plasty of skin incision with stabilization by fixation with K-wires again. The patient is extremely satisfied at eight years follow-up (Figure 5.24a–m).

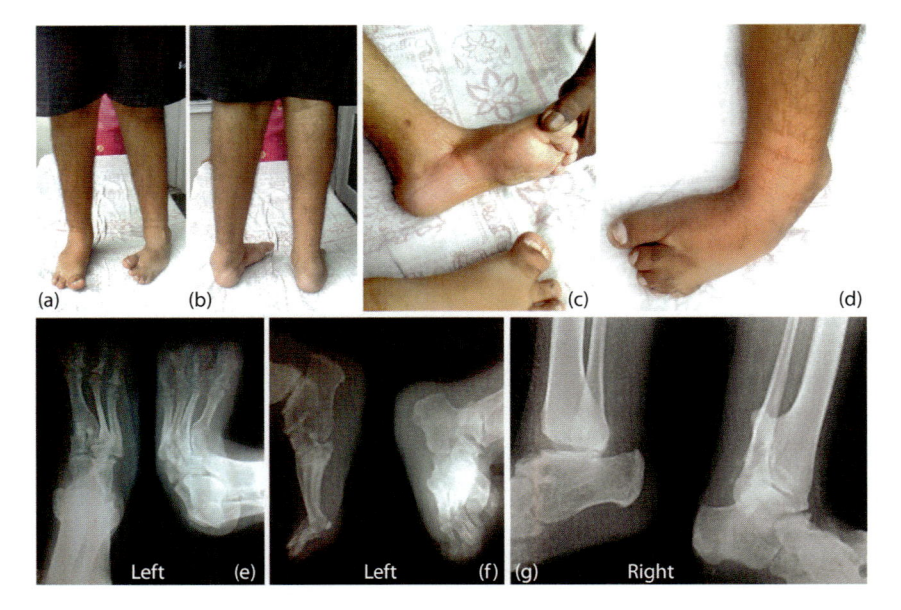

Figure 5.24 **(a,b)** Very severe rigid left clubfoot with other congenital defects as described as seen from front and back. **(c)** Adherent extensive scar of previous surgery. **(d)** Close-up of deformity from dorsal side. **(e–h)** X-rays and CT scan showing congenital fusions, absent ray and exostosis.

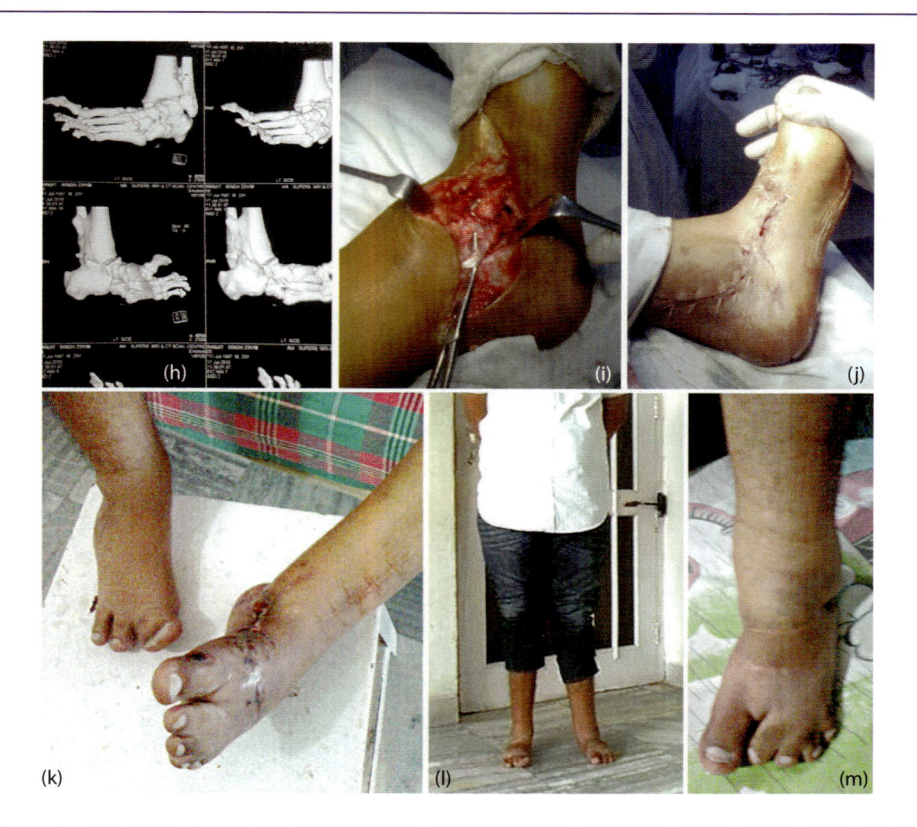

Figure 5.24 (Continued) **(i)** Tibialis posterior insertions are being released. **(j)** After the first stage surgery, incision mark of rotation and triple Z flap and partly corrected foot. **(k)** After first stage seen from different angle. **(l)** Patient standing with corrected deformity after second stage surgery of corrective intertarsal fusion at follow up. **(m)** Close-up of corrected foot at follow-up with rotation flap heeled scar. (Reprinted/adapted by kind permission courtesy from Springer Nature and Copyright Clearance Center's RightsLink. From author's own published article; Mittal RL. *Int Orthop (SICOT)*; June 2018;42(6):1297–1306; For the book *Clubfoot: A Comprehensive Approach* for the publisher Taylor & Francis Group by Dr. Mittal R. L. 2018–2019.)

CASE 23: ADULT CLUBFOOT WITH A STRESS FRACTURE OF THE FIFTH METATARSAL

PS, a 24-year-old male had bilateral rigid clubfoot deformities, the right more severe than left. His father also had bilateral clubfoot deformities. The patient had surgery on both feet at three and six months of age. There were residual deformities on both sides, which further increased with age, with the right foot more deformed. He had very rigid deformity with EQ4 and cock-up of the big toe. He was resigned to his fate, as he was only offered triple arthrodesis to correct the deformities, which was not acceptable to him. He started brisk walking to lose some weight. After about three weeks of this unaccustomed activity, he started getting pain in the right foot on the lateral border. He still continued walking and the pain became unbearable, making walking extremely difficult. He was referred to the author at that stage. A clinical diagnosis of stress fracture of the fifth metatarsal was not difficult to make. On detailed examination, the patient had severe, rigid bilateral clubfoot, the right side much more severe and fracture tenderness (specific point) about the middle of the fifth metatarsal shaft. The deformity on the fracture side (right) was more severe with genu recurvatum and even backache. He was overweight. His right foot was operated on through the DOLARZ-E approach (multiple Z plasties, from wherever skin could be mobilized, with rotation flap) and very extensive deeper dissections (SSR), heel cord Z plasty, and conjoint posterior capsulotomy, releasing abductor hallucis, flexor hallucis, all insertions of tibialis posterior, flexor digitorum, and flexor hallucis longus at Henry's knot, Steindler's, spring, and all other plantar ligaments remaining close to bones, and the interosseous talo-calcaneal ligament. A dorsolateral wedge was excised from the cuboid and cuneiforms. The deformity could be corrected by fixation with multiple K-wires and the wound was closed with adjusting various flaps in corrected position.

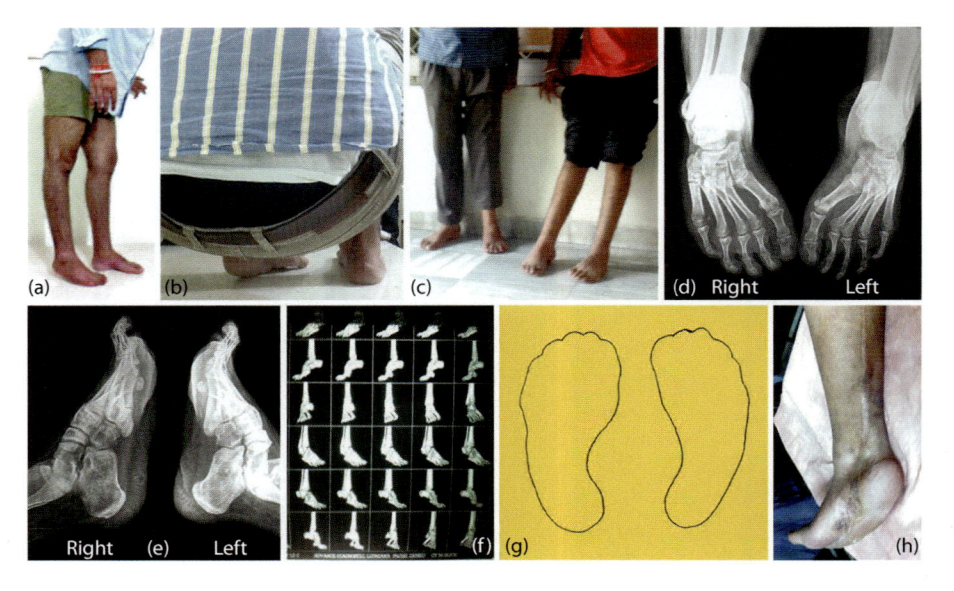

Figure 5.25 **(a)** Patient standing with caution, with support of wall to avoid pain of stress fracture in the deformed foot. **(b)** Patient sitting, showing hidden equinus. **(c)** Patient standing with his father on his right, who also had bilateral congenital clubfeet of lesser degree. **(d–f)** X-rays, AP and lateral views, and CT scan, showing the deformities and stress fracture on the right foot as highlighted. **(g)** Footprints of weight-bearing areas showing bilateral deformities. **(h)** Extensive posterior and medial scars in a close up of the right foot.

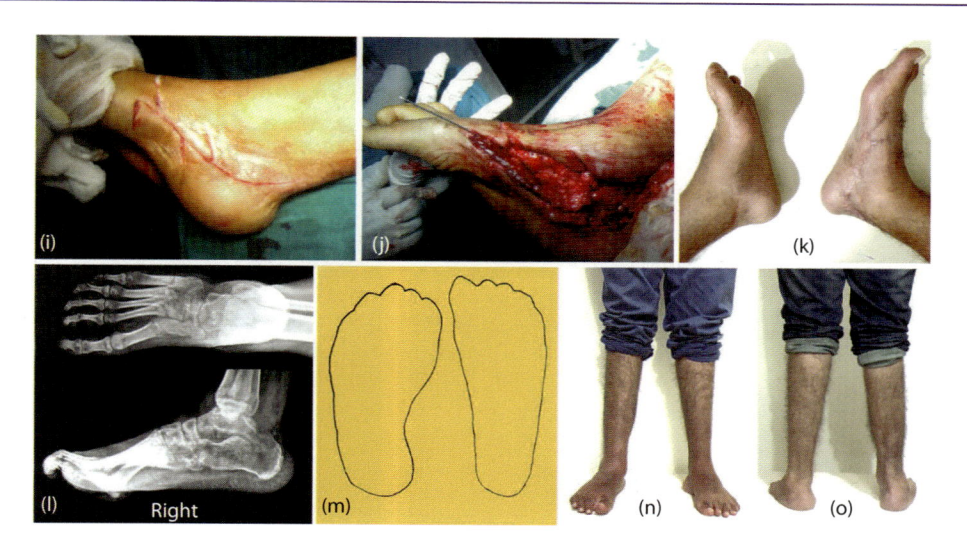

Figure 5.25 (Continued) **(i)** DOLAR + Z plasties initial incision mark. **(j)** Closing the wound with a gap on medial side by a V-Y flap. A K-wire seen in first metatarsal to correct cock-up deformity. **(k)** Close-up showing corrected deformity with well-healed scars **(l)** X-rays showing correction and fracture also healed. **(m)** Footprint of operated foot in good shape compared with other. **(n,o)** Showing very good correction with full patient satisfaction after 2.5 years. (Reprinted/adapted by kind permission courtesy from Springer Nature and Copyright Clearance Center's RightsLink. From author's own published article; Mittal RL. *Int Orthop (SICOT)*; June 2018;42(6):1297–1306; For the book *Clubfoot: A comprehensive approach* for the publisher Taylor & Francis Group by Dr. R. L. Mittal. 2018–2019.)

A well-padded plaster cast was given in undercorrected position to forestall circulatory problems, and the entire deformity was corrected in stages by plaster cast changes every two weeks. Nothing was done to the stress fracture itself. The deformity was well corrected and the stress fracture also healed with three months immobilization in a plaster cast with high patient satisfaction at 2.5 years follow-up. A stress fracture is an extremely rare event in association with congenital clubfoot, with only occasional reports.[9] In clubfoot, the obvious cause of this fracture is altered biomechanics due to the deformity and abnormal stress on the lateral border due to unaccustomed activity. The site of the fracture will be at the maximum stress site. It is not common but occurs when there is some inherent weakness or diathesis. Whenever there is pain in clubfoot on walking without subsiding, stress fracture should be ruled out. The deformity has to be corrected to remove the cause of pain or if there is a stress fracture. Correction is also necessary to prevent other complications and osteoarthritis of proximal joints. Being overweight was also one of the factors leading to this complication, putting more stress on the deformed bones and joints (Figure 5.25a–o).

150 Extreme clubfoot deformities and their management

CASE 24: AN ADULT WITH ARTHROGRYPOSIS MULTIPLEX CONGENITA WITH CLUBFOOT WITH PLANTAR HORN AND OTHER UNIQUE COMPLICATIONS

MK, a male child, first presentation at eight years of age, a patient of arthrogryposis multiplex congenita with bilateral rigid clubfoot (extreme grade 3), as well as club hands. His foot joints of both sides had mobility, but the right foot joints were much less mobile than the left. He was operated

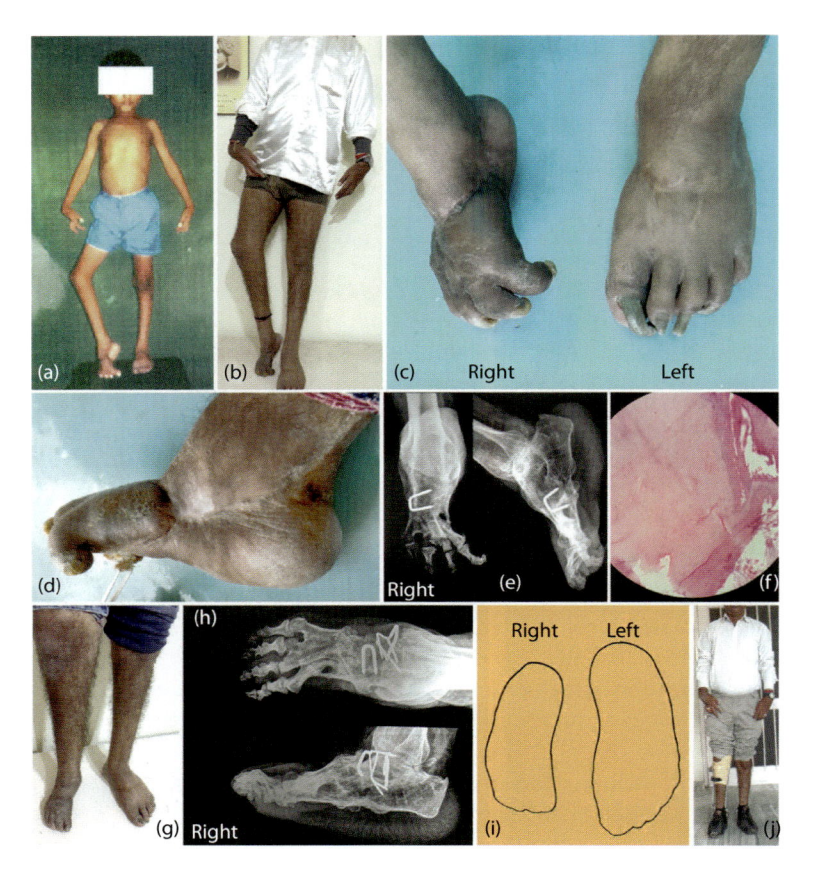

Figure 5.26 **(a)** Patient at eight years of age after the first surgery by DOLAR technique in childhood with residual deformity of right foot. **(b)** Same patient at 33 years of age in standing position with absent great toe ray. **(c)** Close-up of both feet, seen from dorsum, with horny nails not able to cut due to hand deformities, right foot with four toes and old scar. **(d)** Right foot seen from side with hammer second toe and a plantar horn projecting down from ball of foot. **(e)** Skiagrams showing all foot and ankle bones fused with metatarsus varus and flexed toes. **(f)** Cornified horn on histology. **(g)** Corrected deformity at two-years follow-up. **(h)** X-rays showing correction with fused foot joints and ankle with multiple staples in place. **(i)** Footprints of weight-bearing areas with good shape at follow up. **(j)** Patient standing with a PTB brace and padded shoe with compensated heel, walking about fully satisfied. (Reprinted/adapted by kind permission courtesy from Springer Nature and Copyright Clearance Center's RightsLink. From author's own published article; Mittal RL. *Int Orthop (SICOT)*; June 2018;42(6):1297–1306; For the book *Clubfoot: A Comprehensive Approach* for the publisher Taylor & Francis Group by Dr. Mittal R. L. 2018–2019.)

on 25 years ago by the DOLAR technique on both sides with very extensive deeper dissections (SSR). His left foot had excellent correction with high patient satisfaction, and the right foot had only partial correction, because there were congenital tarsal coalitions. He was advised a second surgery for the right foot, which his parents refused due to poverty. The child managed to walk about with that partially corrected right foot.

This patient again came to the author after 25 years, now aged 33 years, with complete inability to walk, with only four toes, the great toe ray absent with a scar present, and an excrutiatingly painful cornified plantar horn (projecting callosity) over the inner side of the ball of the right foot under the second and third metatarsal heads. The extraordinary history of the past 25 years was described by the patient like this: As he could walk with the corrected left foot and partial weight bearing on the undercorrected right foot, his parents did not get the second surgery done due to poverty and unworkable repeated visits from a far-off place of residence. So, he reconciled and continued walking like that for almost 20 years with a callosity and a recurrent chronic ulcer under the deformed great toe subsiding with padding underneath. Gradually, this chronic ulcer also became uncomfortable and painful. He consulted some orthopedic surgeon, who amputated his great toe ray with its callosity. The patient was without a job due to hand deformities as well. He managed for a couple of years, but again started getting a callosity under the ball of the left foot. This callosity was shaved off by a barber, and he continued for about a year further like that, until it projected more and more with unbearable pain. He came to the author crawling in early 2016, as he could not use crutches with club hands. He could no longer put weight on the right foot due to excruciatingly painful horny projection even to the slightest touch. The foot was completely rigid at all foot joints from the toes to the ankle. The remaining four toe joints had flexion deformities and were rigid, with a scary and alarming deformity, showing a scar from the previous surgery. Skiagrams showed bony fusions of all foot joints from the ankle joint to the toes as well with a staple used for fixation at the surgery 25 years ago still there. Capillary circulation was all right with pulsating anterior and posterior tibial arteries. Surgery was performed under tourniquet with the primary aim of obtaining a plantigrade foot. With minimum invasive approaches over the dorsum of the toes and on the dorsolateral side of the foot, without disturbing old scars, corrective fusions of the tarsal joints with appropriate wedge resections were carried out. K-wires were used for the toes to maintain correction and staples to stabilize the intertarsal area. The tourniquet was removed and hemostasis secured. Circulation was good and wounds were closed. A well-padded plaster cast was given and immobilization was continued for three months with a couple of changes. Subsequently, given the complete fusion of every joint of the foot as well as the ankle, with a hard callosity at the ball of the foot and decreased weight-bearing surface area of the foot, the patient was given a Patellar Tendon Bearing (PTB) brace with a padded shoe and heel raise for walking. The patient is highly satisfied and walking about comfortably at two years follow-up. All photographs before and after operation and with the PTB brace are given (Figure 5.26a–j).

CASE 25: CLUBFOOT DEFORMITIES INCREASED AFTER FRACTURE OF BONES IN BOTH LEGS, AND COMPARTMENT SYNDROME (ISCHEMIC)

SS, a 35-year-old adult male with untreated bilateral severe clubfoot deformities, happily married with family and children, walking about in elephant shoes, and not bothered about deformities. He met with a serious accident and fractured the bones in both legs. The fractures united after interlocking nailing of both sides, but his deformities of the feet increased. This made his life difficult

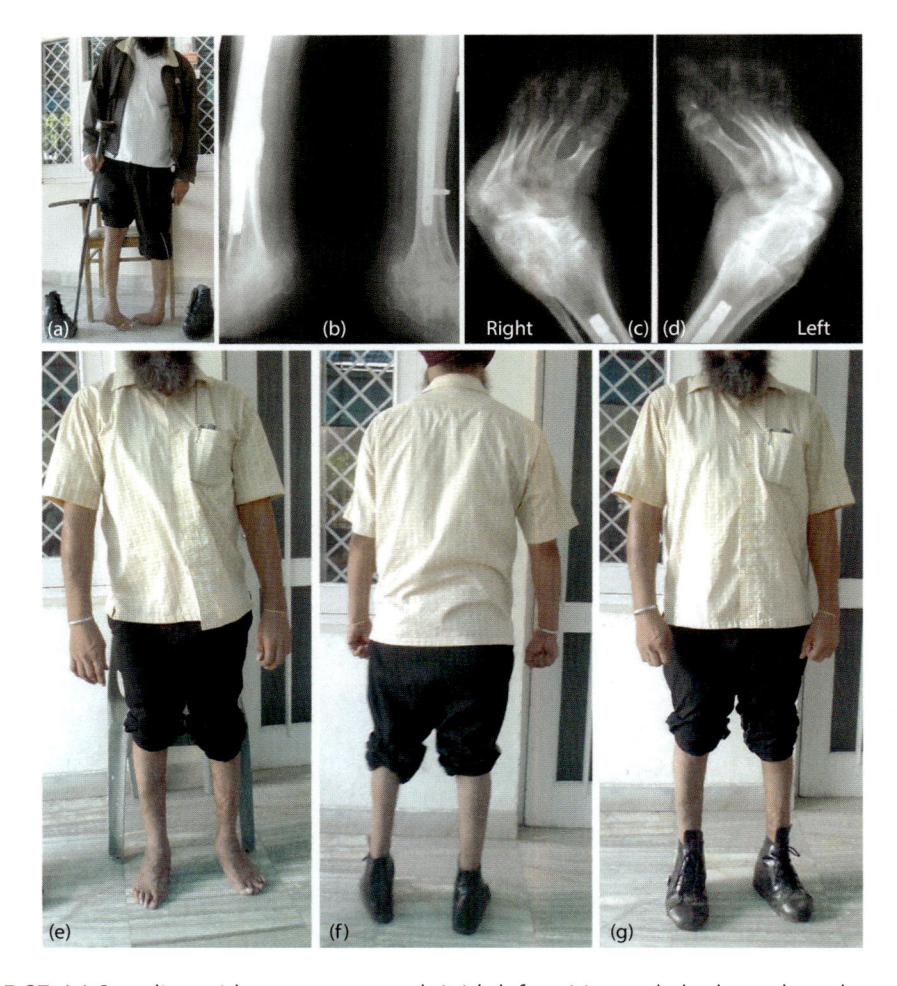

Figure 5.27 **(a)** Standing with very severe and rigid deformities and elephant shoes kept on side, right more deformed. **(b–d)** X-rays showing united fractures both legs with interlocking nails in place, X-rayed feet show grotesque deformities. **(e)** Both feet corrected with patient standing after three stage triple fusion surgeries, each side preserving length. **(f,g)** Seen with shoes from the back and front at 13-years follow-up. Patient is fully satisfied. (Reprinted/adapted by kind permission courtesy from Springer Nature and Copyright Clearance Center's RightsLink. From author's own published article; Mittal RL. *Int Orthop (SICOT)*; June 2018;42(6):1297–1306; For the book *Clubfoot: A Comprehensive Approach* for the publisher Taylor & Francis Group by Dr. Mittal R. L. 2018–2019.)

even for ADL, and he was thus forced to seek treatment. He was referred to the author for correction of these deformities. The deformities were extremely rigid, grade 3, with very slight movements at the foot joints. X-rays showed EQ5, and interlocking nails of the old surgery were visible in the X-rays of the legs in the lower end of both tibiae. His pulse at the ankle was good. After thorough preoperative assessment of these long-standing deformities, he was offered a three-stage triple arthrodesis for both feet in order to achieve the longest possible feet with corrected deformities. The first stage was soft-tissue correction with requisite skin expansion by a limited rotation flap incision with Z plasty of the heel cord, abductor hallucis release, tibialis posterior insertions release, dividing knot of Henry, releasing the spring, other medial and plantar ligaments, the interosseous talo-calcanean ligament, and even releasing the inferior tibiofibular syndesmosis to correct the grade 5 equinus (EQ5). The second stage of triple fusion was done with minimum possible osseous resections and further skin expansion by rotation and Z plasty incision. Plaster immobilization was done, keeping the foot undercorrected. The third stage was done with some more osseous resections and some more skin expansion, thus achieving full correction. First, one foot was operated on and then the second foot, taking about a year for the six surgeries and keeping the patient somewhat mobile on one foot. Excellent corrections have been achieved on both sides with an extremely satisfied patient at about 13 years follow-up. His preoperative and follow-up photographs are shown (Figure 5.27a–g).

CASE 26: UNILATERAL CLUBFOOT AFTER 20-YEAR-OLD BAD CRUSH INJURY, HEALED WITH EXTENSIVE SCAR AND BONY FUSIONS

KR, a 45-year-old male, presented with a right-sided clubfoot, very rigid grade 3, met a roadside accident 20 years previously with a bad crush injury to the lower part of the leg and foot, which was treated, and it healed with an extensive scar all over the foot and ankle area, but repeatedly breaking down on the dorsolateral side of the foot. For 20 long years he continued like this with a recurrent ulcer on the dorsolateral aspect on posterior side, and when it became painful, he came to the author for treatment because of recurrent ulcer as well as pain. Examination revealed scars on the medial side of the lower leg and ankle, but more extensive on the dorsolateral side, adherent with a recurring chronic ulcer near the ankle. Dorsalis pedis was absent, but posterior tibial pulse was normal. There was good vascular supply in the foot and ankle area on color doppler study. X-rays showed fusion of tarsal bones and a screw showing an old united medial malleolus fracture, but mobility at the ankle and tarsometatarsal joints was present. A well planned, extensive, and meticulous surgery had to be done for such a scarred old-standing deformity, so as to obtain the longest possible foot, with triple arthrodesis. A limited medial and posterior incision with a Z plasty was given. Z-lengthening of the heel cord and conjoint posterior capsulotomy were done to correct heel equinus, the malleolar screw was removed, tibialis posterior insertions, flexor hallucis, and flexor digitorum longus were divided, Steindler's release was performed, and spring and other plantar ligaments were released, thus procuring adequate soft-tissue release. After that, through a limited incision through the scar on the dorsolateral aspect, remaining close to bones, triple arthrodesis was performed with appropriate wedge resections, and correction of the deformity was achieved with multiple staples fixation. Hemostasis was secured after removing the tourniquet. Only partial wound closure was possible on the medial and posterior part of the leg over the tendoachilles, leaving a big gap unclosed. A unique double V-Y plasty incision for expanding

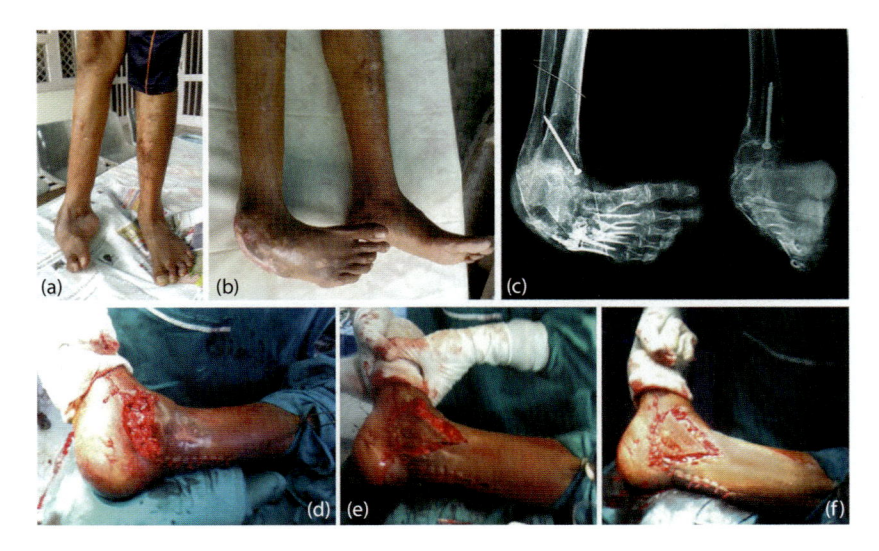

Figure 5.28 **(a)** Patient standing with the severe deformity, right foot. **(b)** Close-up of foot showing adherent scar and ulcer on dorsolateral aspect in posterior part. **(c)** X-rays showing the deformity with a screw in medial malleolus and fused tarsals. **(d)** Showing a big gap below and medial to ankle after straightening the foot. **(e)** One V-Y plasty with base downward. **(f)** Showing the other V-Y plasty in tendoachilles area with base proximal.

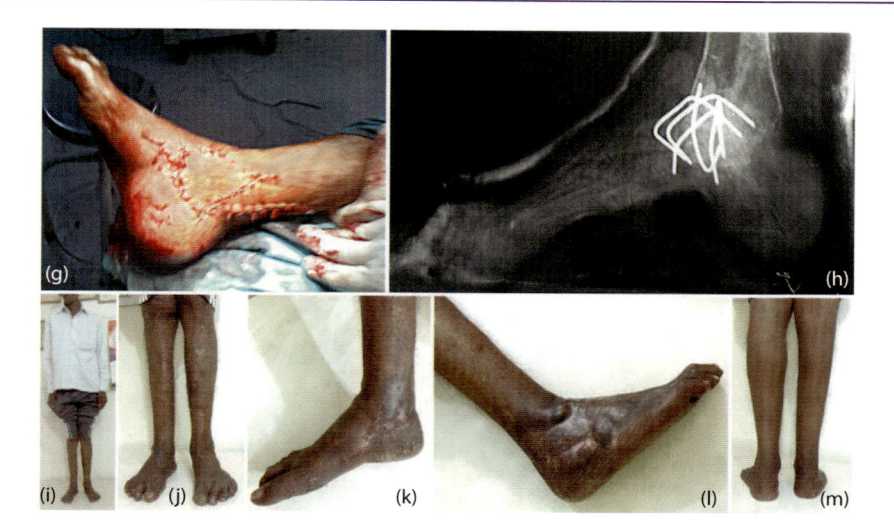

Figure 5.28 (Continued) **(g)** After complete wound closure of both Z plasties with good circulation. **(h)** Showing multiple staples in X-rays with deformity corrected. **(i,j)** Patient standing with corrected deformity with a close up. **(k,l)** Showing the scars from medial and lateral side. **(m)** Showing correction from back. (Reprinted/adapted by kind permission courtesy from Springer Nature and Copyright Clearance Center's RightsLink. From author's own published article; Mittal RL. *Int Orthop (SICOT)*; June 2018;42(6):1297–1306; for the book *Clubfoot: A Comprehensive Approach* for the publisher Taylor & Francis Group by Dr. R. L. Mittal 2018–2019.)

the skin was performed, with the base of one below and in front of the ankle and the base of the other proximal in tendoachilles. The skin was mobilized meticulously to protect the microcirculation. The wound could be closed without tension with circulation intact. A well-padded plaster cast was given in plantar flexion at the ankle for three weeks under cover of antibiotics. At three weeks, an unprecedented wound healing was achieved. Stitches were removed and further immobilization in a plaster cast was given for an additional six weeks. There was about an inch of raw granulated area on the dorsolateral side, which was covered with a partial thickness skin graft with a further plaster cast for three weeks with a window in plaster over the skin graft site for dressings. The healing was uneventful after that, beyond expectations. All the photographs show this unique case with excellent results at 1.5 years follow-up (Figure 5.28a–m).

CASE 27: A 6-YEAR-OLD FEMALE CHILD WITH A UNIQUE COMPLICATION OF CALCANEOVARUS AFTER OVER-ENTHUSIASTIC PONSETI CASTING TREATMENT WITH HEEL CORD TENOTOMY, NEVER SEEN BEFORE

A six-year-old female child, weighing 40 kg, presented for treatment recently in May 2018, having a calcaneovarus right-foot deformity with a painful callosity after Ponseti's casting and heel cord tenotomy treatment. **This case is being shown only to showcase this new complication, not seen earlier, as well as to stress "following the Ponseti method of treatment strictly as recommended by him to get the desired results" and avoid such mishaps. All its do's and don'ts must be observed strictly to get the best results.** On detailed history, it was revealed that the child was born with deformities of both feet. The right foot had a severe rigid equinovarus deformity with partial syndactyly and varus of toes with a broad, hourglass, congenital constriction band in the lower part of the leg. Her left foot was also deformed, having congenital partial amputation of the great toe with varus deformity of all toes. At the age of 1.5 years, the parents started with a 7–10 day serial plaster-casting treatment at an orthopedic clinic, which continued for about a year. At about 2.5 years, percutaneous heel cord tenotomy was done, and after that, about 10 serial casts in full dorsiflexion were given. The child started walking, and the deformity gradually increased over two years, and now the child has presented with a severe and rigid calcaneovarus foot. On examination, inspection of the feet from different aspects revealed many findings. The child was overweight and stood on the lateral side of the heel and the posterior part of the lateral border of the right foot with the medial and anterior part of the foot lifted off ground. From behind, in standing position, there was a visible scar from the percutaneous heel cord tenotomy (enlarge with a magnifying lens and see). On inspection, the tendoachilles was wavy in outline in reflected day light, even after the calcaneus foot indicating the heel cord was still loose, whereas the unaffected side outline was straight. There was an hourglass appearance of the leg in the lower part, indicating a mild broad congenital constriction band. On dorsiflexion in the lying-down position, the right foot could be dorsiflexed much more than the left foot, again indicating loose tendoachilles. Looking at the soles of both feet, there was an oval weight-bearing area wider at the heel and tapering at the fifth metatarsal base with a well-marked thick callosity present. The left foot toes showed varus deformities. Palpation revealed a fixed dorsiflexion inversion and adduction deformity with contracture of the tibialis anterior with calcaneus position, besides a tender callosity at the base of the fifth metatarsal. On X-rays, there was talo-navicular dislocation with calcaneum more horizontal than the left foot, besides some subluxation at other intertarsal joints as compared to the left foot which had typical intertarsal relations. CT angiography showed good collateral circulation on both sides. Corrective surgery was been performed on the right foot through a DOLAR incision initially, but it had to be supplemented with V-Y plasty during closure of the stretched part of the wound on medial side. The tibialis anterior tendon and anterior capsule, neurovascular structures, and other tendons were exposed on anterior aspect after dividing the extensor retinaculum. Anterior capsulotomy of the ankle was done, and the contracted tibialis anterior tendon was lengthened by Z plasty to correct the fixed dorsiflexion deformity. After that, the tendoachilles tendon was exposed and it was found to be involved in dense adhesions with a dull white scar in the lower part and shiny white tendon in the upper part. The tendon was quite loose and, after releasing the adhesions, it became looser. The tendoachilles was shortened by Z plasty excising part of the length from both sides. The abductor hallucis muscle was released and the tibialis posterior tendon insertions were released. The spring ligament and all other intertarsal ligaments, the first tarsometatarsal, and interosseous talo-calcanean ligaments were released. A dorsolateral wedge was excised from the cuboid. Talo-navicular dislocation was reduced as well as cuboid wedge closed, and multiple K-wires were used for fixing them. Hemostasis was secured and circulation of the foot ensured. Wound closure necessitated a V-Y plasty skin flap also, along with the rotation flap in the beginning. A well-padded cast was given in plantar flexed position. This patient has now been seen in August 2018 at three months follow up with good correction (see photographs in Figure 5.29a-v).

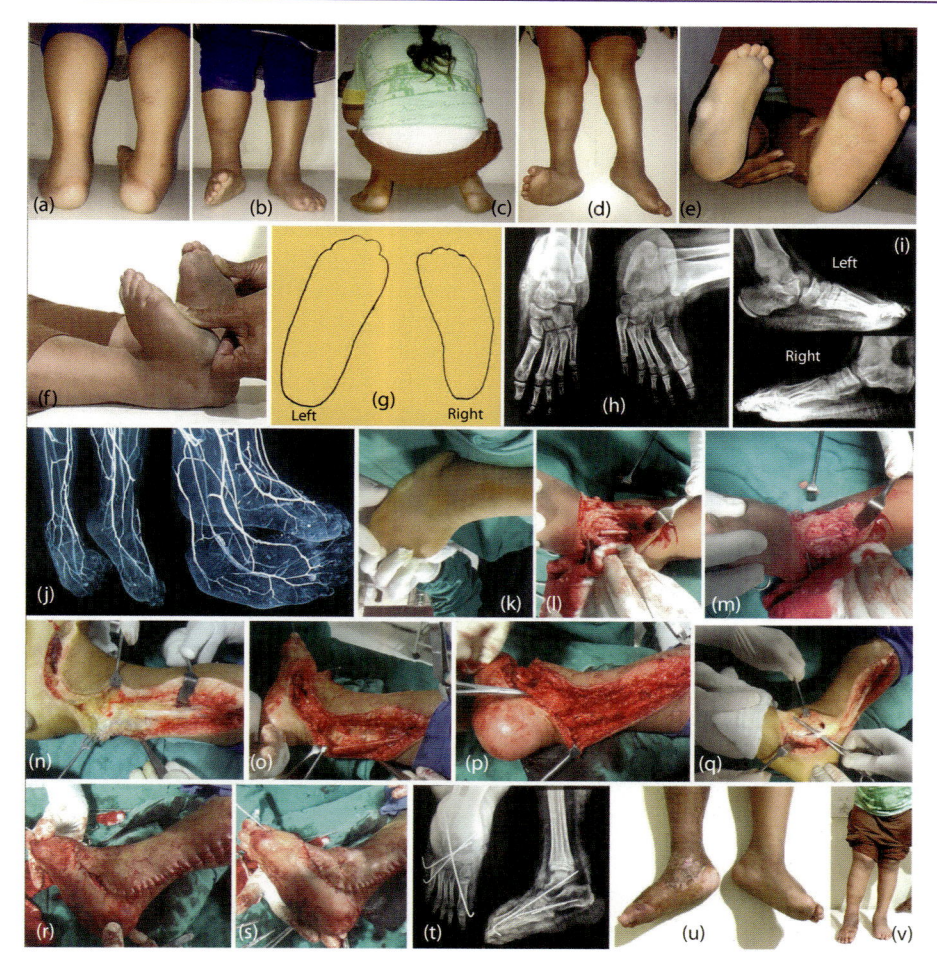

Figure 5.29 (a) Seen from behind with both feet in standing position, there is a well-marked heel cord tenotomy scar. There is also a curved heel cord outline in spite of calcaneus position as compared to straight outline on other side. (b) Seen from front, there is calcaneovarus deformity with an hourglass-shaped broad constriction band and forefoot lifted up from ground. (c) Sitting position right heel is touching the ground more than left indicating laxity of tendoachilles. (d) Lying down dorsiflexed varus right foot compared with left again indicating heel cord laxity. (e) Looking at the soles, there is an oval weight-bearing area with a callosity about the middle of the lateral border, right foot. Left foot also shows congenital partial amputation of great toe with varus of toes. (f) In lying down position, passive dorsiflexion of both feet with right foot more dorsiflexed indicating loose heel cord. (g) Footprints of soles of both feet, indicating deformity of right foot; (h,i) X-rays showing talo-navicular dislocation with some other intertarsal joints disruptions and a more horizontal calcaneum of right foot as compared to left in lateral weight bearing X-ray. (j) CT angiograms showing good collaterals both sides. (k) At operation, on plantar flexion tight tibialis anterior tendon is standing out under the skin. (l,m) Exposed tibialis anterior tendon and its lengthened position. (n) Showing adhesions of tendoachilles. (o) Released from adhesions retracted loose heel cord is seen. (p) Z-shortened heel cord is seen. (q) Releasing tibialis posterior tendon in the sole. (r) Unclosed tense part of wound after closure of the DOLAR incision. (s) V-Y plasty flap used for closure of this gap. (t) X-rays AP and lateral views with K-wires in corrected position. (u) At 3 months post op corrected deformity compared with the other foot in lying down position. (v) Patient standing with support and corrected deformity.

5.3 CONCLUSIONS

The background leading to this research has been a high prevalence of extreme deformities all over the world, at all ages, from birth to older age, and their neglect for want of good, acceptable surgical treatment. Most often, talectomy or arthrodesis procedures were recommended, leading to a shorter, stiff foot and unacceptable functional results. The author has been researching this gray area for almost half a century. A breakthrough has been achieved with numerous, consistent, national and international recognitions over the years. The most recent ones include a lecture in May 2017 on this research at Global Foot/Ankle congress in China on their invitation; an invitation for writing this book, and original publication of a comprehensive article in *International Orthopaedics*, a reputed international journal, authenticating this work, first online in February 2018 and now its print version in June 2018.

This chapter has been specially crafted, giving all the details of the techniques in general and innumerable surgical steps in particular in a variety of case descriptions, each being different. The author considered this a highly important part of this book with details of everything and being the first such publication. Such details could never have been possible in the journal publication due to strict limitation of space, with a fixed number of words. Many new things in pathoanatomy and surgical treatment have come up in the year since this recent publication process, because **"each clubfoot is different" is a proven fact now**. The background of this research (i.e., What was the need? How has this been achieved? What were the innovations in pathoanatomy? What surgical methods have been innovated to treat the multifaceted extreme deformities?) has all been discussed in detail in this chapter.

To describe briefly, the first and foremost thing was to give **a generic name** to scores of confusing terms of literature for residual, relapsed, and uncorrected deformities despite various available treatments. However, every such differently named problem deformity had one thing in common, and that was the need for a good correction. Their morphology could easily be placed under one generic name of extreme deformities. Further, they could be divided into three grades, that is, three subgroups, unifying them in a single name as **trimorphic extreme deformities**. A common pathoanatomical reason was **discovery of the skin contracture**, which always remained neglected prior to this research and as the most important single factor unifying all problem deformities. If the skin chamber is small, the contents will always be crowded. Based on this concept, **triple surgical skin expanding techniques**, as a single or 2-in-1 or even 3-in-1 incision were innovated, in ascending order of enlargement of the skin chamber. In other words, DOLAR for grade 1, DOLARZ for grade 2, and DOLARZ-E for grade 3, with some overlap. There has been a fourth addition also, successfully used in one case to provide further skin in an unusual deformity as 4-in-1. This was as fillet flap and was used in octopus clubfoot (eight toes) reported in the latest *SICOT* publication, but details of this could not be given there due to space restrictions. This is also an evidence-based procedure used often in plastic surgery as fillet flap in severe crush injuries to limbs, where the bones are removed and viable skin with soft tissues are used to provide cover to the raw area. Here, the principle is the same and preaxial accessory toes were filleted out from a proximal-based pedical, and thick soft tissues with skin were used as an additional skin cover, helping in excellent correction of the deformity. Yet another modification in V-Y plasty skin expansion procedure was a 4-in-1, a **double V-Y plasty**, as the skin was badly damaged as a complication of an old crush injury, providing an excellent correction with good wound healing. This case has also been presented in the table of *SICOT* publications. Recently, another modification of Z plasty as single or multiple lazy-Zs, that is, mini vertical cuts on both margins of the incision at different locations for its elongation and closing them horizontally in a wavy fashion. This facilitates closure by lengthening without tension and will prevent contracture of the scar after wound healing. The number of Z plasties can be increased with a larger foot size and more severe/rigid deformities. A proximal relaxing incision or a small partial thickness graft has also been used to facilitate closing the wound or covering of a small defect, respectively.

In this long-term research, there were many other newer perspectives, which evolved after long-term observations and proved with evidence. An important initial new thinking was that **each clubfoot is different**, which prompted study of the detailed pathoanatomy in anatomical dissections and also other areas. Equinus has been viewed from a different perspective, that is, as plantar flexion deformity not only at the ankle but also at distal joints, because these are present in every clubfoot under different names. This was divided in to 5 hierarchic grades as EQ1 to EQ5, from lowest severity to highest. This was considered important from a correction point of view; because we also need corrections of heel equinus, cavus, cock-up big toe, and plantar flexion of toes, which are in fact guised names of equinus. As a part of this, hidden equinus, that is, EQ2 was given special consideration, because, in India, its correction is important for ADL.

Innumerable types of skin contractures were discovered with very wide variations, leading to many innovative ways of dealing with each. In this category, congenital constriction bands of different types and their correction have also been described. Besides the congenital variety, there were associated acquired scars of previous single/multiple surgeries or modified by trauma, that were also corrected in innovative ways.

A special mention about Ponseti's casting treatment is very important. This is a completely evidence-based and good technique for the right type of patients, at the right age, with the right technique, with the right bracing regimen, and with long-term follow-up, as advocated by Ponseti himself. It is highly labor-intensive, and the vast majority of caregivers are not following it due to its multiple inherent problems. This has led to a high incidence of undercorrections and relapses. Ponseti himself has commented on it. The best thing to do to succeed with the Ponseti technique and to be able to follow his principles, would be that dedicated and total care from start to end should be provided by the surgeon who started it and under his care. Further, we find, in percutaneous tenotomy cases, the bones grow more and the tenotomy area with scar does not grow that much and relapse occurs. Ponseti casting is not meant for older age groups and, in extreme deformities in younger children and many times, talo-navicular dislocation is not present. The author has operated on many of these relapses and has seen unique complications with Ponseti treatment. In a specific operated case, a child of 2.5 years with a very rigid deformity had three heel cord tenotomies during the first year with extensive scarring in heel cord area. This was corrected by excising the scar and replacing the gap with a tendon graft with good result. In yet another case, seen and operated only in May 2018, severe/rigid calcaneovarus in a 6-year-old child as a complication of Ponseti casting and heel cord tenotomy that was wrongly executed. Both these cases have been described in detail with innovative surgical corrections achieving very good results as reported in above case descriptions.

Criteria for assessment of results were also different here. Because each case is different, various criteria described in the literature cannot be applied. The patients are the best judges of the improvements after surgery, as they are the beneficiaries. Therefore, patient satisfaction levels of excellent, good, and fair/poor were used. These techniques offer a longer, good-looking, flexible, and better-functioning foot than previous techniques.

Newer, deeper surgical steps adopted so far in these unique patients, in regard to bones, have been an **innovative sliding osteotomy of cuboid** to correct triple plus dislocation; more extensive opening of intertarsal, tarsometatarsal joints, and resection of appropriate dorsolateral wedges from other tarsals, besides the cuboid, saving the joints. Various soft-tissue releases have been carried out to correct the severe medial cavus with cock-up deformity of the big toe (G3 equinus) by fixing with K-wires, including the great toe from the anterior to posterior into the tarsal area. Some of the long-standing grade 3 extreme deformities with EQ5 equinus, required arthrodesis, which was carried out in two, or even three, stages to preserve maximum foot length. The third-generation techniques, in a large variety of cases, have further strengthened the belief that **each clubfoot is different,** and surgery must be planned and executed accordingly.

Widely different pathoanatomical features are being encountered frequently due to adaptative changes of growth, dynamics of various muscles including tibialis anterior seen many times, and static influence of weight bearing with changes in the bones and joints. In a recent case of Klippel–Feil syndrome with clubfoot, unique pathoanatomy had been discovered. There was an almost complete dorsolateral dislocation of the navicular from the three cuneiforms, calcaneocuboid dislocation, G4 equinus, and without talo-navicular dislocation, which was corrected by the DOLARZ-E technique. There is still radiological undercorrection, but clinically, the correction is highly satisfying to the patient and parents. As more and more extreme cases keep coming, research will continue, being based on need. Ponseti casting will not work in such cases.

Further surgical details: The triple surgical skin expanders, DOLAR, DOLARZ, and DOLARZ-E, have been discovered and expanded, right from their origin to the latest in a distinct timeline, as need-based procedures. With the advent of these techniques and spreading awareness, more and more patients are coming for treatment from all age groups. They are as common in younger ages as in older ages. Technical details of earlier procedures of the author, with diagrams and figures, have been picked up from earlier reputed international publications, with kind permissions from the publishers. Surgeries are highly meticulous and time consuming. Otherwise, they are completely evidence-based, and you can go in with full confidence. Avoid injury to the perforators and remain superficial to deep fascia; while shaping out the V-Y plasty flap, only skin is incised and use blunt dissection to mobilize the skin sufficiently, but not too much. You have other supplementary options also: use of a proximal relaxing incision to close the gap or use a small Thiersch graft in a small raw area. Always try to remain as close to the bones as possible in deeper dissections. This way you will be able to save all vital structures. How to manage these postoperatively has also been outlined. It will be quite pertinent to mention here that, being extensive surgeries, the patient has to be kept under strict personal observation for about three to four months in order to achieve the best results. **Do not leave it to others**, because the other person is not likely to have as much concern as you. Hemostasis must be secured after removing the pneumatic tourniquet and circulation of the foot, and incision margins must be ensured. To further ensure it, the foot may be kept in slight undercorrection initially in the first plaster cast, which is well-padded. Sometimes, slitting of the plaster may be needed after 24 hours to avoid circulatory embarrassment and severe pain to the patient. We need to change the plaster every 2–3 weeks or so and achieve full correction by graduated manipulations, in a couple of plaster changes. Hidden equinus is an important consideration for Indian patients for their ADL position, which has been discussed in detail along with its correction.

The author considered the talo-calcanean index[5] as a good index for judging the results in general. Importantly, clinical and radiological corrections did not correlate. The foot may look normal clinically but not radiologically, and vice versa. However, a good radiological correction did occur in the majority. In the author's experience, there is a wide radiological variation, and this also proves that **each clubfoot is different**. Talo-navicular dislocation may not always be present. Many other joint disruptions are quite often seen. Calcaneocuboid dislocation or cuneo-navicular dislocations have also been seen often, besides some other rare disruptions. Therefore, preoperative radiological assessment is important along with a good individualized clinical assessment, which will guide the surgeon to achieve the best possible correction of pathoanatomy. In this, maximum importance should be given to the correction of skin contracture by the various means described. Deeper correction will only be possible if you have enlarged the space for the deeper structures.

There is such a diversity of operative steps in each case that it has been considered essential to describe the details in a variety of patients, so that the reader understands what different surgical steps may be expected and get tuned to this by repeatedly reading these. In the *SICOT* publication, it would not have been possible due to space restrictions. In that publication, many of these cases were presented in a tabulated form only with brief outlines. All these have now been elaborated. Besides these, almost an equal number of new cases have been included with numerous technical differences. Once you know all the different morbid anatomies in various cases, you should be well equipped with the acumen to deal with any eventuality. An enthusiastic surgeon may even acquire the skill to come out of an enigmatic case successfully, after reading these difficult situations. Long-term follow-up with consistency of satisfied patients has been the greatest strength of these techniques.

REFERENCES

1. Mittal RL, Makhni SS, Sidhu GS; Morbid anatomy of congenital clubfoot; *Ind J Orthop*; 1981;15:129–135.

2. Mittal RL; The surgical management of resistant clubfoot by rotation skin flap and extensive soft tissue release; *Int Orthop*; 1987;11(3):189–192.
3. Mittal RL; Obstinate clubfoot with triple plus dislocation; *J Foot Ankle Surg* (Asia Pacific); 2014;1(2):72–77.
4. Mittal RL; Trimorphic extreme clubfoot deformities and their management by triple surgical skin expanders: DOLAR, DOLARZ and DOLARZ-E (evidence based mega corrections without arthrodesis) Online first in April 2018 and now print version; *Int Orthop (SICOT)*; June 2018;42(6):1297–1306.
5. Beatson TR, Pearson JR; A method of assessing correction in clubfeet; *J Bone Joint Surg*; 1966;48-B(1):49–50.
6. Tarraf YN, Carroll NC; Analysis of the components of residual deformity in clubfoot presenting for reoperation; *J Paediatr Orthop*; April 1992;2(12);207–216.
7. Küntscher MV, Erdmann D, Homann HH, Steinau HU, Levin SL, Germann G; The concept of fillet flaps: Classification, indications, and analysis of their clinical value; *Plast Reconstr Surg*; 15 September, 2001;108(4):885–896.
8. Eliezer S, Shal S, Yoav R, Snir H, Steven V, Alo B; Medial forefoot fillet flap for primary closure of transmetatarsal amputation: A series of four cases; *The Foot*; December 2017;33:53–56.
9. Kurup JKN, Kottamttavida IV, Shah H; Stress fracture in club foot; *Ind Jr Ortho Surg*; 2016;2(2):199–201.
10. Sølund K, Sonne-Holm S, Kjølbye JE; Talectomy for equinovarus deformity in arthrogryposis: A 13 (2–20) year review of 17 feet; *Acta Orthop Scand*; 1991;62(4):372–374.
11. Byington R, Keene S, Verhovsek E, Depew J; Arthrogryposis multiplex congenita: A review of treatment options for the lower extremities; *The Internet Journal of World Health and Societal Politics*; 2012;7(2).
12. Turco VJ; Resistant congenital club foot-one-stage posteromedial release with internal fixation. A follow-up report of a fifteen-year experience; *J Bone Joint Surg. Am* 1979; 61–A(6):805–814.
13. Simon GW; Complete subtalar release in Clubfeet. Part II: Comparison with Less Extensive Procedures; *J Bone Joint Surg*; 1985;67-A(7):1056–1065.
14. Kendrick RE, Sharma NK, Hassler W, Herndon CH; Trasometatarsal mobilisation for resistant adduction of fore part of foot; *J Bone Joint Surg Am*; 1970;52(1):61–70.

6

Future of clubfoot

This is a comprehensive book on clubfoot, describing its past and present, as well as directions for the future. The past is, in fact, the yesterday of today and the future is the tomorrow of today. Therefore, **today** is the most important day of reckoning. Hard work, hard work, and hard work; with a pinch of inspiration, like a trigger for a gun or a catalyst for a chemical reaction, is the only way to success. The writing of this book was destined to happen just like this research, as has been mentioned in the Preface and Introduction of this book. Keeping in mind the unique nature of this book and convenience for readers, there have been some repetitions in order to explain the points being discussed at that moment, rather going back to the pages and wasting time and energy. **The future of clubfoot is very bright for patients in the hands of all their caregivers, who are working hard to improve upon the past for a better hope for the future.** The global clubfoot community, mostly living in low and middle income countries with more than 80% of global population, is looking to us expectantly to improve upon their psycho-physico-socioeconomic conditions, so that they can also feel good and live like their normal fellow human beings.

"Truth must of necessity be stranger than fiction," said Basil, placidly (from the Internet—chrisbrauns.com/2008/05/truth-is-stranger-than-fiction/). "For fiction is the creation of the human mind, and therefore is subservient to it." Mark Twain said "Truth is stranger than fiction. It has to be! Fiction is the creation of human mind and truth just happens itself." (https://www.brainyquote.com/quotes/mark_twain_122865n quote source) This research and this book is yet another example of the veracity of this well-known saying.

The author has been passionately working with clubfoot for more than half a century, since January 1961, to be exact. An orthopedic surgeon by chance, the author was first introduced to clubfoot during his training period (residency) after graduating from medical school. How, incredibly, the things progressed to reach the present stage, has been explained in the Introduction. The decision to leave Patiala for Delhi for better career leading to initiation into this research has proved to be a watershed in the author's career. From then on, doing a master's thesis on clubfoot further strengthened this interest. A major gray area of high prevalence of uncorrected, undercorrected, and relapsed clubfoot deformities, all over the world in LMICs including India, was discovered for this need-based research. This was passionately pursued by the author with consistent awards/rewards, acting as motivational force, and ultimately a landmark research article was prepared for *SICOT* publication of 2018. Finally, about the future of clubfoot management, we should be optimistic and work hard to make the future bright.

Clubfoot is the most common congenital orthopedic deformity with a high prevalence in LMICs, where a major portion of the world population lives. There are two areas on which the future of clubfoot management depends: they are preventive and therapeutic. Once preventive measures have been effectively implemented, then come the therapeutic methods. Research must continue in both to find out better methods to improve the socioeconomic status of this LMICs major section of population, besides their psychological and physical disability impact. For a healthy society, regular follow-up measure is highly important in both areas.

6.1 PREVENTIVE MEASURES

There are a large number of factors responsible for congenital defects including clubfoot, all of which can be controlled with concerted efforts by all concerned. The future approach for relief from clubfoot lies to a great extent in prevention as a long-term strategy so that GBD decreases. The well-known quote **"Prevention is better than cure"** should never be out of sight. This is the only cost-effective golden principle when dealing with any problem. In spite of tremendous development, poverty with its socioeconomic problems of humanity have not improved that much. By preventive methods, if you can reduce prevalence of the disease, it will be much easier to deal with a smaller number by so many brilliant methods already available or which will be innovated in the future. Preventive and therapeutic measures will be discussed now.

6.1.1 Control of global population

This is the most important factor but it is not taken as seriously as needed. Population explosion is having an adverse effect in so many ways. This leads to depletion of resources with increasing consumption by the increasing population. A WHO report[1] reporting the demographic figures, tells us that a total of 94% of congenital anomalies, including clubfoot, occur in LMICs, where the majority of the world population lives. According to a different WHO report,[2] congenital anomalies account for 25.3–38.8 million loss of disability-adjusted life-years (DALYs) worldwide. In a study of WHO of 291 diseases for causes of GBD, congenital anomalies ranked as the seventeenth cause of GBD. This WHO study of GBD also reports 361 DALYs per 1,000 population globally and significantly, congenital anomalies account for up to 120 DALYs per 1,000 children.

Spiedel[3] has reported that growth of the world population poses serious threats to human health, socioeconomic development, and the environment. In only 12 years, the world population has grown from five billion to six billion, a number almost equivalent to India's population. He has further quoted the United Nation's (UN's) projection figure of a population rise to 8.9 billion by 2050 and 9.5 billion by 2100. This is going to have a high toll on the world's environment. Demands created will deplete the natural resources and damage ecology. HICs have a far greater adverse role for this damage with only 20% population of the world living there (US, Canada, Europe, Japan) and they consume 67% of resources and produce 75% of pollutants and waste.

However, that was a projected estimate in the year 2000. The **current world population** is 7.6 billion as of April 2018, according to the most recent United Nations' estimate elaborated by Worldometers[4] and it is increasing every year, but at a slightly lesser rate than previously estimated with improved public-health measures and some population-control measures. Increasing the resources is far more costly, difficult, and time consuming than the measures to slow population growth. The future well-being of humanity depends on family planning and reproductive-health services in LMICs and decreased consumption of resources by rich countries. This is going to help our future generations as a long-term policy. War footing efforts are needed for this. If they really want to save the human race from the scourge of congenital anomalies and, for that matter, for all preventable diseases, initiative has to taken by HICs because they have better means. Indirectly, they will be helping themselves also, because the mother earth is one with the whole human race as its family.

6.1.2 Controlling epidemiological factors

As we have discussed in Chapter 2 on epidemiology, congenital malformations, including clubfoot, are much more common in LMICs, where there are poor socioeconomic and environmental factors, illiteracy, lack of a communication network, maternal infections, and nutritional deficiencies. There are numerous other intrinsic and extrinsic epidemiological factors. All these are interrelated. Increasing the literacy rate, awareness, means of communication in remote areas, and public health measures and building various types of infrastructure will help in tackling these. A typical example of such improvement can be seen in the tremendous decrease in post-poliomyelitis paralytic sequelae, including poliotic clubfoot. Because of a good vaccination program throughout the world, we now have fewer cases of paralytic clubfoot to treat. They are also linked with overpopulation, and a significant check on the rising population will indirectly help in controlling them. If the population is less, the increasing development and resources will be enough and thus help in improving the grim picture.

6.1.3 Genetics

Clubfeet are quite frequently associated with genetic factors, as has already been described in Chapter 2. There is a lot which can be done in this field, and this book is not meant to discuss all of that. A lot of research is being carried out in genetics. However, much more needs to be done in this field. If we know about the role of various genes causing congenital defects, including clubfoot, and there is effective genetic counseling, congenital diseases can be effectively reduced. The genetic factors also have interactions with various extrinsic factors in known and many unknown ways, as already discussed in Chapter 2. A lot of research is needed to explore these areas for firm conclusions. If the influence of extrinsic factors is decreased by preventive measures, pure genetics will then be easier to understand and control. Control of extrinsic factors is a lot easier helping doubly: by eliminating their influence as well as helping in genetics by excluding their interaction. Genetic counseling is an important measure before and during pregnancy in the control of congenital defects. Advancement in Genetics should be able to achieve a big leap in the future, solving many problems of dealing with difficult deformities, which are often genetic in nature. It is a highly complicated multifactorial issue and it is not just pure genetics. There is a complicated interaction of various extrinsic and intrinsic factors, which will also have to be worked out for a complete solution to the problem.

6.2 THERAPEUTIC MEASURES

If concerted efforts are made on the prevention side, things will become easier in the future for treating the fewer patients who are afflicted with clubfoot. There are numerous methods of conservative and surgical treatments available, practiced all over the world, innovated by pioneers of those procedures. As discussed in the review of literature in Chapter 3, there are a large number of these. They are McKay's concept of surgical treatment, Lichtblau's medial and lateral release, Turco's partial subtalar release, Simons' complete subtalar release, Ilizarov's technique and its many modifications, the JESS technique, Umex mini fixator technique, various types of midfoot osteotomies triple arthrodesis, talectomies, Ponseti's casting technique, Kite's casting treatment, early surgery in the first few months, and so forth. Most of them are good procedures, provided proper selection of the procedure for any particular case is made. Choose the right tool from the tool box for that particular job. In the author's research, which has been a lifetime work in three phases, initiated in early 1960s and kick-started in about the mid-nineteen-seventies, named Generation 1–3. There has been a distinct timeline, first phase about 25–30 years, second phase of about 12–15 years, and third phase about 7–8 years, with some overlap. This has been need based with the hierarchy of deformity based on rigidity and severity; grade 1 to 3, with a generic name of trimorphic deformities and innovative triple surgical skin expanding incisions: DOLAR, DOLARZ and DOLARZ-E. All the details have been given in Chapters 4 and 5. A significant new thing has been proved beyond doubt, namely, **each clubfoot is different**. The trimorphic extreme clubfoot deformities, grade 1–3 are seen at all ages, even in a newborn. Heterogeneous skin contractures are an extremely important factor in the etiology of clubfoot. None of the procedures described previously in literature and used commonly all over the world have recognized the importance of correcting skin contractures. This has been recognized by the author and published[5] for the first time. A high incidence of residual deformities and relapses has been reported in the literature, if we try to use any of the previous methods for every clubfoot without taking care of the skin contracture. To improve upon this aspect, we have to keep up our efforts to further consolidate what is being practiced and continue to explore newer, unforeseen problems of the future in the following areas.

6.2.1 Pathoanatomy

It has been clear to the readers by now that clubfoot still remains an incompletely solved problem. The basic cause of this, as has been concluded by the author in his research, is its complex pathoanatomy with the basic discovery of skin contracture, which is well documented. Many other obscure areas of pathoanatomy have been revealed during this lifetime work, but still, a lot more needs to be done. A significant discovery in this research, **each**

clubfoot is different, should always be remembered. This will enable us to discover more in pathoanatomy and the subsequent management in the future. Newer vistas will continue opening up, and we have to be prepared for these in future.

6.2.2 Various imaging techniques

Plane X-rays have their own limitations, giving only uniplanar information of that plane only, which has been X-rayed. Despite that, X-rays are an important tool to get the basic knowledge of the deformity and are highly cost effective. Where skiagrams are inconclusive and extra information is required for diagnosis and treatment, other imaging techniques have their role. Ultrasonography is simple with the added advantage of being without radiation hazards and can give useful information as a prenatal diagnostic tool, besides its prognostic value in treatment. Three-dimensional (3D) imaging by 3D CT and 3D MRI studies has the added advantages of diagnosing the spatial relationship of individual bones and various joints. CT also has its role, especially the CT angiography, which will be useful for diagnosing any vascular abnormalities prior to surgery and better surgical management. There are likely to be improvements on this front in the future.

6.2.3 Orthotics of the future

Bracing is an important tool in the management of clubfoot for maintenance of correction and protection of recently healed surgical cases. There are bound to be improvements in this field as well. **In the casting treatment by Ponseti and others, failure on the bracing protocol front is an important negative force for a good percentage of relapses.** Pneumatic bracing, if they are made cost-effective, may be a future hope in this regard. I say cost-effective because the majority of these deformities are prevalent in LMICs with their economic handicap.

6.2.4 Complications

As time passes with the persistent deformities, there are bound to be many more complications coming up with persisting deformities, in the future. Many times, fear of surgery also plays an important role in keeping the deformity uncorrected, and later the patient is forced to seek treatment due to some troublesome complication. Many of such unusual cases, some of them, **the first of their kind**, have been discussed in Chapter 5. In the future too, such cases will keep on coming; some of them may be the first of their kind, and we have to be prepared to take on even more such challenging cases to give the best possible treatment.

6.3 REHABILITATION IN CLUBFOOT IN THE FUTURE

Clubfoot, as we know, is prevalent in LMICs with tremendous GBD due to its physico-psycho-socioeconomic impact. They have physical disability, psychological inferiority complex with all of its problems, social isolation, and they are unemployed or underemployed. There is fear of surgery due to resulting pain, and this feeling is greater in adults, who end up in surgery due to some complication forcing them for an operation. They need total rehabilitation, which has remained neglected in the past. In the future, we must look to this aspect also, so that they no longer remain a burden on society. By total rehabilitation we mean physical, social, and vocational rehabilitation. They should be physically rehabilitated by surgery in later age groups, for which they have to be persuaded by explaining to them all the disadvantages of keeping the deformity and advantages of getting the deformity corrected. Once they are physically alright, they need social rehabilitation by helping them to become part of the societal group in which they are living. Finally, they should be helped to obtain gainful employment. All these types of rehabilitation aspects are interrelated and one boosts the other. Social self-help groups, along with various government schemes, can prove to be a great help in this respect. That is, the only way to reduce the GBD after their own economic situation improves.

6.4 CONCLUSIONS

Some basic principles in the management of clubfoot should always be remembered:

1. Treatment of clubfoot must be started as soon after birth as possible. Kite's, Ponseti's, or other techniques can vary according to the choice of the head of the unit. A dedicated

team, strict regime and long term dedicated follow up to forestall undercorrections or relapses for further measures are the keys to success of any programme.
2. One method cannot be the panacea for all clubfoot deformities. Choice depends on the type of deformity, age, and choice of care provider. For extreme deformities, as have been defined in this book, a considered choice has to be made. Treatment should be able to achieve a good looking, flexible and longer foot with as normal function as possible over a long period and with best possible satisfied patient.
3. *No early surgery*: At birth until the normal walking age, that is, nine months to one year, conservative treatment should be the choice. Surgery should not be done in this age. A high incidence of relapse has been reported in cases where early surgery is performed. Besides a difficult surgery in a tiny foot for identifying the structures, a reactive healing with exuberant reparative tissue results in more fibrosis and contracture. Maintenance of correction by bracing is also difficult at that age until walking starts, due to practical problems. This, in fact, is one of the pitfalls of Ponseti's technique, that is, a prolonged and cumbersome bracing period not followed in the majority of cases as recommended. This has been reported in the literature many times and even commented on in Ponseti's manual. All mild and moderate deformities will be corrected by manipulations and serial casting and maintained temporarily after that by Denis Brown (DB) splint. Even severe deformities will be partially corrected and the remaining part will be easier to correct with less extensive surgery. However, the presence of skin contracture has always remained neglected, until it was reported by the author.
4. *Ponseti casting technique*: This is a very good method and is being used all over the world. However, it is going into disrepute, because the majority of caregivers do not follow the exact technique recommended by the doyen of this technique. Ponseti and Smoley[6] in their report of 2007, and Lynn, Ponseti, and others[7] in their manual titled "Clubfoot: Ponseti Management Manual 3rd edition", have given all the details, by the masters themselves. They have deliberated that:
  i. Ponseti's method will give the best results, in mild and moderate deformities.
  ii. They recommended that the treatment should be started within the first week of birth or up to one month of age.
  iii. Percutaneous heel cord tenotomy was done by them in 79% in more severe cases.
  iv. Minimum age at tenotomy was five weeks, followed up with a prolonged corrective splintage through 3–5 years of age, which often gets neglected. Even otherwise, with proper splintage, recurrences can occur for unknown reasons.

The recurrences/relapses reported by these authors themselves have been 56% first recurrences, 18% second, 53% third, and even a fourth recurrence as the child grows.

Tarraf and Carroll,[8] reporting 95 residual deformities, becoming more evident with growth. Azarpira et al.[9] reported that the real Ponseti method is highly laborious with a very strict regimen. More failure will be experienced if these principles are neglected. Zhao et al.[10] concluded from a comprehensive review of 19 eligible articles out of 519 recorded reports of the Ponseti method, that good corrections were reported initially in about 90% in all, yet recurrence was very common in the maintenance phase of prolonged bracing and noncompliance with a relapse rate of 62%. Results can only improve if every detail of the Ponseti technique is adhered to, which is laborious, both for the patients as well as caregivers. Bhaskar and Patni[11] reported 91 relapses out of 164 feet (56.50%). Carroll[12] commented about Ponseti's technique in his article about trends in the twentieth century: "Surgeons are now learning the limitations of this method." He has also noted that there may be new developments in the future about preventive measures, classification of clubfoot, and treatment modalities in clubfoot with all the advances in biomechanics, biomaterials, surgical advances, orthotics, and so forth.

5. *Author's Experience*: The author has seen in so many actual cases (Ponseti's treatment cases

in Chapter 5) that the most common cause is in the scar of percutaneous tenotomy of heel cord, which becomes adherent and the heel cord does not grow with age as much as the bones in a child and will result in a relapse increasing with age. In the history also, patients tell that initially correction was good, but gradually it is coming up again. Ponseti also commented about it in his cases of relapses in his reports. The author has performed many procedures due to Ponseti's relapses, which are discussed in Chapter 5. The latest ones presented with new complications, not described in the literature till now and we have to be vigilant about newer things in older treated cases.

A child of 2.5 years with three heel cord tenotomies with extensive scar in the heel cord area, was corrected by replacing the gap with a tendon graft with good result. In yet another recent case seen and operated only in May 2018, a unique case of calcaneovarus due to over enthusiasm with Ponseti's casting treatment and percutaneous heel cord tenotomy (details given in Chapter 5). The patient had about 40 weekly casts for about a year starting at 1.5 years of age, followed by heel cord tenotomy and 10 more casts in full dorsiflexion, which resulted in this serious but avoidable complication, which has been treated by ingenuity, and details have been described in Chapter 5.

It can therefore be concluded that Ponseti is a good, evidence-based, technique if the five R's are followed: **Right** age, **Right** type of deformity, **Right** technique, **Right** bracing regime, and **Regular** follow-up. However, the problem is that the vast majority of caregivers are not following what Ponseti recommended, because it requires time and patience, with complete commitment. The surgeon himself has to take the whole responsibility until the end of treatment, and the parents also have to follow instructions for total compliance. This requires dedicated teamwork, which is difficult in general for the medical personnel. For the patients, too, it is difficult because this deformity is mostly seen in LMICs with their numerous socioeconomic limitations. Moreover, Ponseti's method, as clarified by the master himself, is not meant for the **Extreme Deformities**, which have been defined by the author of this book in Chapter 4. These extreme deformities are commonly seen at birth; continue in older children, adolescents, and adults. Ponseti does not correct skin contracture to increase the size of the inner chamber, for the deeper structures to spread out. As commented by the masters themselves, relapses occur commonly due to scars in the tenotomy area and thin calf muscles; there is more growth of the bones than soft tissues. Besides this, dynamic action of muscles, especially tibialis anterior, also contributes to relapse. Heterogeneous skin contracture of three hierarchic grades 1–3, each in three dimensions, has been proved by the author beyond doubt with generous evidence, and the Ponseti technique is unlikely to succeed in such cases.

6. An important discovery from the author's research, that **each clubfoot is different**, has been proved with ample evidence; this must always be on the mind. Each case has to be assessed carefully regarding various causative factors of pathoanatomy, clinically as well as radiologically, and proper planning is done beforehand. If any other more sensitive investigation like CT, MRI, or angiography is needed, it should be done before. A foot print of the plantar aspect of foot or weight-bearing area can be taken before operation and compared with postoperative follow-up foot print to judge the improvement in shape.

7. All moderate and moderately severe deformities can be treated by various other surgical techniques like posteromedial release, Ilizarov, JESS, etc., depending upon the experience of the surgeon. In experienced hands, even some selected lesser extreme deformities can be treated successfully by these techniques.

8. However in more extreme deformities with or without scars of earlier surgeries, skin contracture plays a significant role in the pathoanatomy of the deformity, and skin expanding techniques are the answer: single (DOLAR), 2-in-1 (DOLARZ) or 3-in-1 (DOLARZ-E) techniques. They are evidence-based and quite safe to perform. These techniques have to be learned and practiced to gain confidence. Strict postoperative care,

with commitment, for 3–4 months is very important in every case to achieve the desired results.

9. Research will continue as newer problems will keep on coming and they too have to be looked into. As an example, even in this book, a new pathoanatomical feature of a rigid calcaneovarus, resulting from over enthusiasm with Ponseti's technique and discovered only a couple of weeks before submitting the draft of this book, has been recorded as the last case in Chapter 5. Hard work by all concerned in the present is very important, because the past was the present earlier and the future too will become the present soon. You must remember that it is the present only that is under your control, and controlling the present to the best of your ability will help you to control all three: the past, the present, and the future.

10. Long-term follow-up of the cases operated by the three surgical techniques have shown continued excellence in results with high patient satisfaction. Some of them may even have been radiological undercorrections with nice clinical results. The bones and joints seem to adjust in their new anatomical positions in such cases while maintaining normal weight-bearing alignment, and thus they maintain good functional result on long-term bases.

11. The future will definitely be guided by evidence-based medicine. Whatever can be proved by ample evidence will naturally be more authentic, rather than empirical. Evidence is always based on scientific principles and hence will always be acceptable.

12. It has been argued time and again that various assessment protocols, including those of Pirani and Demiglio, cannot be universally applicable. Such a protocol, which is universally applicable, is yet to be discovered. At least, in clubfoot and more extreme deformities, where each clubfoot is different with innumerable variables, it may be difficult to apply these.

6.5 TO SUMMARIZE

Each clubfoot is different is a very important discovery, proved by evidence as described in Chapter 4. This difference is present even at birth and persists throughout life. Many of the differences may be seen in future and be prepared for them too. If you discover a problem, the solution also becomes available. The human mind has infinite potential and nothing is impossible. Treatment must start as soon after birth as possible. All mild and moderate deformities can be treated by serial manipulations and casting treatments. Ponseti's technique is a good method for treating such cases, provided his instructions and protocol are carried out to the letter and spirit, as recommended by him. Literature has reported high incidence of residual deformities and relapses, even up to 95%, because of a casual approach to a good technique, bringing it into disrepute. A dedicated and committed teamwork is essential for desired results. Use it where indicated and not in every case indiscriminately. It is not a panacea for all.

In this regard, discovery of heterogeneous skin contractures with very wide variation (primary alone or in combination with secondary scars) is a reality, proved on ample evidence. It is an essential prerequisite to correct it first to make the room bigger by triple surgical three-dimensional skin expanders before any deeper correction. This landmark new approach is going to be a future strategy in the surgical management of clubfoot. Improvements over the past are always to be expected in the future, as research never stops. Realigning the bones with a good shape of the foot without fusion and a better satisfied patient can be possible only if the room is bigger for a comfortable spread of its contents.

A highly important pathoanatomical feature in clubfoot is equinus, seen in a new perspective and so also its correction, which would translate to correcting all plantar flexions up to the toes. Based on this, a new perspective for equinus has been proposed. That is, a generic name for many different names for plantar flexion at the ankle, hindfoot (heel), intertarsal and tarsometatarsal joints (midfoot), and toe joints (forefoot) but with the common aim of correcting all, which has been documented in a recent publication of *SICOT* journal (2018). A comprehensive classification of equinus with five grades: EQ_1–EQ_5 in increasing hierarchy has been suggested. One or more or all may be present in varying proportions in innumerable combinations. Greater details have been described in Chapter 4.

About 20 complications, hitherto neglected, and many newer ones not reported earlier, have been recognized. They have psycho-physico-socioeconomic problems and need to be corrected to overcome these problems. To name them, they are social stigma, inferiority complex, awkward gait, physical handicap for running and jumping, painful walking (due to inflamed bursa, bunion, infection, scar, ulcer), painful and unstable genu recurvatum with locking and other knee problems, stress fracture of the fifth metatarsal, heterogeneous myriad scars of earlier surgeries, marital problems (before and after), additional congenital defects (coalitions, polydactyly, etc.) and complications due to them, complicated arthrogryposis multiplex congenita, plantar horn, hallux varus, early osteoarthritis in foot, knee and spine, post-trauma problems, the latest case of calcaneovarus after Ponseti casting, and so forth. Many times, fear of surgery also plays an important role in keeping the deformities remaining untreated until late age, which has been seen as a cause for late complications. Nothing concrete is available in the literature about these, except a few anecdotal references here and there, which advise arthrodesis of foot joints, resulting in shortened stiff foot. In the present techniques, triple arthrodesis can be avoided in most of the cases with maximum foot length with preserved flexibility.

Various additional skin procedures, besides those in the basic third-generation triple skin expanders are a proximal relaxing incision, limited partial thickness skin graft, fillet flap, double V-Y plasty, a separate V-Y plasty at M.P. joint for hallux varus; multiple lazy-Z plasties instead of major Z plasties, etc. In addition to added skin procedures, there are numerous newer procedures, which fit in with the new name of DOLARZ-E or EXTENDED to cover even the still to adopt newer procedures. All these multiple procedures make it more than DOLARZ, being multiple in nature depending upon case to case, and hence the name: DOLARZ-E; E stands for extended. This was earlier called the DOLARZ PLUS technique and even documented in December 2014 in *Asia-Pacific JFAS*. However, later on, this was modified to DOLARZ-E, which is more descriptive. Not only skin, but many new procedures in the deeper tissues, involving soft tissues and bones, have also been done, depending upon the pathoanatomy. Even the yet to be innovated newer procedures will be covered by this.

Newer, deeper surgical steps adopted so far in these patients have been an innovative sliding osteotomy of cuboid to correct triple plus dislocations; more extensive opening of intertarsal, tarso-metatarsal joints, resection of appropriate dorsolateral wedges from other tarsals, besides cuboid, **saving the joints**, tendon grafting in tendoachilles gap, lengthening of tibialis anterior with anterior capsulotomy, Z-shortening of tendoachilles in a case of stretched and loose tendoachilles were done in unique cases. Some of them were due to complication due to Ponseti's casting treatment with percutaneous heel cord tenotomy. The Robert Jones procedure (a well-known surgical procedure) is sometimes required to maintain correction of severe medial cavus with cock-up deformity of the big toe (G3 equinus). However, mostly the cock-up big toe can get corrected with extensive plantar release of hallucis brevis, plantar capsulotomies of intertarsal and tarsometatarsal joints and K-wire fixation of the first metatarsal ray to the tarsals from the front for 6–8 weeks. Some grade 3 extreme procedures where triple arthrodesis is indicated, are done in two or even three stages to preserve maximum foot length; the first stage is maximum soft tissue correction; the second stage is some more soft tissue release and undercorrected triple arthrodesis with removing articular cartilage only from the treated joints, and the third stage is full correction with limited additional osseous resection. This is done to preserve maximum length of the foot, which has its own advantages later in life by providing more weight-bearing surface area and lesser weight per unit area of foot. Three stage triple arthrodesis was done in one case on both sides in Case 25 described in Chapter 5. The third-generation techniques have further strengthened the belief that **each club foot is different** and surgery has to be planned and executed accordingly. In a recent case of Klippel–Feil Syndrome with clubfoot, yet another unique pathoanatomy was discovered. This was an almost complete dorsolateral dislocation of navicular from the three cuneiforms, calcaneo-cuboid dislocation, G4 equinus without talo-navicular dislocation, which was corrected by the DOLARZ-E technique. Obviously, there had been radiological undercorrection in this case, but the clinical result was excellent at 1 1/2 years follow up. As more and more extreme cases keep coming, research will continue to depend on the requirements.

As this is a comprehensive book on clubfoot, it covers not only congenital clubfoot but acquired varieties also. Congenital clubfoot is by far the most common type of clubfoot, and by convention, the word congenital is not prefixed in its name. However, all others have to be prefixed with its cause. All other varieties are very uncommon. In the literature also, congenital clubfoot dominates. The same principles of treatment apply to all the cases of acquired clubfoot also, except that arthrodesis procedures and tendon transfers are much more often needed in these cases than in the congenital type. One has to look to the cause, which may be affecting the other parts of the lower also and besides the correction of foot deformity, other surgeries may also have to be done to restore foot function. As an example: in a child with cerebral palsy clubfoot deformity may be bilateral with spastic scissoring and flexion deformity at knees and considered for surgery; we have to correct all to make the feet functional.

REFERENCES

1. World Health Organization; 2012; Congenital anomalies: Fact sheet N 370. http://www.who.int/mediacentre/factsheets/fs370/en/
2. World Health Organization; *The Global Burden of Disease: 2004 Update.* Geneva: WHO Press; 2008.
3. Speidel JJ; Environment and health: 1. Population, consumption and human health; McCally M, ed. *CMAJ*; 2000;163(5):551–556.
4. www.worldometers.info/world-population/ World Population. November 3, 2017. Retrieved April 24, 2018, from http://worldpopulationreview.com/continents/world-population/
5. Mittal RL; The surgical management of resistant clubfoot by rotation skin flap and extensive soft tissue release; *Int Orthop*; 1987;11(3):189–192.
6. Ponseti IV, Smoley EN; The classic congenital club foot: The results of treatment; *Clin Orthop Relat Res*; 2009;467:1133–1145.
7. Lynn S, Ponseti I, Others; *Clubfoot: Ponseti Management Manual*, 3rd ed. 32 pages, 2009; 8.5″ × 11″, Four-Color, English & Others, ISBN-13 #978-1-60189-002-3
8. Tarraf and Carroll (1992) quoted by; Huang YT, Lei W, Zhao L, Wang J; The treatment of congenital club foot by operation to correct deformity and achieve dynamic muscle balance; *J Bone Joint Surg*; 1999;81-B(5):859–862.
9. Azarpira MR, Emami MJ, Vosoughi A R, Rahbari K; Factors associated with recurrence of clubfoot treated by the Ponseti method; *World J Clin Cases*; 2016 16;4(10):318–322.
10. Zhao D, Li H, Zhao Li, Liu J, Wu Z, Jin F; Results of clubfoot management using the Ponseti method: Do the details matter? A systematic review; *Clin Orthop Relat Res*; 2014;472(4):1329–1338.
11. Bhaskar A, Patni P; Classification of relapse pattern in clubfoot treated with Ponseti technique; *Ind. J Orthop*; July–August 2013;47(4):370–376.
12. Carroll NC; Clubfoot in the twentieth century: Where we were and where we may be going in the twenty-first century; *J Pediatr Orthop B*; January 2012;21(1):1–6.

Index

A

Abductor hallucles, 88; *see also* Muscular abnormalities
ACE, *see* Angiotensin Converting Enzyme
Activities of daily living (ADL), 88
ADF, *see* Ankle dorsiflexion angle
ADL, *see* Activities of daily living
AEDs, *see* Anti-epileptic drugs
Angiotensin Converting Enzyme (ACE), 16
Ankle dorsiflexion angle (ADF), 54
Ankle joint anatomy, 67–68; *see also* Congenital clubfoot pathoanatomy
Anteroposterior (AP), 53
Anti-epileptic drugs (AEDs), 13
AP, *see* Anteroposterior
Arthrogryposis multiplex congenita, 150–151

B

Bensahel's functional method of conservative treatment of clubfoot, 40
Benzene, toluene, ethylbenzene, and xylene (BTEX), 19
Bilateral clubfoot, 133
 with callosities, 133
 with multiple congenital constriction bands, 110
BMI, *see* Body mass index
Body mass index (BMI), 11
BTEX, *see* Benzene, toluene, ethylbenzene, and xylene

C

Calcanean osteotomy, 47
Calcaneo-cuboid angle (CCA), 55
Calcaneo-cuboid distance (CCD), 55
Calcaneo-cuboid joint, 69
Calcaneovarus, 156–157
Calcaneum, 69
Callosities in bilateral clubfoot, 133
Canadian Early and Mid-Trimester Amniocentesis Trial group (CEMAT), 17
CAP, *see* Clubfoot Assessment Protocol
CAs, *see* Congenital anomalies
Cavus, 46, 87
CCA, *see* Calcaneo-cuboid angle
CCBS, *see* Congenital constriction band syndrome
CCD, *see* Calcaneo-cuboid distance
CEMAT, *see* Canadian Early and Mid-Trimester Amniocentesis Trial group
Central nervous system (CNS), 10
CHD, *see* Coronary heart disease
Chorionic villous sampling (CVS), 18
Chronic obstructive pulmonary disease (COPD), 12
CINHAL, *see* Cumulative Index to Nursing and Allied Health Literature
Clubfoot, 169–171
 with additional plantar fascio-myocutaneous contracture of forefoot, 108
 arthrogryposis multiplex congenita with, 150–151
 bilateral, 133
 with callosities, 133
 with coalitions and adherent scars, 146–147
 complications, 91–95, 166
 controlling epidemiological factors, 164–165
 control of global population, 164
 deformities after fracture of and compartment syndrome, 152–153
 with extreme equinus, 124–125
 future of, 163
 genetics, 165
 global community, 163
 grades of, 51
 heterogeneous skin contractures, 169
 imaging techniques, 166
 isolated deformity, 5
 Klippel–Feil syndrome with multiple deformities and, 126–127
 in LMICs, 163, 166
 management of, 166–169
 with multiple congenital constriction bands, 110
 neglected, 34
 octopus, 94, 134–136
 orthotics, 166
 pathoanatomy, 165–166
 preventive measures, 164
 rehabilitation, 166

Clubfoot (*Continued*)
   with stress fracture of fifth metatarsal, 148–149
   treatment of, 40, 165
Clubfoot Assessment Protocol (CAP), 51, 52
Clubfoot pathoanatomy, 71–72; *see also* Congenital clubfoot pathoanatomy
   abnormality in talus, 75
   anatomical dissections in stillborn foetuses, 74
   anterior length increase and posterior length decrease, 74
   biomechanics of abnormalities, 82–83
   cadaver clubfoot, 80
   casting treatment, 78–79
   confusion on location of defect, 73
   defective cartilage anlage, 75
   deltoid ligament shortening, 73
   fibrosis beyond medial malleolus, 73
   heel inversion, 73
   in idiopathic clubfeet in aborted foetuses, 77–78
   literature review, 73–79
   observations, 80–82
   study, 79–80
   subtalar complex anatomy, 77
   surgical procedures and postoperative management, 76
   and surgical techniques, 79–80
   talo-navicular dislocation, 76
   unilateral deformity, 81
Clubfoot scoring system, 52
CNS, *see* Central nervous system
Collateral operation, 41; *see also* Contemporary techniques
Colossal dorsal callosity, 144–145
Combined medial and lateral release, 41; *see also* Contemporary techniques
Compartment syndrome, 152–153
Complete subtalar release (CSTR), 42, 95; *see also* Contemporary techniques
Computed tomography (CT), 93

Congenital anomalies (CAs), 11
   malnutrition, 15
Congenital clubfoot, 5, 6–8, 73, 171; *see also* Epidemiology of clubfoot
   bizarre, 92
   idiopathic, 15
   varieties of, 20
Congenital clubfoot pathoanatomy, 67, 71–83, 95–97; *see also* Surgical technique evolution
   normal anatomy of foot and ankle, 67–71
   planes and axes of movements, 71, 72
Congenital constriction band syndrome (CCBS), 22–23
Congenital disorders, 46
Conjoint posterior capsule (CPC), 67, 84
Contemporary techniques, 40, 57–58
   abnormal subtalar rotation, 40
   collateral operation, 41
   combined medial and lateral release, 41
   complete subtalar release, 42
   French technique, 40
COPD, *see* Chronic obstructive pulmonary disease
Coronary heart disease (CHD), 14
CT, *see* Computed tomography
CT scanning, 55; *see also* Imaging techniques
Cuboid, 69
Cumulative Index to Nursing and Allied Health Literature (CINHAL), 39
Cuneiforms, 69
Cuneo-navicular joints, 69
CVS, *see* Chorionic villous sampling

D

DALYs, *see* Disability-adjusted life-years
DB splint, *see* Denis Brown splint
Deformities at toes, 88
Denis Brown splint (DB splint), 167

DGI, *see* Dietary glycemic index
DGL, *see* High dietary glycemic load
Dietary glycemic index (DGI), 16
Dimeglio scoring system, 51, 52
Disability-adjusted life-years (DALYs), 11, 164
DOLAR, *see* **DO**rso-**LA**teral **R**otation
DOLARZ-E surgical technique, 85, 87; *see also* Third-generation research; Triple surgical techniques
   second-generation research and, 104–105
   third-generation research and, 105
Dorsolateral hump, 90–91
DOrso-**LA**teral **R**otation (**DOLAR**), 85, 101–103; *see also* Triple surgical techniques
   skin flap, 2, 96

E

EA, *see* Early amniocentesis
Early amniocentesis (EA), 17
Edwards syndrome, 22
Epidemiology, 8
Epidemiology of clubfoot, 5, 23–26
   amniocentesis and uterine factors, 17–18
   classification, 5–8
   congenital clubfoot, 5, 6–8
   congenital constriction bands, 22–23
   distal amputations and deformities, 22–23
   equinovarus deformity, 6
   factors in, 8–11, 18–19
   genetics and clubfoot, 20–22
   in LMICs, 11
   maternal diseases, 16–17
   medications, 13–14
   nomenclature, 5
   nutritional deficiency, 14–16
   pathogenesis theories, 20
   post-polio paralysis with equinovarus deformity, 6
   effect of smoking, 11–13

Equino-cavo-varus, *see* Equinovarus
Equinovarus, 5
    left and valgus right foot, 6
Equinus, 87–88
    clubfoot with very extreme, 124–125
    deformity, 73
    hyperacute equinus, 90
    residual equinus, 91
Extreme clubfoot deformities, 96, 99, 158
    evolution of triple surgical techniques, 101
    first-generation surgical technique, 101
    second-generation research and DOLARZ surgical technique, 104
    third-generation research and DOLARZ-E surgical technique, 105
    variations in, 100
Extreme deformities, 88
    grade 3, 109–110
    with extensive scars, 122
    uncorrected, 123

F

FAO, *see* Foot Ankle Orthosis
FBS, *see* Fetal blood sampling
Fetal blood sampling (FBS), 18
Fetal constraints, 11
First-generation surgical technique, 101; *see also* Triple surgical techniques
    criteria for grading results, 104
    hidden equinus, 103–104
    postoperative management, 103
    rotation-flap incision details, 103
    steps, 101–103
Fluconazole, 13
Foot anatomy, 67, 68; *see also* Congenital clubfoot pathoanatomy
    arches, 71
    bones, 68–69
    calcaneo-cuboid joint, 69
    calcaneum, 69
    capsules, ligaments, and joints, 69–70
    cuboid, 69
    cuneiforms, 69
    cuneo-navicular joints, 69
    intercuneiform joints, 69
    metatarso-phalangeal joints, 69
    muscles and tendons, 70
    navicular, 69
    subtalar joint, 69
    talo-calcaneo-navicular joint, 69
    talus, 68–69
    tarsometatarsal joints, 69
Foot Ankle Orthosis (FAO), 40
Forefoot, 49; *see also* Residual deformities
French technique, 40; *see also* Contemporary techniques

G

GBD, *see* Global burden of disease
Genu recurvatum
    with painful locking and instability, 137–138
    pre-adult residual/relapse with, 130–132
Global burden of disease (GBD), 3
Grade 3 rigid foot, 139–141

H

Heel cord tenotomy
    calcaneovarus, 156–157
    highly rigid deformity, 114–115
    Ponseti higher, 118
    residual deformity, 116–117
HFCS, *see* Hindfoot Contracture Score
Hibb's angle, 47
High dietary glycemic load (DGL), 16
High dome smaller foot, 142–143
Highly rigid deformity, 114–115
Hindfoot Contracture Score (HFCS), 52
Human genetics, 20
Hyperhomocysteinemia, 14

I

Idiopathic congenital clubfoot, 5
Ilizarov techniques, 42, 58
    distraction osteotomies, 44
    distractor, 43
    frame, 58
    Joshi's external skeletal system, 43
    mini external fixator, 44
    relapsed clubfeet, 44
    treating rigid equino-cavo-varus foot deformities, 44–45
    treatment with ring fixators, 42
Imaging techniques, 53, 59–60
    CT scanning, 55
    MRI, 55–56
    skiagrams, 53–54
    ultrasonography, 54–55
Intercuneiform joints, 69
Interphalangeal joints (IP joints), 88
Intrauterine growth restrictions (IUGRs), 18
IP joints, *see* Interphalangeal joints
Isolated clubfoot deformity, 5
IUGRs, *see* Intrauterine growth restrictions

J

Japas midfoot osteotomy, 47
JESS, *see* Joshi's external skeletal system
Joshi's external skeletal system (JESS), 43, 58; *see also* Ilizarov techniques

K

Kite method, 34
Klippel–Feil syndrome
    with clubfoot, 159
    with multiple deformities and clubfoot, 126–127

L

Lapidus procedure, 47
Lateral tibio-calcaneal angle (LtiC), 54

Literature review on clubfoot, 33
  assessment protocols, 51–52, 59
  calcanean osteotomy, 47
  contemporary techniques, 40–42, 57–58
  Dimeglio scoring system, 51, 52
  early surgery, 51, 59
  historical perspective, 33–35, 56–57
  Ilizarov and allied techniques, 42, 58
  imaging techniques, 53–56, 59–60
  Japas midfoot osteotomy, 47
  Lapidus procedure, 47
  midfoot osteotomy, 46
  older children and adults, 45–47, 59
  Pirani clubfoot scoring system, 52
  Ponseti's technique, 35–39, 57
  residual deformities, 48–51, 59
  scoring system, 51–52
  talectomy, 48, 59
  triple arthrodesis, 47
LMICs, see Low-and middle-income countries
Low-and middle-income countries (LMICs), 3
LtiC, see Lateral tibio-calcaneal angle

M

MA, see Midterm amniocentesis
Magnetic resonance angiography (MRA), 56
Magnetic resonance imaging (MRI), 7, 55–56; see also Imaging techniques
Malleolar to navicular distance (MMN), 55
Meary's angle, 47
Metatarso-phalangeal joint (MP joint), 69, 88
Metatarsus adductus, 49–50; see also Residual deformities
MFCS, see Midfoot Contracture Score
Micronutrients, 16

Midfoot
  cavus, 90
  osteotomy, 46
Midfoot Contracture Score (MFCS), 52
Midterm amniocentesis (MA), 17
Mini external fixator, 44
Mini open technique, 39
MMN, see Malleolar to navicular distance
Moebius syndrome, 21
Morbid anatomy, 95, 96
MPRs, see Multiplanar reconstructions
MRA, see Magnetic resonance angiography
MRI, see Magnetic resonance imaging
Multiplanar reconstructions (MPRs), 56
Multiple congenital constriction bands
  bilateral clubfoot with, 110
  unique clubfoot with, 112–113
Muscular abnormalities, 88
  abductor hallucis, 88
  tendoachilles percutaneous tenotomy scar, 89–90
  tibialis anterior, 88–89

N

Navicular, 69
Neglected clubfoot, 34
Neural tube defects (NTDs), 9
  causes, 16
Neuroleptics, 14
Nonsteroidal anti-inflammatory drugs (NSAIDs), 14
NSAIDs, see Nonsteroidal anti-inflammatory drugs
NTDs, see Neural tube defects

O

Octopus clubfoot, 94
  in adult, 134–136
OFCs, see Orofacial clefts
Oligohydramnios, 18
180° everted foot, 144–145
Orofacial clefts (OFCs), 18

P

Paralytic equinovarus deformities, 6
Patio syndrome, 21
Pirani clubfoot scoring system, 52
Plantar flexion, 87
Plaster casting, 34
Plaster of Paris (POP), 39
PMSTR, see Posteromedial subtalar release
Poland–Moebius syndrome, 22
Ponseti method, 34, 35, 57
  advantages of mini open technique, 39
  age of start of treatment, 35
  casting treatment, 36–37, 156–157, 159
  higher heel cord tenotomy, 118
  highly rigid deformity after, 114–115
  noncompliance reasons, 36
  obstacles in Uganda, 38
  pitfalls of, 37
  recurrences, 35, 36
  residual and relapsed deformity after, 119
  residual deformity after, 116–117
POP, see Plaster of Paris
Posteromedial subtalar release (PMSTR), 53
Post-polio paralysis with equinovarus deformity, 6
Pre-adult residual/relapse, 130–132

R

Repeated stretching technique of Arcaeus, 33
Residual deformities, 48, 59
  double column osteotomy, 48
  double tarsal wedge osteotomy, 49
  forefoot, 49
  metatarsus adductus, 49–50
  after Ponseti adherent heel cord tenotomy, 116–117
  after posteromedial release, 51
  and relapsed deformity, 119
  resistant bean-shaped clubfeet, 49
  results of revision surgeries, 49

Residual hallux varus, 90
Rigid foot, 139–141

S

Scarpa's shoe, 33
Scars
　　extreme deformity with extensive, 122
　　failed surgery, 120–121
　　heterogeneity of, 88, 96
Second-generation research, 104–105; *see also* Triple surgical techniques
Selective serotonin reuptake inhibitor (SSRI), 13, 24
SES, *see* Socioeconomic status
Skiagrams, 53–54; *see also* Imaging techniques
Skin contracture, 83, 96, 159
　　classification, 84–85
　　evidence of, 84
　　heterogeneous, 169
Socioeconomic status (SES), 18
SSR, *see* Subtotal Subtalar Release
SSRI, *see* Selective serotonin reuptake inhibitor
Subcutaneous Achilles tenotomy, 33
Subtalar joint, 69
Subtotal Subtalar Release (SSR), 142
Surgical technique evolution, 83; *see also* Congenital clubfoot pathoanatomy
　　deformities at toes, 88
　　DOLARZ-E, 87
　　DOLARZ technique, 85
　　dorsolateral hump, 90–91
　　equinus, 87–88
　　first-generation surgical techniques, 83
　　generic name, 86
　　heterogeneity of scars, 88
　　muscular abnormalities, 88–90
　　second-generation surgical technique, 85
　　skin contractures, 83–85
　　symptomatic genu recurvatum, 91
　　third-generation technique, 85–86
　　trimorphic extreme deformities, 86
　　types of clubfoot, 86
　　unusual pathoanatomical problems with morbidity, 91–95
Symptomatic genu recurvatum, 91

T

TAL, *see* Talar length
Talar length (TAL), 55
Talar neck angle (TNA), 56
Talectomy, 48, 59
Talipes equinovarus, 5
Talo-calcaneal index (TCI), 53, 160
Talo-calcaneo-navicular joint, 69
Talo-navicular (TN), 92
　　subluxation, 53–54
Talus, 68–69
TARP syndrome, 21
Tarsometatarsal joints, 69
TCI, *see* Talo-calcaneal index
Tendoachilles percutaneous tenotomy scar, 89–90; *see also* Muscular abnormalities
Thiersch graft, 105
Third-generation research, 105–107; *see also* DOLARZ-E surgical technique; Triple surgical techniques
　　arthrogryposis multiplex congenita, 150–151
　　bilateral clubfoot with multiple constriction bands, 110
　　bilateral extreme clubfoot with callosities, 133
　　calcaneovarus after Ponseti treatment, 156–157
　　clubfoot deformities and compartment syndrome, 152–153
　　clubfoot with additional plantar fascio-myocutaneous contracture, 108
　　clubfoot with extensive coalitions and adherent scars, 146–147
　　clubfoot with stress fracture of fifth metatarsal, 148–149
　　clubfoot with very extreme equinus, 124–125
　　criteria for assessment and grading, 106–107
　　extreme deformity with extensive scars, 122
　　extreme grade 3 with unusual pathoanatomy, 109–110
　　extreme uncorrected deformity, 123
　　failed surgery scars, 120–121
　　genu recurvatum with painful locking and instability, 137–138
　　grade 3 rigid foot, 139–141
　　high dome, smaller foot with psychosocial problem, 142–143
　　Klippel–Feil syndrome, 126–127
　　octopus clubfoot, 134–136
　　180° everted foot and colossal dorsal callosity, 144–145
　　Ponseti higher heel cord tenotomy, 118
　　pre-adult residual/relapse with genu recurvatum, 130–132
　　residual and relapsed deformity, 119
　　residual deformity after Ponseti adherent heel cord tenotomy, 116–117
　　rigid deformity after Ponseti, 114–115
　　shaping of VY-plasty flap, 106
　　surgical steps, 107
　　triple plus dislocations, 128–129
　　unilateral clubfoot, 154–155
　　unique clubfoot with multiple constricting bands, 112–113
3D imaging, *see* Three-dimensional imaging
Three-dimensional imaging (3D imaging), 166
3D micro-CT system, 55
Tibialis anterior, 88–89; *see also* Muscular abnormalities
　　intraoperative abnormal, 90
　　overactive tibialis anterior, 90
Tibialis posterior, 88

TN, *see* Talo-navicular
TNA, *see* Talar neck angle
Tobacco, 12
Total Pirani Score (TPS), 52
TPS, *see* Total Pirani Score
Traumatic equinovarus deformity, 6
Trimorphic extreme clubfoot deformities, 100, 158; *see also* Extreme clubfoot deformities
Triple arthrodesis, 35, 47
Triple plus dislocations, 128–129
Triple surgical techniques, 101; *see also* Extreme clubfoot deformities
   cutting edge concept, 101
   extremely rigid clubfoot, 105
   first-generation surgical technique, 101–104
   second-generation research and DOLARZ surgical technique, 104–105
   skin expanders, 160
   skin expanding techniques, 158
   third-generation research and DOLARZ-E surgical technique, 105
   triple surgical skin expanders, 160

U

Ultrasonographic diagnosis, 54–55, 166; *see also* Imaging techniques
Unilateral clubfoot, 154–155
Unique clubfoot with multiple constricting bands, 112–113
United Nation's (UN's), 164
UN's, *see* United Nation's
Uterine-constraining factors, 18

V

VY-plasty flap shaping, 106

W

WHO, *see* World Health Organization
World Health Organization (WHO), 11

X

X-rays, 166